HEALTH LITERACY
IN CANADA

HEALTH LITERACY IN CANADA

A PRIMER FOR STUDENTS

Laurie Hoffman-Goetz, Lorie Donelle, and Rukhsana Ahmed

Canadian Scholars' Press Inc.

Toronto

Health Literacy in Canada: A Primer for Students
Laurie Hoffman-Goetz, Lorie Donelle, and Rukhsana Ahmed

First published in 2014 by
Canadian Scholars' Press Inc.
425 Adelaide Street West, Suite 200
Toronto, Ontario
M5V 3C1
www.cspi.org

Every reasonable effort has been made to identify copyright holders. CSPI would be pleased to have any errors or omissions brought to its attention.
Canadian Scholars' Press Inc. gratefully acknowledges financial support for our publishing activities from the Government of Canada through the Canada Book Fund (CBF).

Library and Archives Canada Cataloguing in Publication

Hoffman-Goetz, Laurie, author
      Health literacy in Canada : a primer for students / Laurie Hoffman-Goetz, Lorie Donelle, and Rukhsana Ahmed.

Includes bibliographical references and index.
Issued in print and electronic formats.

ISBN 978-1-55130-559-2 (pbk.).--ISBN 978-1-55130-560-8 (pdf)--
ISBN 978-1-55130-561-5 (epub)

      1. Health literacy--Canada. I. Donelle, Lorie, author
II. Ahmed, Rukhsana, author III. Title.

RA440.3.C2H64 2014   613'.0971   C2013-908452-5   C2013-908453-3

Text design by Aldo Fierro
Cover design by Em Dash Design

Printed and bound in Canada by Webcom.

Canada

MIX
Paper from
responsible sources
FSC
www.fsc.org   FSC® C004071

CONTENTS

LISTS OF FIGURES, TABLES, AND BOXES

FIGURES

TABLES

BOXES

HEALTH LITERACY IN CANADA: A UNIQUE AND SIGNIFICANT RESOURCE FOR STUDENTS AND PRACTITIONERS IN CANADA AND INTERNATIONALLY

I would like to thank the authors for asking me to write the foreword for this outstanding book on health literacy. Not only did I learn a great deal more about health literacy than I knew before, in spite of the fact that I have been in the field for more than a decade, but I also thoroughly enjoyed reading it, particularly the many real-life examples that are included. I am sure that others who are involved or interested in health literacy will have the same experience. In particular, undergraduate and graduate students in a wide range of health- and education-related fields, whether in Canada or other countries, will benefit hugely from this book, as it provides a comprehensive and insightful overview of the field that is valid beyond the boundaries of this country. It also includes many features that will make it especially useful to students, including examples of exemplary initiatives, periodic summaries of key points, questions for reflection, learning exercises, a glossary of important terms, descriptions of potentially useful resources, informative tables and figures, an index, and well-chosen quotations to introduce chapters.

In addition to students, this book will be of considerable interest to practitioners and policy-makers in a number of fields both within and outside of health, partly because its tone and use of language align with a diverse readership, and partly because of its unique content. Most obviously, it is the only book that I am aware of that provides a uniquely Canadian perspective on health literacy. Not only does it adhere to a widely used Canadian definition of health literacy endorsed by the Canadian Expert Panel on Health Literacy (Rootman & Gordon-El-Bihbety, 2008, p. 11), but it also presents many Canadian examples of research and practice, some of which are unique in the world (for example, comic books on health issues affecting Aboriginal youth developed by the Healthy Aboriginal Network). However, it is not limited to Canadian examples, but draws examples from other parts of the world, particularly the United States.

Health Literacy in Canada also explores a range of topics that are not usually covered in depth in books on health literacy. For example, Chapter 4 is devoted to discussing the social determinants of health in relation to health literacy. It links health literacy to the Ottawa

Charter for Health Promotion, as well as to the less well-known, but relevant, Toronto Charter for a Healthy Canada. This chapter also clearly and convincingly links health literacy to social justice and health equity, suggesting that "there should be equal opportunity for individuals to attain optimal health potential," and that supporting people to become more health literate may make an important contribution to achieving optimal health. This chapter also introduces intersectionality theory as a useful tool for analyzing and understanding the role of health literacy in the context of the determinants of health; this is the first time that I have encountered the use of this perspective in a book on health literacy. Intersectionality theory is also applied to understanding the impact of the determinants of health, including literacy and health literacy, on Aboriginal populations.

In Chapter 5, a unique examination of culture and health literacy, the authors discuss the concepts of acculturation and assimilation, cultural competency and safety, and multiculturalism and the effect of culture on health literacy. I was particularly impressed by the discussion of cultural competency, which goes far beyond standard notions of cultural competency in its approach to health literacy. This chapter also contains many concrete examples of the role that culture plays in relation to health literacy, including during interactions between health professionals and patients. It is truly an important contribution to understanding the importance of culture in relation to health literacy, which is not covered as comprehensively in other books on the topic.

Chapter 6, on information technology and health literacy, also makes a significant contribution to our understanding of health literacy, both in Canada and elsewhere. Among other topics, it covers eHealth literacy, the online culture of health and health care, the relationship between information literacy and health literacy, and the role of social media in health literacy. I found the section on social media particularly interesting, perhaps because I have not seen it discussed to any great extent in other books on health literacy. I was especially fascinated by the discussion of the semantic web and medical ontologies and their potential.

Health Literacy in Canada also contains a very interesting chapter (Chapter 7) on the mass media and health literacy, which is, again, unusual in a book on health literacy. Drawing on work and examples from Canada and elsewhere, it makes a strong case for paying more attention to the mass media in relation to health literacy. As the authors note, "considering media in the light of health literacy is essential"; they also suggest that "media literacy education can address a variety of relevant health literacy concerns." This chapter also introduces the concept of critical media health literacy, which has been the focus of some recent research in Canada. It draws attention to the significant opportunities for public media to promote health literacy, implying that the media has the potential to become a strong partner in this endeavour.

Although the book has a strong emphasis on health promotion as it relates to health literacy—as opposed to health care, which is the case with many other books on the subject—it does not neglect health care. Chapter 9, which addresses clinical health literacy, provides practical suggestions for health care providers. Chapter 10, with a focus on health literacy interventions, also provides suggestions for health care providers regarding how to communicate effectively with patients who have different levels of health literacy, as well as means to obtain further training to improve their ability to do so. This chapter also covers interventions that are appropriate for different stages of the life course, which is a concept that has only recently been applied to health literacy, partly because of work done in Canada.

The main contribution of this book will likely be to inform and educate students and people working in health and related fields about health literacy, and to provide them with tools that will improve their knowledge and practice. Another possible contribution may be to convince policy-makers in health and related areas of the relevance of health literacy in addressing inequities in health and society, and to persuade them to consider the need for a rights-based approach. A third contribution may be to lead people interested in health literacy to reflect on its current state.

In the latter regard, I can attest to the fact that reading this book has led me to reflect on the development of the field since the release of the report of the Canadian Expert Panel on Health Literacy (which I co-chaired with Deborah Gordon-El-Bihbety) five years ago. The panel's main recommendation was that "a comprehensive, coordinated, coopera-tive and integrated Pan-Canadian Strategy on Health Literacy be developed, funded and implemented to improve the level of health literacy in Canada and the extent to which people receive the support they need to cope with the health literacy demands they en-counter" (Rootman & Gordon-El-Bihbety, 2008, p. 39). It is encouraging to note that in Canada over the past five years some developments have moved us closer to such a strat-egy; some of these developments are addressed in this book. For example, the Canadian Public Health Association, in partnership with the Canadian Council on Learning and the Public Health Agency of Canada, developed terms of reference for the establishment of a Canadian Health Literacy Council, which was one of the panel's suggestions. The Public Health Agency of Canada established a senior advisor position in health education and literacy to develop a program on health literacy. As a result, numerous health literacy resources have been developed, including a discussion paper titled "An Intersectoral Ap-proach for Improving the Health Literacy of Canadians" (Mitic & Rootman, 2012) that has been made available in English and French through the website of the National Col-laborating Centre for Determinants of Health. Elements of this paper were included in the publication on health literacy recently released by the European Office of the World Health Organization (Kickbusch, Pelikan, Apfel, & Tsouros, 2013)

In addition, research on health literacy has continued in Canada with some new investigators entering the field, including one of the authors of this book. The Canadian Medical Association has become more involved in health literacy work, passing two resolutions to promote it and developing an online credit course for physicians and other health professionals. A number of other non-governmental organizations in the health sector, such as the Healthy Living Alliance and the Canadian Cancer Association, have also become involved by endorsing health literacy as a priority and offering sessions on health literacy at their conferences. In addition, several new measurement tools have been developed (see, for example, Sabbahi, Lawrence, Limeback, & Rootman, 2009; Wu et al., 2010). A number of health literacy networks, Lawrence, Limeback, & Rootman focused on different dimensions of health literacy (e.g., mental health), population groups (e.g., older adults), or information sources (e.g., librarians) have also formed.

Canadians have also continued to contribute to international work in the field of health literacy. Canadians have recently presented at several roundtables, conferences, and other scholarly venues to advance the health literacy agenda. For example, a snapshot of Canadian health literacy milestones, and examples of the pockets of innovative health literacy programs, initiatives, and activities that are taking place across our country, were shared during the 2012 Institute of Medicine Roundtable on Health Literacy (Vamos, 2013), which highlighted timely international health literacy efforts and featured international presentations and global discussions. Canadian contributions were also made at the Institute for Healthcare Advancement Conference and the 2013 World Conference of the International Union for Health Promotion and Education.

It is apparent that we have made significant progress toward achieving many of the recommendations of the Canadian Expert Panel on Health Literacy as Canada continues on the journey toward health literacy that began in the late 1980s. It has clearly become a field of research and practice that is both exciting and challenging, and is open to the contributions of students and practitioners in many fields. I anticipate that the publication of this excellent and important book will re-energize the field of health literacy in Canada by building the health literacy knowledge and skills of students and practitioners in a wide variety of health and other fields. I hope that you will be one of them.

Irving Rootman, PhD
Vancouver, British Columbia
September 2013

REFERENCES

Kickbusch, I., Pelikan, J.M., Apfel, F., & Tsouros, A.D. (2013). *Health literacy: The solid facts.* Geneva: World Health Organization.

Mitic, W., & Rootman, I. (2012). *An intersectoral approach for improving the health literacy of Canadians: Discussion paper.* Victoria, BC: Public Health Association of British Columbia.

Rootman, I., & Gordon-El-Bihbety, D. (2008). *A vision for a health literate Canada: Report of the Expert Panel on Health Literacy.* Ottawa, ON: Canadian Public Health Association.

Sabbahi, D.A., Lawrence, H.P., Limeback, H., & Rootman, I. (2009). Development and evaluation of an oral health literacy instrument for adults. *Community Dentistry and Oral Epidemiology, 37,* 451–462.

Vamos, S. (2013). Health literacy policy and programs: Health literacy in Canada. In Institute of Medicine, *Health literacy: Improving health, health systems and health policy around the world: Workshop summary* (pp. 37–41). Washington, DC: The National Academies Press. Retrieved from http://www.iom.edu/Reports/2013/Health-Literacy-Improving-Health-Health-Systems-and-Health-Policy-Around-the-World.aspx

Wu, A.D., Begoray, D.L., MacDonald, M., Wharf Higgins, J., Frankish, J., Kwan, B., Fung, W., & Rootman, I. (2010). Developing and evaluating a relevant and feasible instrument for measuring health literacy of Canadian high school students. *Health Promotion International, 25*(4), 444–452.

ACKNOWLEDGEMENTS

Health literacy draws from many fields, and the writing of this book was made possible with the help and encouragement of our colleagues at the University of Waterloo, Western University, and the University of Ottawa. We thank Dr. Jose F. Arocha, Associate Professor in the School of Public Health and Health Systems at the University of Waterloo, who contributed to Chapter 6; his knowledge and research expertise in medical decision making and health informatics were essential. We are also indebted to Dr. Maria Thomson, Assistant Professor in the Department of Social and Behavioral Health at Virginia Commonwealth University, who co-authored Chapter 5. Her insights and expertise in patient–provider communication in cancer care provided much-appreciated context and relevance. We thank Dr. Irving Rootman for being a tireless champion of health literacy in Canada and an inspiration to the authors.

We gratefully acknowledge Dr. Joan Wharf Higgins and Dr. Lynne Robinson for their review of the manuscript and their thoughtful suggestions and advice. You have helped us to craft a more comprehensive and insightful book. At Canadian Scholars' Press Inc., our sincere thanks go to Daniella Balabuk for her skilful work as project editor, to Caley Baker for excellence as production editor, to Elizabeth Phinney for thorough copy-editing, and to Lily Bergh, who provided enthusiastic support at the book proposal stage.

We are especially appreciative of our students, past and current, who provided the motivation for us to write a textbook on health literacy in Canada. We acknowledge Kristina Schmidt for help with the initial formatting of the book and Benjamin Deignan for his help preparing the glossary.

Finally, we could not have written this book without the patience, support, and encouragement of Wendel, Rich, and Hasan. We dedicate this book to you.

CHAPTER 1

WHY A BOOK ON HEALTH LITERACY FROM A CANADIAN PERSPECTIVE?

Taking positive action to provide all Canadians with the opportunities they
need to obtain a solid education and achieve adequate literacy skills is one of the
best ways to foster healthy citizens and a prosperous, competitive nation.
—Federal, Provincial, and Territorial Advisory Committee on
Population Health, "Toward a Healthy Future," 1999

CHAPTER LEARNING OBJECTIVES

- Introduce health literacy as a public health issue in Canada
- Introduce the importance of studying health literacy in a Canadian context
- Introduce key milestones in the health literacy movement in Canada
- Introduce health literacy as a human rights and social justice issue

SETTING THE STAGE

There is extensive and compelling evidence that shows that literacy is one of the major factors influencing health status. However we define or measure health, people with limited health literacy are much worse off than those with better health literacy. Not only is health literacy critical for individuals, but it is also critical for both health care providers and health systems: low health literacy is associated with greater use of health care resources. More than just enhancing health, it makes good economic sense to focus on health literacy as a priority issue. By addressing the needs of Canadians with limited literacy skills, *all* Canadians benefit (Perrin, 1998).

Every day we receive health information, most of which leaves us with more questions than answers: Is coffee good for me or bad for me? How many insulin injections do I take a day? Can I go to any doctor or hospital I want? Should I take vitamin D supplements? Is H1N1 still a threat? Health information can be useful in helping us to make important health decisions. However, for those who cannot access, read, or understand messages at the most basic level, it can be confusing and overwhelming. And while people with low literacy skills can find health information puzzling, even those with advanced literacy skills can find health information challenging to grasp.

Information about health is constantly changing as a result of major advances in medical science, new and emerging research findings, and rapid technological advancements (U.S. Department of Health and Human Services [DHHS], n.d.). So even though limited literacy skill is endemic, particularly in developing countries, limited health literacy is a global problem. For example, 90 million people in the United States find it difficult to understand and correctly use health information (Institute of Medicine, 2004). In Canada, 60 percent of adults do not possess a level of health literacy adequate to manage their own health and health care needs (Canadian Council on Learning [CCL], 2008a). This means that, without the required level of health literacy, large populations may encounter difficulty finding health care services, sharing personal medical history with health care providers, adopting preventative health and health-promoting behaviours (e.g., exercise, health screening), engaging in self-care for chronic disease management (e.g., medical regimens, monitoring blood sugar level), responding to emergency medical situations, and so on (DHHS, n.d.; Zarcadoolas, Pleasant, & Greer, 2006).

In this chapter we introduce the main themes of the textbook: literacy as a fundamental determinant of health; adequate health literacy as essential for the public health of Canadians; health literacy as an issue of human rights and social justice; and literacy and health literacy as critical for the prosperity and well-being of the country. We begin with select definitions of health literacy to best situate this concept within a public health perspective. We then consider the leadership role Canada has had in spearheading the health literacy movement. We conclude the chapter with a consideration of why health literacy is linked to human rights and social justice.

SOME KEY DEFINITIONS

Although health literacy is considered a public health goal (Nutbeam, 2000), lack of agreement on the meaning of the term "has become a source of confusion and debate" (Baker, 2006, p. 878), challenging the promotion of health literacy efforts. Even decades after the term *health literacy* first appeared in print, scholars still identify it as a complex and multi-faceted construct (Weiss et al., 2005; Zarcadoolas, 2011) that is difficult to define and measure (Baker, 2006; Mancuso, 2009). As noted by Mancuso (2009),

> Health literacy has originated from the necessary skills of reading and numeracy to one of critical thinking, problem-solving, decision-making, information-seeking, and communication, along with a multitude of social, personal, and cognitive skills that are imperative in order to function in the health-care system. In addition, health literacy has expanded into the realm of culture, context, and language. (p. 78)

Despite the considerable amount of research that has been undertaken on health literacy over the past decade (Gazmararian, Curran, Parker, Benhardt, & Debuono, 2005), gaps and debates still exist in attempts to define this concept (Rootman & Gordon-El-Bihbety, 2008). The World Health Organization defined health literacy as "the cognitive and social skills which determine the motivation and ability of individuals to gain access to, understand and use information in ways which promote and maintain good health" (as cited in Nutbeam, 2000, p. 264). Nutbeam

(2000) expanded the concept of health literacy by linking it to empowerment—that is, improving people's access to health information increases their capacity to use that information effectively and enables them to influence health at the individual, community, and societal levels. Underscoring the importance of health contexts and the implications of health literacy over the course of people's lives, the Canadian Council on Learning and the Canadian Expert Panel on Health Literacy offered a comprehensive definition of health literacy as one's "ability to access, understand, evaluate and communicate information as a way to promote, maintain and improve health in a variety of settings across the life-course" (Rootman & Gordon-El-Bihbety, 2008, p. 11). *The Calgary Charter on Health Literacy* (Coleman et al., 2008) indicates that a health literate person is one who is able to read, write, listen, speak, calculate, critically analyze, communicate, and interact; skills that help develop her or his ability to utilize information to promote good health. This all-inclusive definition adds greatly to our understanding of the primacy and complexity of health literacy in promoting health across the lifespan. Chapter 2 of this book offers an expanded discussion of health literacy definitions and theoretical frameworks.

HEALTH LITERACY IS CRITICAL TO PUBLIC HEALTH

The challenges in today's health care system—reduction in health care funding, an aging population, increased immigration, cultural diversity, shortages in personnel, patient waiting times, managed care, home health care, long-term care, and growing use of technology—make health literacy an urgent public health issue. We can think of health literacy as a critical component of quality health care (Nielsen-Bohlman, Panzer, & Kindig, 2004). Fundamentally, adequate health literacy is a public right for all Canadians, regardless of differences in age, gender, culture, ability, and sexual orientation among and between population groups. A large body of research indicates an association between low literacy and adverse health outcomes, and demonstrates how health literacy can improve public health.

The health of a population reflects a multiplicity of factors, many of which are outside the conventional health care system. These factors are often referred to as the social determinants of health (Wilkinson & Marmot, 2003). As explained by Kickbusch (2004), "Access to health information and utilization of health knowledge play a crucial role for the fulfillment of personal and societal expectations and for enabling citizens to make healthy choices" (p. 1). As such, the notion of health literacy extends well beyond the health care system and is "an active process" that influences individuals' activities of everyday living (p. 4). In this sense, health literate individuals become consumers in the health marketplace, patients in the health care system, voters on health issues, and social actors in health movements. Hence, health literacy is critical to public health because it can empower individuals to actively, confidently, and fully participate in multiple life roles (e.g., parent, employee, patient, consumer, citizen, and so on) so that they can "continually learn new information and unlearn outdated information in order to maintain good health and act as informed patients" (p. 5). Chapter 4 will expand on the concept of health literacy as an important determinant of health.

Increasing health literacy can be "transformative" for individuals, communities, and the entire population. This transformative power can be seen in the links to citizen engagement in civil society to issues related to health. For example, Kickbusch (2004) identified several factors that underscore health literacy as critical to health, social, and economic development. These factors include citizens' expectations and goals related to health information and health care; an aging society; an expansive health care system that requires complex decision making by patients; increased marketing of health information and products, using both traditional and new media channels (e.g., TV, newspaper, Internet); the free movement of persons, goods, and services, giving rise to culturally diverse perceptions and practices of health; low levels of health literacy affecting the health care system by limited use of preventive services; and knowledge of disease management. These factors demonstrate a shared concern about the impact of health literacy, making health literacy critical to public health care.

WHY HEALTH LITERACY FROM A CANADIAN PERSPECTIVE?

Health literacy, different from general literacy, involves the simultaneous use of a more complex and interconnected set of abilities: to read and act upon health information, to communicate needs to health professionals, and to understand health instructions (Canadian Council on Learning, 2008a). Health literacy is one of the most important components in achieving and maintaining health. Canadians with low health literacy skills may not always understand the information they read or what health professionals tell them. Petch, Ronson, and Rootman (2004) underscored the link between literacy and health, emphasizing both direct and indirect effects (see Table 1.1).

TABLE 1.1: DIRECT AND INDIRECT EFFECTS OF LOW LITERACY ON HEALTH

Type of Effect on Health	
Direct	Difficulty finding and understanding health information
	Having more health-related problems
	Making more medication errors
	Having more accidents in the workplace
Indirect	Occupying lower paying jobs and/or being unemployed
	Feeling more stress and being more vulnerable when things go wrong
	Practicing unhealthy behaviours, such as smoking and getting less exercise
	Paying more visits to the hospital and staying in the hospital longer
	Facing more difficulties in navigating the health care system

Source: Adapted from Petch, E., Ronson, B., & Rootman, I. (2004, p. 11). Literacy and health in Canada: What have we learned and what can help in the future? A research report. Clear language edition. Canadian Institutes of Health Research. Retrieved from www.cpha.ca/uploads/portals/h-l/literacy_e.pdf [accessed: 15 June 2013].

There are many research studies showing that low literacy (and low health literacy) is linked to poor health outcomes. Importantly, DeWalt and colleagues (2004) undertook a systematic review of the published literature on literacy and health outcomes. Health literacy was assessed using a number of instruments (such as the Test of Functional Health Literacy of Adults) with a variety of populations drawn from many countries (including Canada, the United States, Australia, and European nations). The health outcomes considered were also diverse—ranging from parental knowledge about child health care to hospitalization rates, smoking rates, adherence to antiretroviral therapy, and many others. What these researchers showed was that low health literacy is consistently associated with numerous adverse health outcomes.

Further support for the association between low health literacy and poor health outcomes comes from work by the Canadian Council on Learning (CCL, 2007a). The studies and reports from the CCL indicated that 60 percent of Canadians lack the skills and ability to make appropriate health decisions. The CCL findings stress the importance of health literacy to the clarity and comprehension of communication within health care encounters. Being health literate can improve communication between the provider and the patient, with a greater likelihood of attaining a desired health outcome. Chapter 7 ("Mass Media and Health Literacy") and Chapter 8 ("Risk Communication and Health Literacy") outline the importance of health literacy in understanding health (risk) information from diverse information sources.

The CCL findings also emphasize the Canadian data collected from a number of international surveys known as the International Adult Literacy Skills Survey or IALS survey. The IALS surveys will be considered in detail in Chapter 3. However, what is important to note here about the IALS survey results is that just under half (48 percent) of Canadian adults do not have the skills needed in prose, document, and quantitative literacy to function effectively at work (much less thrive) in a knowledge-based economy. The low literacy levels were especially troubling as they were not uniformly distributed throughout all segments of the population. Particularly concerning was the prevalence of low literacy skill among seniors, immigrants, Aboriginal people, and those with limited income and education. We will explore why the unequal distribution of the burden of low health literacy is an essential one for us to consider in Chapter 3.

Health literacy has important health and social implications. Individuals with limited literacy may find it difficult to adequately manage their own health and/or the health of their family members. In a study of Canadian adults with limited literacy and chronic illness, King and Taylor (2010) found that participants felt powerless, fearful, and isolated because of both their chronic illness and limited literacy. Limited health literacy levels have detrimental effects on one's physiological well-being and can also adversely affect one's self-concept. King and Taylor (2010) discovered through their analysis that participants were "very much aware of their responsibility for their own health, but their feelings of powerlessness were often barriers to taking a more active role" (p. 15). It is challenging for family members to step in and take a more active role as caregiver if the patient in question feels isolated or stigmatized by their literacy levels. Limited health literacy is a barrier that can go unnoticed by both family members and health care providers alike. The researchers found that, of their participants in the study, "67% admitted to problems with reading and had not shared this knowledge with a spouse because they were ashamed" (p. 2). Moreover, participants expressed their belief that their role as competent adults would be questioned if their literacy levels were brought to the attention of others. Laverack (2005) provides further insight into the relationship between information and personal power, especially for individuals and families with limited resources (e.g., income, education). He challenges our notion that "knowledge is power" in describing conditions where the lack of personal or community resources prohibits individuals and/or families from carrying out health-enhancing behaviours. For example, despite knowing the importance of healthy food choices to promote and maintain positive health, a sense of powerlessness may be generated among those with little income who live in neighbourhoods without convenient access to healthy food in reasonably priced grocery stores.

Why should we consider health literacy from a Canadian reference point? Are the factors mediating low health literacy in this country different from other jurisdictions? Are the challenges unique to Canada, or are they shared by other countries? In Chapter 3, we will look closely at how Canada performs relative to other countries in population measures of literacy and health literacy. However, it is important to realize here that broad systems in Canada shape the health literacy issues and national debates. These system factors include immigration patterns, cultural and ethnic composition, minority language rights and culture, emphasis on social justice and health equity, and Internet use and broadband penetration.

Consider the factor of immigration trends and how this might affect health literacy. In 2006, 20 percent of the Canadian population was born outside of Canada; in Toronto, the largest urban centre in the country, one in two residents was foreign-born (Statistics Canada, 2008). Of these immigrants, the largest group was from Asia, including the Middle East (see Figure 1.1 below). This can be compared with patterns in the United States, where the largest group of immigrants (41 percent) came from Latin America and the Caribbean between 2000 and 2005 (although immigration from Asia was also important, at 32 percent) (Martin & Midgley, 2006). Why would immigration patterns be relevant to health literacy issues for Canada (and indeed for any country)? The effects of immigration patterns on population health literacy are likely multi-factorial, but we often tend to consider only one variable, that of language. Many immigrants have a primary or first language different from that of their new countries. Using the 2006 Canadian Census data, it has been estimated that 70.2 percent of the immigrant population had a mother tongue other than one of the two official languages. And, of those whose first language was neither English nor French, the largest proportion spoke Mandarin, Cantonese, or other Chinese dialects. Arabic and Punjabi were also spoken by a significant number of immigrants to Canada from Asia and the Middle East (Statistics Canada, 2006). In the United States, the immigration patterns differed from Canada, and the primary language of immigrants from Latin America and the Caribbean was Spanish. While all English- or French-as-a-Second-Language immigrants to Canada and the United States face significant cultural and linguistic barriers, the specific barriers and challenges vary between countries. These in turn have important consequences for health literacy and the types of interventions that are needed.

Language and culture are intimately related. They have independent, interdependent, and interactive effects on health and health literacy. Culturally bound beliefs, values, preferences, and the linguistic frame provide the experiential context for health literacy and interpretation of health information (Andrulis & Brach, 2007). To add even more complexity, differences in provincial and territorial health care systems also affect access to health information and health resources for immigrants to Canada. Many countries share the vision of improving the health literacy of their populations. Chapter 5 discusses in detail important considerations related to cultural aspects of health literacy.

FIGURE 1.1: PERCENTAGE OF IMMIGRANTS TO CANADA BY REGION OF BIRTH, 1971–2006

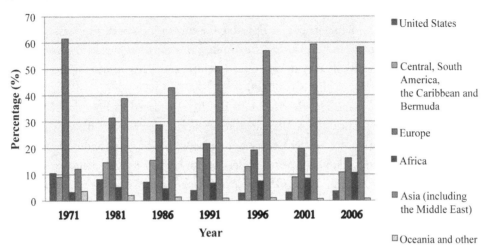

Note: "Other" includes Greenland, St. Pierre and Miquelon, the category "Other country," and a small number of immigrants who were born in Canada.

Source: Modified from Statistics Canada. (2009). *Censuses of population, 1971–2006*. Chart 13.1. Retrieved from http://www41.statcan.ca/2008/30000/grafx/htm/ceb30000_000_1-eng.htm [accessed: 13 June 2013].

REVIEW AND REFLECT

Identify direct and indirect effects that low health literacy has on health.

If you were charged with recommending a province-wide public health strategy to improve health literacy, which of these factors would you focus on? Why?

THE HEALTH LITERACY MOVEMENT IN CANADA

Through its nationwide, province-wide, and local health literacy initiatives, Canada is recognized as an international leader in the field of health literacy. For a comprehensive review of the milestones in literacy and health research in Canada, the reader is referred to Rootman and Ronson (2005). The following section is a brief introduction to key developments and initiatives in understanding the Canadian path to health literacy, and additional detail is provided in Chapter 2. Although there have been many milestones in the literacy movement (such as Frontier College, which is highlighted in Chapter 3), here the focus is on milestones of *health literacy* initiatives in Canada.

The Canadian Public Health Association (CPHA), a national not-for-profit voluntary association, has been a chief proponent and at the forefront of health literacy efforts. CPHA offers and produces a range of programs and support materials in the area of health literacy, such as a directory of plain language health information, a plain language and clear verbal communication training manual for health professionals, and an easy-to-use guide to work with low-literacy youth and seniors, among others (see www.cpha.ca).

In 2006, with funding from the Health and Learning Knowledge Centre of the Canadian Council on Learning, CPHA formed the Expert Panel on Health Literacy, which was charged with assessing the nature and scope of health literacy levels in Canada, identifying barriers to creating a health literate public, assessing the effectiveness of existing interventions to improve health literacy, and evaluating the implications of the evidence for policies and programs to improve health literacy through the development of recommendations (CPHA, 2007; Rootman & Gordon-El-Bihbety, 2008).

The National Literacy and Health Program (NLHP), established in 1994 by CPHA and funded by the Secretary of State's new National Literacy Secretariat, fostered partnerships with national health associations to raise awareness among health professionals about the links between literacy and health and to improve health services for consumers with literacy difficulties (Rick Wilson Consulting Inc., 2004). These partnerships resulted in projects, conferences, and the publication and dissemination of plain language materials. As noted by Rootman and Ronson (2005), "The NLHP is considered to be a model for raising awareness, exploring issues, developing resource materials and building partnerships in this field" (p. S62).

The Literacy and Health Project, Phase One: Making the World Healthier and Safer for People Who Can't, jointly sponsored by the Ontario Public Health Association and Frontier College, has been instrumental in demonstrating the literacy and health connection, fostering partnerships between literacy and health organizations, and creating a clearing house on literacy and health information (Perrin, 1989, 1998).

The Centre for Literacy (www.centreforliteracy.qc.ca/) offers one of the largest and most comprehensive special collections on literacy and related topics in Canada. By holding workshops; publishing newsletter articles; integrating evidence-based literacy research, policy, and practice; and establishing an extensive network of local, national, and international partners, the Centre has been an avid advocate for health literacy initiatives since 1995. For example, the Health Literacy Project is a joint health literacy initiative of The Centre for Literacy and the Department of Nursing of McGill University Health Centre (MUHC), which has examined the complex set of factors associated with health and literacy, and attempted to identify ways to recognize and address barriers to patient communication. The Centre has also been actively involved in creating a health literacy curriculum module for university nursing students, a training model for health care providers, and patient navigation kits on breast and prostate cancer, participating in national and international panels on health literacy policy, and collaborating on *The Calgary Charter on Health Literacy: Rationale and Core Principles for the Development of Health Literacy Curriculum* (Coleman et al., 2008).

Initiated by CPHA's National Literacy and Health Program, the first Canadian Conference on Literacy and Health ("Charting the Course for Literacy and Health in the New Millennium") was held in Ottawa in 2000. The conference brought together health professionals, government representatives, researchers and academics, literacy providers, health administrators, policy-makers, adult learners from both Canada and the United States, and representatives of pharmaceutical companies to consider literacy as a critical health issue and to develop literacy and health partnerships. The conference revolved around five themes, including making health services and health information easy to use for all Canadians, looking for ways to improve the training of health professionals, learning more through research, learning from learners, and building literacy and health partnerships, and offered 37 workshops related to issues of health literacy within Canada. Not only did the conference address "the problem of access to health information and services that low-literacy health consumers require to be healthy," it went beyond by also exploring "the specific challenges that people who have low literacy skills and disabilities and/or cultural differences face in accessing the health services they need" (CPHA, 2001, p. 52).

Created in 2004, the Canadian Council on Learning (CCL) is an independent, non-profit corporation, funded by Human Resources and Social Development Canada, to promote and support evidence-based research to improve learning across all walks of life in Canada. CCL has been a champion of health literacy initiatives as well. Its 2007 and 2008 *Health Literacy in Canada* reports (CCL, 2007a, 2008a) were pivotal documents that stressed the importance of health literacy as a public health goal in Canada. The strikingly high prevalence of low levels of health literacy among adult Canadians sparked the development of research priorities and focused interventions to improve health literacy levels in communities and population groups across the country (see www.ccl-cca.ca/CCL/Home/index.html). Similarly, Copian, known as the one-stop information centre for adult literacy programs, resources, services, and activities across Canada, contains a large collection of references to literacy and health (see www.en.copian.ca).

Canadian librarians have also championed health literacy initiatives. Library initiatives to promote health literacy demonstrate the role librarians can play in improving health information access, processing, and understanding for the general public (S. Murray, 2008). These initiatives have included listing health literacy outreach as one of the job responsibilities for librarians, and collaborating with educational institutions and non-profit, community, and public health organizations. For example, the Irving K. Barber Learning Center in British Columbia partnered with telecommunication companies to develop online tools to support health literacy. These partnerships led to the development of links to reliable online health information and the development of a Consumer Health Information website that includes information literacy tools and consumer health stories archives (S. Murray, 2008). Chapter 6 of this text challenges readers to consider the important relationship between health literacy skills and information technology (e.g., the Internet). With funding from the Ontario Ministry of Health Promotion, the Consumer Health Information Service (CHIS) was developed by the City of Toronto Reference Library; CHIS provides a range of services to address health literacy barriers faced by newcomers to Canada and those with limited literacy skills. Some of these services include hands-on courses in English and French on how to locate reliable online health information, hosting various health talks, and presenting workshops on health literacy (S. Murray, 2008).

REVIEW AND REFLECT

Libraries are an important partner in promoting the health literacy of Canadians. Explain.

Some other province-wide and local health literacy initiatives that provide promising practices include the Health Literacy Network, the Healthy Aboriginal Network, and the Healthy Living Performance Standards for Schools in British Columbia; the Literacy Audit Kit in Alberta; "It's Safe to Ask" Project and Literacy and Health Project in Manitoba; To Be Born Equal—To Grow to Health Programme in Quebec; Health Literacy in Rural Nova Scotia Research Project; discussion paper for Inuit communities on literacy and health in Nunavut; Hispanic Health Literacy Video Project and Farsi-speaking TV series on health in Vancouver; Health and Literacy Committee in Prince Albert, Saskatchewan; Diabetes Management project (Ottawa), Literacy and Health project (North Bay), Patient Education project (Hamilton) in Ontario; "Going to the Doctor" resource prepared by Yukon Learn; "It's Your Health" resource prepared through the Nova Scotia Heart Health Partnership; and the Manitoba Cervical Cancer Screening Program (CPHA, 2006a; Rootman & Gordon-El-Bihbety, 2008). See Chapters 9 and 10 for an expanded discussion of health literacy interventions within Canada.

TABLE 1.2: TIMELINE OF HEALTH LITERACY ACTIVITIES IN CANADA

Growing interest in literacy in the late 1980s
OPHA/Frontier College Literacy and Health project (1989–1993)
National Literacy and Health Program (1994–present); CPHA Clear Language Service (1997–present)
National conferences on Literacy and Health (2000, 2004)
National Literacy and Health Research Project (2002–2006)
CPHA Expert Panel on Health Literacy (Rootman & Gordon-El-Bihbety, 2008)
In-depth analysis of National Health Literacy data (CCL, 2007b, 2008a)
International health literacy experts, co-hosted by The Centre for Literacy of Quebec and the Calgary Institute on Health Literacy Curricula (2008), create the Calgary Charter on Health Literacy (2009)
Centre for Chronic Disease Prevention and Control, Public Health Agency of Canada (PHAC-British Columbia) National Health Literacy Workshop (2011)
International Health Literacy Workshop hosted by Public Health Agency of Canada (PHAC-British Columbia) (2012)
International Roundtable on Health Literacy hosted by University of British Columbia (UBC) Institute for Heart and Lung Health and Peter Wall Institute (2013)

These promising health literacy initiatives add greatly to our understanding of the leadership role Canada has in health literacy. Unfortunately, these efforts are not enough to enable every Canadian to read, write, listen, speak, analyze, communicate, interact, and use numbers and information to meet the demands of everyday life. In later chapters, we consider why a strong case can be made for developing more multidisciplinary and multi-sectorial partnerships for promoting health literacy.

HEALTH LITERACY, HUMAN RIGHTS, AND SOCIAL JUSTICE

Low health literacy is no longer a hidden public health concern in Canada. As identified earlier in this chapter, a large proportion of adult Canadians performed very poorly on measures of prose, document, and quantitative literacy according to the International Adult Literacy Skills Survey. An even greater percentage cannot find, understand, and use health information and services to make proper health decisions by themselves (CCL, 2008a). The low levels of health literacy tend to be concentrated among the most vulnerable Canadians—seniors, immigrants, Aboriginal peoples, and the unemployed. It is important for us to consider, therefore, why health literacy (and literacy more broadly) should be positioned as an issue of equity and social justice.

What is meant by social justice, equity, and human rights in the context of health literacy? Whitehead (1992) defined health inequities as differences in health that are unnecessary, avoidable, unfair, and unjust. Building on Whitehead's work, Braveman and Gruskin (2003) defined equity in health as the "absence of systematic disparities in health (or in the major social determinants of health) between groups with different levels of underlying social advantage/disadvantage—that is, wealth, power, or prestige" (p. 254). As Mary Robinson, former United Nations High Commissioner for Human Rights, commented,

> The right to health does not mean the right to be healthy, nor does it mean that poor governments must put in place expensive health services for which they have no resources. But it does require governments and public authorities to put in place policies and action plans which will lead to available and accessible health care for all in the shortest possible time. To ensure that this happens is the challenge facing both the human rights community and public health professionals. (World Health Organization, 2002, p. 11)

The Universal Declaration of Human Rights and other major international human rights treaties, such as the 1966 International Covenant on Economic, Social and Cultural Rights, the 1989 Convention on the Rights of the Child, the 1979 Convention on the Elimination of All Forms of Discrimination Against Women, and the 1965 International Convention on the Elimination of All Forms of Racial Discrimination, among others, recognize that the right to health is a basic human right. According to the World Health Organization's (2002) rights-based approach to health, health systems should be accessible to all, especially to the "most vulnerable or marginalized sections of the population, in law and in fact, without discrimination on any of the prohibited grounds" (p. 18). Consequently, health literacy—the ability to read, write, listen, speak, calculate, critically analyze, communicate, and interact, skills that help develop one's ability to utilize information to promote good health—becomes an integral element of the human right to health. According to the Ottawa Charter for Health Promotion's social justice perspective (World Health Organization, 2012), addressing low health literacy calls for the provision of equal rights to accessible health information and understandable health services across different population groups.

Canada has an important role to play nationally and internationally in addressing low health literacy issues and in demonstrating how improved health literacy can affect the provision of health care. As an international leader in the health literacy field, through research, initiatives, and other activities (Rootman & Ronson, 2005), Canada has been recognized for its hard work in this area and its capacity to establish a vision for a health literate Canada (McNeil-Mulak, 2004; Rootman & Gordon-El-Bihbety, 2008). However, this vision will only be realized through undertaking additional research, strengthening existing initiatives and other activities, and harnessing political will; increasing community development, organizational development, and partnership building between health and literacy sectors; and combining the efforts of practitioners, public policy-makers, and the public (Perrin, 1998; Rootman & Gordon-El-Bihbety, 2008; Rootman & Ronson, 2005).

The Expert Panel on Health Literacy has summed up a vision for a health literate Canada, further emphasizing a social justice perspective:

> All people in Canada [should] have the capacity, opportunities, and support they need to obtain and use health information effectively, to act as informed partners in caring for themselves, their families and communities, and to manage interactions in a variety of settings that affect health and well-being. (Rootman & Gordon-El-Bihbety, 2008, p. 23)

This vision assumes shared responsibility by individuals and society in enhancing health literacy; by making Canada a health literate country, government and individuals can reduce inequities in health information access, which can translate into better informed health decision making and health care use. Thus, we should view health literacy through multiple lenses: as an important determinant of health, as a fundamental human right, and as a foundation of social justice.

Health information can be puzzling for anyone seeking to lead an active and healthy life to obtain, understand, assess, communicate, and apply. While reading, writing, listening, speaking, calculating, critically analyzing, communicating, interacting, and utilizing information to promote good health depend on a person's abilities, these are also subject to health care professionals' ability to communicate health information to health care consumers. In other words, following instructions after a doctor's visit, managing a chronic illness, or taking medication properly on the part of patients depends on health care providers using clear and easy-to-understand language, directions, and presentations of materials when communicating with patients. As such, just as everyone has the right to understand health information, everyone has the responsibility to clearly communicate health information. Chapter 4 provides a more detailed discussion of health literacy as a human right and a social justice issue.

Taking the task seriously, our goal in this textbook is to provide students and practitioners in health communication, health promotion, public health, nursing, medicine, health informatics, health education, cultural studies, library science, and, indeed, in any field where there is a focus on health, with deeper insights into and a better understanding of issues related to health literacy in Canada.

KEY LEARNING POINTS

The Expert Panel on Health Literacy and the Canadian Council on Learning (CCL) have defined health literacy as a person's ability to access, understand, evaluate, and communicate information in a way to promote, maintain, and improve health in a variety of settings across the life course. Low health literacy is strongly associated with poor health outcomes for individuals, communities, and health systems. Improving health literacy is an active and transformative process. Canada has been a leader in health literacy initiatives, drawing on partnerships with many organizations, including the Canadian Public Health Association, the CCL, the Centre for Literacy, public libraries, and literacy networks across the provinces. The health literacy of Canadian adults is low, with more than half of the population having difficulty finding and using health information to support their health decision making. Low health literacy is particularly concerning for seniors, immigrants, Aboriginal people, the unemployed, and those with limited education. Given this burden among vulnerable subgroups of Canadians, health literacy must be seen as a public health issue and as one of social justice.

A CANADIAN MILESTONE

With funding from the Social Sciences and Humanities Research Council of Canada, researchers and practitioners from St. Francis Xavier University and community organizations developed a community–university participatory action partnership to explore the link between literacy and health. The project involved the lived experiences of people with low literacy in three rural Nova Scotia counties. People were asked how they found and used health information, services, and supports. Among the compelling findings from this study was that low health literacy is a public health and social justice issue in Canada. This understanding of health literacy is found in the voice of one of the participants:

It is not that I did not try. I tried everything that there is to try. I ran out of options.... I can't go to work wherever I try.... I'm a high-risk injury, they won't hire me. I got no education ... I've tried to put my life together so I could support myself and my son. I can't put this together ... I'm in the middle of a puzzle. There's a piece that don't fit in there, can't get it to fit.... If you were me, how could you make it better? That is my question to you. (Unemployed fish plant worker)

Source: Gillis, D., Quigley, B., & MacIsaac, A. (2005, p. 28). Responding to the challenge of literacy and health. *Literacies,* 5. Retrieved from http://www.literacyjournal.ca [accessed: 7 August 2013].

ADDITIONAL RESOURCES OF INTEREST
Decoda Literacy Solutions
http://decoda.ca/resources/library/library-materials-by-topic/health-literacy-materials/
This website of Decoda Literacy Solutions, a literacy organization in British Columbia, lists health

literacy materials intended for use by adult learners, health care practitioners, teachers and tutors, and anyone interested in health literacy issues. Categorized into six sections, the listed materials are accessible online or through the library. The content includes research articles, government sites, documents and reports, online videos, interactive tutorials, podcasts, stories, and so on.

Health Sciences North
http://www.hsnsudbury.ca/PortalEn/ProfessionalResourcesandNetworks/HealthLiteracy-Resources/tabid/672/Default.aspx
This website of Health Sciences North, a regional hospital serving the residents of the City of Greater Sudbury and northeastern Ontario, lists health literacy materials that are categorized into seven sections for use by patients and their families, health care consumers, health care professionals, and anyone interested in health literacy issues. The listed materials—web links, articles, books, reports, videos—are accessible online or through the Health Sciences Library.

Health Literacy Council of Canada
http://www.healthliteracy.ca/en/welcome-healthliteracyca-website.html
The website of the Health Literacy Council of Canada lists health literacy materials that will be useful to the public and professionals alike. The listed materials—health literacy information, resources, and tools—offer an interactive space for users to learn and share.

CHAPTER 2

WHAT IS HEALTH LITERACY?

To be a health literate society, we need a health literate public, health literate health professionals and health literate politicians and policy-makers.
—ILONA KICKBUSCH, SUZANNE WAIT, AND DANIELA MAAG,
NAVIGATING HEALTH, 2005

CHAPTER LEARNING OBJECTIVES
- Differentiate health literacy from literacy and health communication
- Define health literacy
- Provide an overview of health literacy frameworks
- Provide an overview of tools and approaches to measure individual health literacy skills

INTRODUCTION

We begin this chapter with a consideration of the similarities and differences between the broad topics of health communication, literacy, and health literacy. We will outline a number of definitions of health literacy. We will also present important conceptual frameworks for thinking about how to intervene to improve individual (and population) health literacy. Select health literacy measurement tools will be described, together with a discussion of the benefits and limitations associated with these assessments and a few examples of how these tools have been used in the Canadian context.

HEALTH COMMUNICATION, LITERACY, AND HEALTH LITERACY
HEALTH COMMUNICATION

Health communication is an intriguing and multifaceted field of study that encompasses the disciplines of communication and health promotion. It is "an area of study that simultaneously allows one to look at the creation of shared meaning and at the impact of messages on health and health care delivery" (Thompson, Dorsey, Miller, & Parrott, 2003, p. 1) As a field of inquiry, health communication focuses on four main levels of communication analysis: intrapersonal, interpersonal, group/organizational, and societal (Kreps, Bonaguro, & Query, 1998). At each of these levels, health communication scholarship has contributed to our understanding of how communication plays a powerful and complex role in health care and health promotion. As a field of study, health communication is large in its mandate and scope; *health communication* serves as an umbrella term describing strategies used to inform people about personal and public health issues and risks. As a set of strategies, health-based messages are directed toward improving the health status of individuals, communities, and populations. Thus, we can describe health communication as a discipline concerned with any type of information exchange and information strategies about health. Health communication strategies can include the use of

- edutainment (e.g., storytelling, puppet shows, or television shows, such as the children's television show *Sesame Street*);
- health journalism (e.g., journalists specializing in health issues, such as André Picard from *The Globe and Mail*);
- interpersonal communication (e.g., a dyadic encounter between patient–provider);
- media advocacy to shape health issues in ways that build support for and influence healthy public policy (e.g., dangers of using tobacco products);
- risk communication, whereby information is provided to individuals and communities to inform decision making in support of positive health (e.g., information regarding flu vaccination);
- social communication (e.g., communicating with friends/family about health through face-to-face interactions and social media); and
- social marketing to change values, motivation, and behaviours regarding health issues (e.g., information campaigns advising against texting while driving).

REVIEW AND REFLECT

The next time you watch television, read a magazine, or go online, notice the number and format of the health information messages provided to you through mass media sources.

Health communication messages are deliberate in how they are constructed. These purposefully designed messages take into account issues of accuracy (e.g., evidence informed), readability level (e.g., grade 6–8 ability), audience appeal (e.g., threat versus humour message), format/audiovisual display (e.g., pamphlet, social media), cultural appropriateness (e.g., language, pictorial representation), and dissemination or delivery channels (e.g., mass media, social media, pamphlet) (National Cancer Institute, 2004). All health communication strategies are based on the assumption and expectation that the intended audience has the literacy and health literacy skill needed to access and understand the health message(s). This chapter and other chapters in this book will challenge the widely held assumptions regarding literacy and health literacy competency among Canadians.

LITERACY

According to the United Nations Educational, Scientific and Cultural Organization (UNESCO), literacy was historically understood as the status of being "well educated or learned" (UNESCO, 2005). Although it may seem conventional, it is important to note that early literacy education was not considered to be a basic human right until the right to education was recognized in the 1948 Universal Declaration of Human Rights. Literacy was taught as a set of technical skills that included reading, writing, and calculating. These technical skills, described later in this chapter, served as a foundation for what is now known as "functional literacy." Despite the importance of well-developed functional literacy skills, beginning in the early 1970s, there was a monumental shift in how educators thought about literacy development. Much of the impetus for this shift came from Paulo Freire's (2000) work in education and specifically on literacy development within underprivileged communities in Brazil. What Freire observed and reported in his writings on literacy education (including his seminal work *Pedagogy of the Oppressed*) was that literacy training should include skill development and self-efficacy in advocacy and political action. The Freirian model of literacy education encouraged individuals, mostly impoverished and disenfranchised, to question why things have to be the way they are and to collectively consider how to create change for the better. This model of literacy acknowledges the social dimensions of acquiring and applying literacy. Chapter 3 in this text, "Population Measures of Literacy and Health Literacy," highlights the influence of income, employment, age, and education as important social dimensions in literacy knowledge and skill development. Chapter 5, "Culture and Health Literacy," will help you to understand that literacy knowledge and skill development is culturally and linguistically defined. What is important to recognize is that literacy is not a stand-alone skill, but a social practice contributing to lifelong learning. This skill and practice influence one's "entire spectrum of daily life from the exercise of civil and political rights through matters of work, commerce and childcare to self-instruction, spiritual enlightenment and even recreation" (UNESCO, 2004, p. 10). As you will learn later in this chapter, this way of conceptualizing literacy is reflected in many (but not all) of the frameworks describing health literacy.

In agreement with this cognitive/social/cultural model of literacy, Human Resources and Skills Development Canada defines literacy as "the ability to understand and employ printed information in daily activities, at home, at work and in the community, to achieve one's goals and to develop one's knowledge and potential" (Statistics Canada, 1997). Similarly, the Canadian Council on Learning (CCL) defines literacy as "the ability to analyse things, understand general ideas or terms, use symbols in complex ways, apply theories, and perform other necessary life skills—including the ability to engage in the social and economic life of the community" (CCL, 2007c, p. 86). The Centre for Literacy, located in Montreal, is even more explicit in incorporating the cognitive/social/cultural components in the definition provided on its website (see www.centreforliteracy.qc.ca/). It is especially noteworthy that the Centre uses a values-based approach in its definition:

> [A] complex set of abilities needed to understand and use the dominant
> symbol systems of a culture—alphabets, numbers, visual icons—for per-

sonal and community development.... [I]n a technological society, literacy ... include[s] multiple literacies such as visual, media, and information literacy ... [that create] the capacity of individuals to use and make critical judgements about the information they encounter on a daily basis. (Centre for Literacy, n.d.)

Another important perspective that has emerged in recent years about functional literacy is that it is a practice-based skill. Essentially what this means is that the more a person reads, the better he or she becomes at reading. The Committee on Learning Sciences stressed that literacy as a complex skill requires thousands of hours of practice to develop and maintain (National Research Council, 2012). Population measures of adult literacy skill provide strong evidence that many Canadians are not engaging (or not engaging often enough) in practice activities (e.g., reading) that maintain adequate literacy ability. In fact, Canadian statistics indicate that only 14 percent of leisure activity is devoted to reading (see Figure 2.1). Yet adequate literacy skill has taken on greater importance in managing everyday activities. Both newspapers and television news broadcasts highlight the increase in societal complexity and global communication that has become a part of our everyday functioning.

FIGURE 2.1: CANADIANS' LEISURE ACTIVITIES

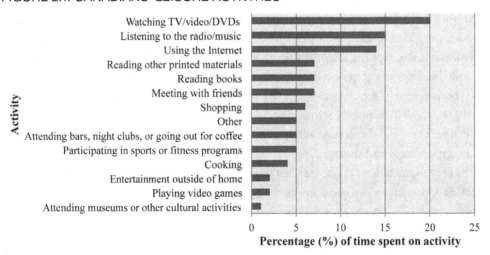

Source: Modified from Canadian Publishers Council. (2004). Book buying attitudes and behaviours. Figure 1. Retrieved from http://www.pch.gc.ca/eng/1290026184681/1305115272786 [accessed: 13 June 2013].

The most commonly cited population measures of literacy are from the International Adult Literacy Survey (IALS), which include an assessment of prose, document, and quantitative proficiency (Statistics Canada, 1997, 2005). What we know from the population-based surveys is that approximately 48 percent of Canadian adults have difficulty with very simple reading materials.

Numeracy skill is another key element of basic literacy. Numeracy refers to the ability to use simple mathematical concepts to effectively budget and manage finances, to maintain health (i.e., understand health-related information related to decision making around medications, health risks, diet, and exercise), and to manage a household (i.e., home repairs/renovation, mortgage, shopping) (Bunker, Houghton, & Baum, 1998; Dingwall, 2000; Epstein, Alper, & Quill, 2004). Approximately 55 percent of Canadian adults lack the numeracy skill to meet the complex demands of everyday life (Statistics Canada, 2005). Chapter 3 discusses in detail the population measures of literacy and health literacy abilities of Canadians.

As we pointed out earlier in this chapter, it is of concern that many Canadians function below the expected minimum level of prose and numeracy skill and are challenged by increasingly complex information. Literacy proficiency is essential for the facilitation of personal, community, social, and civic development. People also need specialized skill in the areas of scientific, technological, cultural, media, computer, and health literacies (Kickbusch, 2001). In fact, we are witness to one of the most significant labour shifts in the workplace in the movement from labour-intensive to knowledge-based economies (OECD, 2001). The Organisation for Economic Co-operation and Development (OECD) emphasizes high levels of education and literacy skill as key competencies needed to function within our knowledge-based economies (see Box 2.1).

BOX 2.1: THE ORGANISATION FOR ECONOMIC CO-OPERATION AND DEVELOPMENT (OECD)

The Organisation for Economic Co-operation and Development (OECD) is an organization of 34 member countries. Canada is one of the original 19 founding member countries of the OECD. Representatives of the OECD member countries meet to advance ideas and review progress in specific policy areas, such as economics, trade, science, employment, education, or financial markets.

Source: Adapted from the Organisation for Economic Co-operation and Development (OECD). Retrieved from http://www.oecd.org/ [accessed: 18 June 2013].

Similarly, in health care, we are witnessing increased knowledge demands that coincide with the rise in chronic diseases. For example, diabetes tends to involve greater individual participation to self-manage the disease. Successful self-care is, for the most part, dependent on access to accurate health information. While a number of traditional health information sources (e.g., health professionals, family and friends, television, newspapers, magazines) remain important, the Internet is steadily becoming a primary resource for health information (see Figure 2.2).

FIGURE 2.2: PERCENTAGE OF CANADIANS WHO CONSULT EACH SOURCE OF HEALTH-RELATED INFORMATION

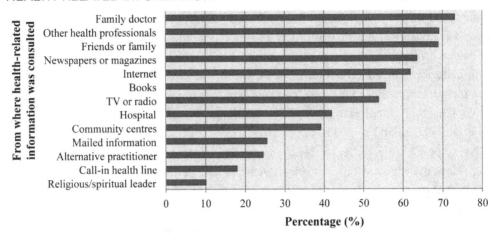

Source: Modified from Canadian Council on Learning. (2008, p. 44). Survey of Canadian attitudes toward learning. Figure 33. Retrieved from http://www.ccl-cca.ca/pdfs/SCAL/2009/SCAL2008_EN.pdf [accessed: 13 June 2013].

Yet widespread online information access has created a paradoxical situation. On the one hand, the general public has ever-increasing access to greater amounts of health information; on the other, the complexity of this health information makes access to it increasingly limited. The remainder of this chapter focuses on how Canadian adults' health literacy skill is measured in individuals. Chapter 3 will address literacy and health literacy skill and measurement at the population level.

WHY SHOULD WE CARE ABOUT DEFINING AND MEASURING HEALTH LITERACY?

As consumers of health care and health services, each of us is bombarded with the literacy demands of the "information age" in which we live. Today, more than ever before, we are expected to understand increasingly sophisticated information about health issues and health care systems (Statistics Canada, 2000). Furthermore, we are encouraged to become involved in health-promoting activities that are often dependent on high levels of literacy proficiency.

Health promotion is defined as the process of enabling people to increase control over, and to improve, their health (World Health Organization, 1986). The principles that guide the practice of health promotion and literacy skill are based on empowerment, collaboration, and social justice and equity, which will be discussed in greater detail in Chapter 4. More often than not, the public's understanding of health promotion is that of individual responsibility for personal lifestyle enhancement (e.g., reduce salt intake or increase physical activity). While behavioural change activities are an important component of health promotion, many other determinants of health influence the health of Canadians (Public Health Agency of Canada, 2003). Broadly speaking, health promotion is enhanced through the availability of supportive environments, equitable access to information and services, the development of effective life skills, and the opportunity to control choices about health.

In addition, the burden of disease within Canada is chronic in nature (and we would argue that this is true across North America) and better suited to management strategies rather than to curative ones. With the increased prevalence of chronic diseases, Canadians are routinely advised by the government and the health care community to take on greater accountability for their own health (Raphael & Curry-Stevens, 2004). At the same time, "person-centred" care is the preferred model advocated by health care providers. The person-centred model is characterized by shared communication, personalized interactions, and collaborative decision making about health care and treatment (Berry, Seiders, & Wilder, 2003; Institute of Medicine [IOM], 2001). This model of care is based on the active participation of the health care recipient as part of the health care team.

Recognition of the information demands and the movement toward a person-centred model of health care has heightened our awareness of the need for improved health literacy (IOM, 2004). Access to and understanding of health information are integral components of decision making within this model of health care. Much of the success in managing chronic disease is reliant on public access to and understanding of verbal or written information, participation in decision making, and a commitment to an established treatment plan that accommodates the life context (e.g., limited income) of the individual or family. Fundamental to self-health promotion and chronic disease management are the literacy and health literacy skills that individuals have or which they need to acquire to access reliable health information and make informed decisions. But as you may suspect from our discussion on literacy proficiency, individuals' limited literacy skill remains a significant barrier to health information access for approximately 50 percent of Canadian adults (Health Canada, 2003).

HEALTH LITERACY DEFINITIONS

Building on our knowledge of health promotion, health literacy similarly stems from the understanding of health and literacy as fundamental human rights. While health literacy is not identical to general literacy, there is significant overlap (Gillis & Quigley, 2004). What is clear is that general literacy skill and health care experience(s) are necessary components of health literacy skill development (Speros, 2005). If you, or a friend, or a family member have experienced an illness or are managing a chronic disease, you can appreciate that information gained from prior health-related experiences provides the "building blocks" for developing greater health care knowledge. Past health care experiences help a person to develop a mental picture or set of expectations that can be drawn on in future health care situations (Speros, 2005). What this means is that if you have knowledge about a specific topic, such as heart disease or diabetes, it increases your understanding of new information. Why should this be the case? Previous knowledge about a health issue provides a mental link and acts as a bridge to new information about a topic from what you have previously learned. The breadth of your vocabulary and your knowledge about a topic are also significant components that contribute to your ability to comprehend information (Beier & Ackerman, 2005; Hirsch, 2003; Reid,

Kardash, & Robinson, 1994; Samuelstuen & Braten, 2005; Spires & Donley, 1998). As Hirsch (2003) has stated, "[K]nowledge about the topic speeds up basic comprehension and leaves working memory free to make connections between the new material and previously learned information" (p. 3).

Technical words or unfamiliar medical or health care terminology affect our understanding of health information. Simply put, people with greater vocabulary skills have an easier time understanding information that is presented to them (Reid, Kardash, & Robinson, 1994). Your level of literacy directly impacts your ability to obtain information relevant to your personal health, to understand the significance and relevance of that information, and to apply that information to promote your own health or that of your family and community (Mitic & Rootman, 2012). In effect, the relationship between lifelong learning, literacy, and health literacy is particularly strong.

As health care trends shift from an emphasis on acute illness to chronic disease management and health promotion (e.g., self-health management), the concept of health literacy has evolved as well. Yet, despite ever-increasing research on health literacy over the past several decades, we still do not have a single, unanimously accepted definition of this term (Sorensen et al., 2012). In 2008, a group of international scholars on health literacy met in Canada and concluded that health literacy skills are based on reading, writing, listening, speaking, numeracy, and critical analysis, as well as communication and interaction skills (Coleman et al., 2008). Despite this, the primary components that make up health literacy do not have universal agreement. There are some important consequences of the lack of consensus on what constitutes adequate (let alone optimal) health literacy. For health literacy students, educators, and researchers who try to operationalize health literacy beyond the functional skills of information access and comprehension, significant challenges occur. We will return to this issue of challenges later in the chapter when we discuss the measurement of health literacy.

In a recent systematic review, Sorensen et al. (2012) identified 17 definitions of health literacy that have been used in the research literature. Students are encouraged to read this systematic review for a more comprehensive listing of health literacy definitions. In this chapter we will highlight some of the most commonly used definitions. Definitions of health literacy have evolved from simply being "the ability to read, understand, and act on healthcare information" (Potter & Martin, 2005) into multifaceted, comprehensive models (Nutbeam, 2000; Zarcadoolas, Pleasant, & Greer, 2005). Early definitions of health literacy focused on *functional skills* that included the ability to manage words (prose and document literacy) and numbers (numeric literacy) in a *medical context*. One of the early definitions of health literacy from the Ad Hoc Committee on Health Literacy in 1999 described it as a functional skill set that includes the ability to perform basic reading and numerical tasks specific to the health care environment. Experts in the field suggest that adequate functional health literacy enables individuals to understand oral and written information about health care issues, follow written and numerical directions regarding their therapeutic regimens and diagnostic tests, ask pertinent questions of health care providers, report past medical history, and contribute to problem solving related to their care (Parker, Baker, Williams, & Nurss, 1995). One of the most often cited definitions of health literacy comes from the U.S. Institute of Medicine (2004), which defines health literacy as "the degree to which individuals have the capacity to obtain, process, and understand basic health information and services needed to make appropriate health decisions" (p. 4).

Other definitions of health literacy incorporate a broader, more complex, and interconnected set of abilities, such as reading and acting upon written health information, communicating needs to health professionals, and understanding health instructions, all linked to the core value of citizen/public empowerment (Coleman et al., 2008; Sorensen et al., 2012). The following definitions reflect this shift from specific individual abilities to more of a *population* perspective. For example, the Canadian Expert Panel on Health Literacy defines health literacy as "[t]he ability to access, understand, evaluate and communicate information as a way to promote, maintain and improve health in a variety of settings across the life-course" (Rootman & Gordon-El-Bihbety, 2008, p. 11). This definition draws attention to the dynamic nature of health literacy and the influence of the everyday life context and an individual's stage in life in shaping health literacy skills.

Kickbusch and Maag (2008) provide another influential definition of health literacy: "The capacity to make sound health decisions in the context of everyday life—at home, in the community, at the workplace, in the health-care system, in the market place and in the political arena. It is a critical empowerment strategy to increase people's control over their health, their ability to seek out information, and their ability to take responsibility" (p. 206). This definition draws on the need for diverse skills and competencies that promote empowerment and engagement (see Box 2.2).

BOX 2.2: HEALTH LITERACY DOMAINS OF COMPETENCY

Home/Community/Workplace: *Basic health competencies* and the application of health-promoting, health-protecting, and disease-preventing behaviours, as well as self-care.

Health Care System: *Patient competencies* to navigate the health system and act as an active partner to professionals.

Marketplace: *Consumer competencies* to make health-related decisions in the selection and use of applicable goods and services and to act on consumer rights if necessary.

Political Arena: *Citizen competencies* through informed voting behaviours, knowledge of health rights, advocacy for health issues, and membership of patient and health organizations.

Source: Adapted from Kickbusch, I., & Maag, D. (2008, p. 207). Health literacy. Table 1. In K. Heggenhougen & S. Quah (Eds.), *International Encyclopedia of Public Health* (Vol. 3). San Diego: Academic Press, pp. 204–211. Retrieved from http://www.ilonakickbusch.com/kickbusch-wAssets/docs/kickbusch-maag.pdf [accessed: 18 June 2013].

An additional definition of health literacy is provided by Zarcadoolas and colleagues (2005). From their perspective, health literacy represents an intersection of different literacies that extend beyond the health sector. These literacies include fundamental literacy, science literacy, civic literacy, and cultural literacy. Specifically, health literacy is "the wide range of skills and competencies that people develop to seek out, comprehend, evaluate and use health information and concepts to make informed choices, reduce health risks and increase quality of life" (Zarcadoolas et al., 2005, p. 197). As we will learn in Chapter 8, scientific literacy (which overlaps with health literacy and numeracy) is distressingly low among Canadian adults.

Finally, we cannot leave the challenge of defining health literacy without considering the perspective offered by Nutbeam (2000). He defines health literacy as "the cognitive and social skills which determine the motivation and ability of individuals to gain access to, understand, and use information in ways which promote and maintain good health (p. 264). This definition of health literacy also implies the achievement of a level of knowledge, personal skills, and confidence to take action to improve *personal and community health* by changing personal lifestyles and living conditions (Nutbeam, 2000). Nutbeam's multifaceted definition attributes cognitive and social as well as behavioural aspects to health literacy and addresses the broader determinants of health—the social, economic, and environmental determinants—to improve personal and community health.

As a component of health literacy, health numeracy is also an elusive concept. It has been defined as "the degree to which individuals have the capacity to access, process, interpret, communicate, and act on numerical, quantitative, graphical, biostatistical, and probabilistic health information needed to make effective health decisions" (Golbeck, Ahlers-Schmidt, Paschal, & Dismuke, 2005, p. 375). As proposed by Golbeck and her colleagues (2005), health numeracy consists of four components: basic, computational, analytical, and statistical skill. Basic health numeracy involves the ability to identify numbers and comprehend quantitative data with no number manipulation (e.g., correctly identify the date of a health care appointment). Computational numeracy involves skill in simple arithmetic. Analytical skill requires interpretive skills characteristic of the ability to determine whether scores fit within an established range (e.g., what is a "normal" blood pressure?). Statistical numeracy requires an understanding of basic biostatistics (i.e., probability, life expectancy, risk). We use numeracy skills each day when reading nutrition labels while grocery shopping, when calculating the correct dose of over-the-counter medications for relief from cold symptoms, or when deciding whether we can afford to enrol our children in extracurricular community activities such as sports programs. Think back over the last 24 hours and consider how many times and for how many different activities health numeracy skills were needed. Health numeracy is especially important in effective self-health care, in managing chronic disease, and in helping individuals to understand and participate in decision making regarding their health.

REVIEW AND REFLECT

Review the information below from the National Cancer Institute (www.cancer.gov) about breast cancer risk. Assess how well this information serves people who want to know more about breast cancer and consider the level of prose and numeric skill needed to comprehend this important public health prevention message.

BREAST CANCER RISK

Anything that increases the chance of developing a disease is called a risk factor. Risk factors for breast cancer include the following:

- age
- age at the start of menstruation
- age at first live birth
- number of first-degree relatives (mother, sisters, daughters) with breast cancer
- number of previous breast biopsies (whether positive or negative)
- at least one breast biopsy with atypical hyperplasia

Other risk factors, such as age at menopause, dense breast tissue on a mammogram, use of birth control pills or hormone replacement therapy, a high-fat diet, drinking alcohol, low physical activity, obesity, or environmental exposures, are not included in risk estimates with the Breast Cancer Risk Assessment Tool for three reasons: evidence is not conclusive or researchers cannot accurately determine how much these factors contribute to the calculation of risk for an individual woman, or adding these factors does not increase the accuracy of the tool appreciably. Breast cancer may also be caused by inherited gene mutations. Hereditary breast cancers account for approximately 5% to 10% of all breast cancers.

To summarize this point, there are commonalities among what is meant by the terms *health communication*, *literacy*, and *health literacy*. General literacy and health literacy share similarities but are also distinct. For example, people with higher education and advanced literacy skills can still experience difficulty in obtaining, understanding, and using health information. We have also reviewed the multiple and evolving definitions of health literacy, which tend to fall into one of two dimensions: the medical/individual dimension or the public/population dimension. Common to the medically based health literacy definitions are reading, writing, listening, speaking, numeric, and cultural knowledge and skill; that is, the ability to comprehend health information for informed decision making. These definitions emphasize functional abilities for health literacy. Definitions of a public/population perspective also include the above-mentioned components but extend the scope of health literacy from the individual to include community- and civic-level engagement within the broader social determinants of health.

HEALTH LITERACY FRAMEWORKS

In this section, we introduce frameworks of health literacy. The Merriam-Webster dictionary (2012a) defines a *frame of reference* (or "framework") as "a set of ideas, conditions, or
assumptions that determine how something will be approached, perceived, or understood."
Frameworks are helpful in providing us with an organized and structured way of looking at
an issue and its related concepts. Frameworks can be simple or quite complex and reflect the
conceptual perspective or understanding of the developer(s).

One of the most influential frameworks for health literacy was put forward by the U.S. Institute of Medicine (2004). This framework includes a variety of components: reading and writing,
numeracy, listening, speaking, and cultural and contextual knowledge. In this framework, individual literacy skill is an important contributor to health literacy development. This framework
proposes that health literacy has a significant impact on health care outcomes and costs (see Figure
2.3). And, as influential as this framework has been in the development of the health literacy field,
it is important to note the limited perspective on the social determinants of health.

FIGURE 2.3: INSTITUTE OF MEDICINE HEALTH LITERACY FRAMEWORK

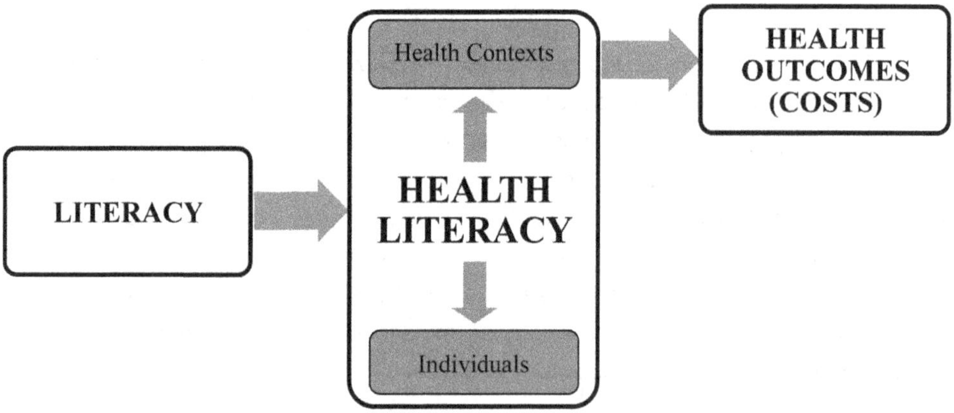

Source: Modified from Institute of Medicine. (2004, p. 33). *Health literacy: A prescription to end confusion.* Figure 21.
Washington, DC: The National Academies Press.

There are other frameworks of health literacy that go beyond reading, writing, and numeracy
skills to include the wider spectrum of knowledge domains of the social determinants of health.
A widely accepted framework of health literacy is one offered by Nutbeam (2000), who frames
health literacy as a typology with functional, interactive, and critical skills components. *Functional* health literacy skill consists of basic reading, writing, and numeric skill for everyday use.
This category comprises the comprehension and communication of health facts, awareness of
health services, and use of the health system. *Interactive* health literacy involves advanced cognitive, social, and literacy skills that contribute to the development of personal skills in a supportive
environment. For example, participants in weight management group programs demonstrate
interactive health literacy skills. Interactive health literacy is directed at improving individual
motivation and self-confidence to act in ways that enhance health. *Critical* health literacy consists

of advanced analytical, advocacy, and social skills that are geared toward critiquing broader social and political structures with the goal of creating positive change within communities and at the societal level. An example of critical health literacy is the advances made by the Mothers Against Drunk Driving (MADD) organization. MADD is a group of people who have successfully organized to advocate for social and legislative change in drinking and driving behaviours. The different typologies of functional, interactive, and critical health literacy represent knowledge, skills, and attitudes that support greater self-sufficiency and control in personal health management, but extend health literacy to include collective engagement (e.g., groups and communities) with a wider range of health knowledge and skills (e.g., activism and advocacy) to act on the social determinants of health (Nutbeam, 2000; Sorensen et al., 2012).

Nutbeam's framework has been applied within the Canadian context with older Spanish-speaking immigrant women in exploring diet-related colon cancer prevention strategies (Thomson & Hoffman-Goetz, 2012). These researchers suggest that the health literacy framework needs to be thought of as a continuum rather than as discrete categories of skills. At the low functional health literacy level, general problem identification skills might be evident, whereas at a higher level (but still within functional health literacy), specific information identification skills would occur.

Kickbusch and Maag (2008) have proposed a health literacy framework that expands on Nutbeam's typology. This framework incorporates the multiple domains in which health (as a resource for everyday living) happens and includes: (1) the health care system, (2) home and community, (3) the workplace, (4) the political arena, and (5) the marketplace (see Figure 2.4).

FIGURE 2.4: DOMAINS OF HEALTH LITERACY

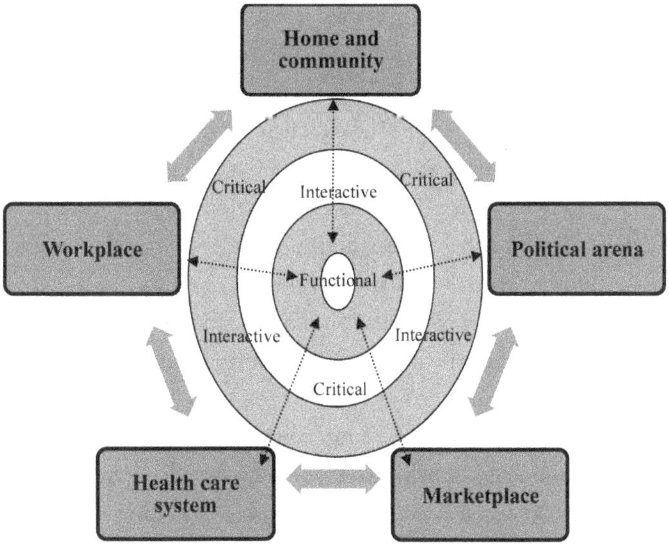

Source: Modified from Kickbusch, I., & Maag, D. (2008, p. 207). Health literacy. Figure 5. In K. Heggenhougen & S. Quah (Eds.), *International Encyclopedia of Public Health* (Vol. 3). San Diego: Academic Press, pp. 204–211. Retrieved from http://www.ilonakickbusch.com/kickbusch-wAssets/docs/kickbusch-maag.pdf [accessed: 18 June 2013].

The development of health literacy is viewed as a shared responsibility that recognizes the individual's role but also acknowledges the responsibility of the "communicator" (i.e., other individuals, health care providers, the health system) to frame health information and services in a way that accommodates educational, cultural, spiritual, and physical diversity (Coleman et al., 2008; Kickbusch & Maag, 2008). *The Calgary Charter on Health Literacy*, originally created as a framework for educational curriculum development, posits the accountability for health literacy with individuals but also with health care providers and systems. The expert group that created the Charter states that "health care professionals can be health literate by presenting information in ways that improve people's understanding and the ability of people to act on information. Systems can be health literate by providing equal, easy, and shame-free access to and delivery of health care and health information" (Coleman et al., 2008, p. 2).

By improving people's access to health information and their capacity to use it in personally meaningful ways, health literacy is crucial to empowerment (greater control of health decisions) and successful personal health care management, and also for creating change at the broader community and societal levels. In its advanced form, health literacy allows individuals to participate in the ongoing public and private conversations about health, medicine, scientific knowledge, and cultural beliefs with a confidence that they have the right to ask for what they need in order to stay healthy.

CANADA'S ROLE IN HEALTH LITERACY EXPERTISE

Canada has been and continues to be a recognized leader in health literacy research and development. Reviewing the timeline of health literacy development within Canada reveals that inquiry and investigation of health literacy issues extends over three decades. Chapter 1 of this book provides a detailed timeline of health literacy activity within Canada. One of the key Canadian health literacy initiatives was the formation of the Expert Panel on Health Literacy. This group of experts was supported in their work by the Canadian Public Health Association and produced a seminal report titled *A Vision for a Health Literate Canada: Report of the Expert Panel on Health Literacy* (Rootman & Gordon-El-Bihbety, 2008). Based on the work of the Expert Panel, the current Canadian definition of health literacy is the "degree to which people are able to access, understand, appraise, and communicate information to engage with the demands of different health contexts in order to promote and maintain good health across the life-course" (Kwan, Frankish, & Rootman, 2006, as cited in Rootman & Gordon-El-Bihbety, 2008, p. 11).

Embedded within this definition is the understanding that health literacy–related tasks simultaneously require prose, document, and numeracy skills. From a Canadian context, health literacy is understood to be a wide range of skills that improve the ability of people to act on information in order to live healthier lives. Health literacy allows the public and personnel working in all health-related contexts to find, understand, evaluate, communicate, and use information. Health literacy applies to all individuals (consumers of health care and providers) and to health systems. The Canadian health literacy framework, similar to others, recognizes the impact of family and community, and societal and global influences on health literacy development (Coleman et al., 2008).

The Expert Panel on Health Literacy reported on the low health literacy among many Canadians and expressed specific concern regarding seniors, immigrants, and unemployed Canadians (see Chapter 3 for greater detail on how Canadians fare on population measures of health literacy). In their report, the Expert Panel put out a "call to action" for policy-makers, government, researchers, health care providers, educators, and other sectors of society that influence health to address the serious disparities in health literacy among the Canadian public. You can see from their "call to action" that they have incorporated a values-based (social justice/ equity) approach to health literacy in demanding action on reducing the reported disparities.

MEASUREMENT OF HEALTH LITERACY

From our review of health literacy definitions and frameworks, we know that health literacy is conceptualized as an individual issue and also as a societal concern. In this section, we will review *individual* health literacy assessment instruments. (A review of *population* measures of health literacy and measurement strategies is found in Chapter 3.) Health literacy skill is related to individuals' ability to gain value from health messages, materials, and conversations. Low health literacy means that a person has difficulty in reading, understanding, and interpreting even the simplest health information. Yet, studies have found that health education material often exceeds the reading levels of the average adult (Friedman, Hoffman-Goetz, & Arocha, 2004; Rudd, 2010). The reading difficulty of health-related material for the general public is often well above a high-school level. Imagine how frustrating it must be for people with low health literacy to be given health education materials written at such a high level that even university professors have difficulty understanding it. As an exercise, try testing the readability level of any written health material you have (a page from this or another textbook, a page from a website, etc.) using the Simplified Measure of Gobbledygook (SMOG), the Flesch Reading Ease or Flesch-Kincaid Grade Level, or the Gunning's Fog Readability (sometimes called the Fog Index) formulas (see Box 2.3: Readability Assessments).

BOX 2.3: READABILITY ASSESSMENTS

Readability tests (e.g., Flesch-Kincaid, SMOG) are based on mathematical formulas designed to assess the suitability of reading materials for different ages or grade levels. Different formulas will assess sentence length, syllable count, and difficult vocabulary. Although different assessment tools are available for use, they cannot be compared and contrasted. Three of the most utilized assessments are provided below.

THE GUNNING'S FOG INDEX (OR FOG) READABILITY FORMULA

Step 1: Take a sample passage of at least 100 words and count the number of exact words and sentences.

Step 2: Divide the total number of words in the sample by the number of sentences to arrive at the Average Sentence Length (ASL).

Step 3: Count the number of words of three or more syllables that are NOT (i) proper nouns, (ii) combinations of easy words or hyphenated words, or (iii) two-syllable verbs made into three with -es and -ed endings.

Step 4: Divide this number by the number of words in the sample passage. For example, 25 long words divided by 100 words gives you 25 Percent Hard Words (PHW).

Step 5: Add the ASL from Step 2 and the PHW from Step 4.

Step 6: Multiply the result by 0.4.

The ideal readability score is 7 or 8. A Fog index score above 12 is too difficult for most people to read.

Source: Readability Formulas. (n.d.). *The Gunning's Fog Index (or FOG) Readability Formula.* Retrieved from http://www.readabilityformulas.com/gunning-fog-readability-formula.php [accessed: 13 August 2013].

SIMPLIFIED MEASURE OF GOBBLEDYGOOK (SMOG)

The SMOG readability assessment is considered to be the most rigorous of the reading assessment tools because it focuses on words and sentences rather than on words alone.

The assessment involves:

- identifying 30 sentences (three 10-sentence samples) of written text;
- counting the syllables in every word and highlighting the words that have three or more syllables;
- estimating the square root of the total number of words with multiple syllables within the 30 sentences of text; and
- adding 3 to the square root value to obtain a reading grade level.

Source: McLaughlin, G.H. (2008). *SMOG: Simple Measure of Gobbledygook.* Retrieved from http://www.harrymclaughlin.com/SMOG.htm [accessed: 18 June 2013].

FLESCH READING EASE/FLESCH-KINCAID GRADE LEVEL*

The Flesch-Kincaid Grade Level is based on word and sentence length. This formula assesses words, syllables, and sentences to determine the minimum reading grade level required by an individual to read the text. Use the link and follow the steps to assess the readability of text.

Source: Flesch, R. (1979). *How to write plain English.* Retrieved from http://pages.stern.nyu.edu/~wstarbuc/Writing/Flesch.htm [accessed: 18 June 2013].

*Microsoft Word is also set up to calculate readability using Flesch Reading Ease and Flesch-Kincaid Grade Level assessments.

As discussed above, health literacy includes a composite of reading, writing, listening, speaking, numeracy, and critical analysis, as well as communication and interaction skills.

Measurement of health literacy skill has been broadly categorized into assessments of prose, numeric, and document assessments. Unfortunately, most measurements of the health literacy of Canadians have been geared to prose literacy only. Arguably, the challenges that exist in finding consensus on a definition of health literacy also exist in the measurement instruments. Existing instruments measuring health literacy tend to reflect *functional health literacy* skill only. In fact, there are no standardized instruments or methods to *comprehensively* assess the full spectrum of health literacy skills (Davis & Wolf, 2004). In addition, the instruments we do have to measure functional health literacy are limited to only a few languages (e.g., English, Spanish, Mandarin or Cantonese). Indeed, a cultural bias may be present in many of the existing instruments (Stewart, Riecken, Scott, Tanaka, & Riecken, 2008), and a critical analysis of current health literacy assessment instruments is both timely and particularly relevant in Canada, given our multicultural and cultural mosaic society.

Still, there are many tests and techniques to measure individual health literacy ability. In this section, we will describe a few of the most common assessment instruments that measure the functional health literacy skills of individuals. These include the Rapid Estimate of Adult Literacy in Medicine (REALM), the Short Assessment of Health Literacy for Spanish Adults (SAHLSA-50), the Test of Functional Health Literacy in Adults (TOFHLA), and the Newest Vital Sign (NVS). It is important to keep in mind that, while these tests and assessments have been applied to research settings, we have far less information about whether they are appropriate for screening in clinical health care settings (Davis & Wolf, 2004). Another approach to measuring individual health literacy involves using open-ended, qualitative approaches, such as "Teach-Back" or "Ask Me 3." These will also be briefly described in this section.

RAPID ESTIMATE OF ADULT LITERACY IN MEDICINE (REALM) AND SHORT ASSESSMENT OF HEALTH LITERACY FOR SPANISH ADULTS (SAHLSA-50)

The Rapid Estimate of Adult Literacy in Medicine (REALM) is an assessment tool designed to measure adults' ability to read common medical, anatomical, or illness terms. This instrument is considered one of the most easily administered tools for assessing health literacy in English. Essentially, REALM and the Rapid Estimate of Adult Literacy in Medicine—Short Form (REALM-SF) are word recognition tests and do not assess reader comprehension. The REALM assessment consists of a list of 66 words that range from simple to increasingly difficult pronunciation (Davis et al., 1993). Individuals score 1 point for the correct pronunciation of each word for a total possible score of 66 points. According to REALM, individuals who receive a score greater than 60 would be able to read most health education materials. REALM-SF is a seven-item word recognition test that provides clinicians with a valid, quick assessment of patient health literacy. It takes approximately 3 minutes to administer and score. The test is administered by providing a copy of the following seven words:

- menopause
- antibiotics
- exercise

- jaundice
- rectal
- anemia
- behaviour

The individual being assessed is instructed to read out loud as many words as they can from the list of seven, beginning with the first word. If the individual is unable to read a word, they are instructed to say "blank" and move on to the next word in the list until they either cannot verbalize any additional words or they complete the list.

A REALM-SF score of 1–3 reflects the need for low-literacy materials, and even those who score 4–6 correct responses will likely struggle with most patient education materials. Individuals who do not pronounce any of the words correctly are not likely to be able to read even the lowest level of literacy materials and would require verbal instructions that are frequently repeated. These individuals would likely do best with educational materials composed of illustrations or audiovisual strategies. Someone with a REALM-SF score of 7 would likely be able to read most health education materials (Agency for Healthcare Research and Quality, 2009). REALM was used to assess health literacy skill among individuals attending a rural health clinic (Wood, 2005). Their REALM scores indicated that nearly half of the individuals who consented to participate in the research would not be able to read most patient education materials. Findings from this research were helpful in developing skill-appropriate health education print and audiovisual resources for the clinic participants.

Similar to REALM-SF, the Short Assessment of Health Literacy for Spanish Adults (SAHLSA-50) is a health literacy assessment tool containing 50 items that is designed to assess a Spanish-speaking adult's ability to read and understand common medical terms. The SAHLSA is based on the Rapid Estimate of Adult Literacy in Medicine (REALM).

TEST OF FUNCTIONAL HEALTH LITERACY IN ADULTS (TOFHLA)

Another widely used health literacy (prose and numeracy) assessment instrument is the Test of Functional Health Literacy in Adults (TOFHLA) and the shortened version (S-TOFHLA) of this same test (Davis, Michielutte, Askov, Williams, & Weiss, 1998; Parker et al., 1995). The TOFHLA is an improvement over the REALM assessment tool because it measures participants' comprehension of text passages based on real health care situations. It consists of two parts: reading comprehension and numeric knowledge. In the prose section of the test, every fifth to seventh word is omitted from the sentences of health information, and the reader must select the correct word to complete each sentence from multiple-choice responses. This process of omitting words and having the reader choose the correct word to finish the sentence is called the "Cloze" procedure, and it measures individuals' comprehension of printed information.

The TOFHLA numeracy items assess a patient's ability to comprehend directions for taking medicines, monitoring blood glucose, keeping clinic appointments, and applying for medical financial assistance. The reading comprehension and numeracy scores are equally weighted in the final TOFHLA score, which ranges from 0–100. Scores of 0–59 represent inadequate health literacy skill, 60–74 indicates marginal health literacy, and 75–100 indicates adequate health literacy. The TOFHLA takes up to 22 minutes to administer and to date is recognized as the most useful health literacy assessment tool (Davis et al., 1998). The TOFHLA is a U.S.-based assessment, and because of this, the instrument may need to be adapted for use in other countries. For example, the TOFHLA asks questions about Medicare, which may not be applicable to English speakers in other countries, including Canada.

Using the S-TOFHLA, researchers examined the relationship between health literacy skill and knowledge of disease among older individuals (65 years and over) who were managing a chronic disease (asthma, diabetes, congestive heart failure) (Gazmararian, Williams, Peel, & Baker, 2003). According to the scores, approximately 25 percent of individuals had inadequate health literacy skill and knew significantly less about their disease than those who tested as having adequate skill. Canadian researchers also used the shortened version of the TOFHLA to assess the health literacy (prose and numeracy skill) of older Canadian adults living independently within the community (Donelle, Arocha, & Hoffman-Goetz, 2008). Interestingly, most (91 percent) of the older adults involved in the study scored as having "adequate" health literacy skill, indicating their ability to read, understand, and interpret most health material.

NEWEST VITAL SIGN (NVS)

The Newest Vital Sign (NVS) health literacy assessment was developed to measure both prose and numeric literacy skill (Weiss et al., 2005). Available in English and Spanish versions, the instrument has six assessment questions based on participant comprehension of an ice cream nutrition label (see Figure 2.5).

REVIEW AND REFLECT

Referring to Figure 2.5 below, answer the following Newest Vital Sign assessment questions to determine your health literacy:

1. If you eat the entire container [of ice cream], how many calories will you eat?
2. If you are allowed to eat 60 grams of carbohydrates as a snack, how much ice cream can you have?
3. Your doctor advises you to reduce the amount of saturated fat in your diet. You usually have 42 g of saturated fat each day, which includes one serving of ice cream. If you stop eating ice cream, how many grams of saturated fat would you be consuming each day?
4. If you usually eat 2,500 calories in a day, what percentage of your daily value of calories will you be eating if you eat one serving?
5. Pretend that you are allergic to the following substances: penicillin, peanuts, latex gloves, and bee stings. Is it safe for you to eat this ice cream?
6. Ask "Why not?" only if the individual responds "no" to question 5.

FIGURE 2.5: NEWEST VITAL SIGN ICE CREAM NUTRITION LABEL

Nutrition Facts

Serving Size	1/2 cup
Servings per container	4

Amount per serving

Calories 250	Fat Cal 120

	%DV
Total Fat 13g	20%
Sat Fat 9g	40%
Cholesterol 28mg	12%
Sodium 55mg	2%
Total Carbohydrate 30g	12%
Dietary Fiber 2g	
Sugars 23g	
Protein 4g	8%

* Percent Daily Values (DV) are based on a 2,000 calorie diet. Your daily values may be higher or lower depending on your calorie needs.
Ingredients: Cream, Skim Milk, Liquid Sugar, Water, Egg Yolks, Brown Sugar, Milkfat, Peanut Oil, Sugar, Butter, Salt, Carrageenan, Vanilla Extract.

NEWEST VITAL SIGN ANSWERS

1. 1,000 calories
2. 1 cup
3. 33
4. 10%
5. No
6. Because it has peanut oil

Source: Weiss, B.D., Mays, M.Z., Martz, W., Castro, K.M., DeWalt, D.A., Pignone, M.P., ... & Hale, F.A. (2005). Quick assessment of literacy in primary care: The newest vital sign. *Annals of Family Medicine, 3*(6), 514–522.

Participants score one point for each correct answer with a response range of 0–6. The average time for test administration is approximately 3 minutes for the English version and slightly longer (approximately 3.5 minutes) for a Spanish version. Those scoring >4 (greater than four correct answers) on the NVS are, by this assessment, considered to have adequate literacy. A score of <4 (less than four) on the NVS signifies the possibility of limited literacy. Cautionary interpretation of NVS scores of <2 (less than two) is recommended. Respondents scoring <2 have a greater than 50 percent chance of having marginal or inadequate literacy skills (Weiss et al., 2005). Of all the health literacy assessment instruments, the NVS may be the most sensitive test for *screening* persons with limited literacy skill.

THE TEACH-BACK TECHNIQUE

The majority of individuals have difficulty in remembering the information given to them by their health care provider (Kessels, 2003). One strategy to enhance individual understanding of health care information is through the use of the "teach-back" technique. It is an effective method for ensuring that individuals understand verbal or written health information (Weiss, 2007). In your own experience with health care providers, you have likely been asked "Do you have any questions?" or "Do you understand?" and most likely your responses were "No" and "Yes" respectively. More often than not, individuals will not request clarification and will often indicate their understanding of the intended message, even if this is not the case. Confusion and a lack of understanding of health information have been frequent consequences of clinical encounters, especially for seniors, English-as-a-Second-Language (ESL) immigrants, and persons with low literacy. The teach-back technique helps individuals and health care providers to avoid miscommunication and misunderstanding by having the provider ask the person receiving the information or instructions to explain or demonstrate what they have heard. Although the teach-back method can be time-consuming, a recent Canadian study suggests that it is a much better measure of health literacy than S-TOFHLA or Cloze-type tests, especially for people with low health literacy. Additional detail regarding this technique can be found in Chapter 10 of this book.

ASK ME 3 TECHNIQUE

Effective communication with others is an extension of a shame-free and culturally safe environment in which individuals are genuinely welcome to ask questions and seek clarification about what they don't understand. In fact, many individuals, even those with well-developed literacy skills, will often claim to understand information or instructions to avoid appearing uninformed in the presence of the clinician. A simple remedy to this common scenario is to encourage individuals to ask questions. The U.S. National Patient Safety Foundation holds the registered trademark license for Ask Me 3 (National Patient Safety Foundation, n.d.), which is a technique whereby an individual is encouraged to ask three basic questions during every health care encounter. The questions asked by the individual are: What is my main problem? What do I need to do (about the problem)? Why is it important for me to do this? This technique encourages a "climate" of inquiry between the individual and health care provider/educator.

The teach-back and Ask Me 3 techniques are not intended to empirically assess the health literacy skill of individuals. Rather, they are easy-to-administer techniques to assess someone's understanding of the health information/instructions "in the moment." Even so, they are useful in determining individuals' comprehension of health information, which is an essential component of functional health literacy. Physicians from the Cleveland Medical Clinic in the United States are strong advocates for the use of the teach-back and Ask Me 3 techniques. Physicians' use of these strategies has been associated with an enhanced understanding of health information among the people they see in their practice, but equally important, the use of these techniques is showing promise in improving cross-cultural communication and minimizing existing health disparities (Misra-Hebert & Isaacson, 2012). We will further discuss the teach-back and Ask Me 3 techniques and their use in clinical settings in Chapter 9.

KEY LEARNING POINTS

Health communication serves as the umbrella concept for literacy and health literacy. Increased prevalence of chronic disease, an aging Canadian population, ease of access to health information—generally and online—and a climate of fiscal restraint within health care have created an expectation for self-health management within contemporary health care. Fundamental to self-health promotion and chronic disease management are the literacy and health literacy skills necessary for individuals to access reliable health information and make informed decisions. The information demands of chronic disease self-management and the movement toward a person-centred model of health care have heightened our awareness of the need for improved health literacy.

Our understanding of literacy skill development in many ways has foreshadowed the evolutionary path of health literacy. Like literacy education, adequate health literacy skill is considered a basic human right. The conceptual development of health literacy has evolved from a focus on individual functional skills to more complex population-based models.

The creation of a health literate Canada is the responsibility of the general public, health care professionals, and government systems. Health literacy, similar to basic literacy, is not a stand-alone skill. It constitutes a social practice that contributes to lifelong learning. While there are several tests and techniques to measure health literacy ability in people, these assessment instruments are criticized for limiting assessment to functional health literacy skills. A research focus on developing comprehensive health literacy assessment instruments is needed.

A CANADIAN MILESTONE

THE NUNAVUT LITERACY COUNCIL

In 1999 the Nunavut Literacy Council (NLC) was created to promote reading and writing in all official languages of Nunavut. The NLC uses community development and intergenerational learning as core strategies to support and ensure the survival and maintenance of Aboriginal languages. The Nunavut Literacy Council offers literacy training and provides resources to community members in all the official languages: Inuktitut, Inuinnaqtun, English, and French. As well, literacy training has been linked with health promotion initiatives, such as Aboriginal Head Start, pre-natal nutrition, and family support programming. The NLC partners with community groups, such as the Elders and the Municipal Council of Pelly Bay (located east of Cambridge Bay), to develop traditionally based Inuktitut programs. Examples from the Pelly Bay community include:

- Creating traditional puppets, and writing and performing a puppet show
- Organizing a traditional sealskin clothing sewing group in which Elders teach younger women Inuktitut language skills
- Distributing illustrated Inuktitut stories through the local grocery store and reading the stories over the local radio

Source: Nunavut Literacy Council. (n.d.). *Home page.* Retrieved from http://www.nunavutliteracy.ca/home.htm [accessed: 18 June 2013].

ADDITIONAL RESOURCES OF INTEREST

ABC Canada

http://www.abc-canada.org/

ABC Life Literacy Canada is a non-profit organization with a goal of inspiring Canadians to increase their literacy skills. The organization offers online literacy resources and provides programs and initiatives to support literacy skill among Canadians. This organization strongly advocates for business, unions, government, communities, and individuals to support lifelong learning.

AlphaPlus

http://alphaplus.ca/

AlphaPlus is an online organization that strives to increase adult literacy skills using digital technologies. Online resources, tools, and training are available through this site. The mandate of this organization stems from a values-based approach to literacy development whereby all Canadians have the literacy and digital skills to enable them to participate actively in the social, political, cultural, and economic life within their communities and country.

Canadian Literacy and Learning Network

http://www.literacy.ca

Canadian Literacy and Learning Network (CLLN) is the national hub for research, and information and knowledge exchange, increasing literacies and essential skills across Canada. CLLN, a non-profit charitable organization, represents literacy coalitions, organizations, and individuals in every province and territory in Canada.

Canadian Public Health Association—Health Literacy Portal

http://www.cpha.ca/en/portals/h-l.aspx

This website is designed to provide easy access to information about health literacy in Canada for health professionals, researchers, and interested individuals. It features the Expert Panel on Health Literacy's final report as well as links to other key Canadian and international health literacy resources.

Health Literacy

http://healthliteracy.ca/

Created by the Canadian Public Health Association, this website is dedicated to promoting health literacy in Canada and around the world. It provides health literacy information, resources, and tools for both the public and professionals. In addition, the online site provides organizations, governments, and employers with a virtual space to engage each other; share resources, tools, and expertise; and strengthen health literacy collaboration across jurisdictions. The goal is to improve the health of all Canadians by improving health literacy.

Copian—Connecting Canadians in Learning

http://www.en.copian.ca

Originally the National Adult Literacy Database (NALD), Copian is a Canadian non-profit registered charity with a mission to provide Internet-based literacy and essential skills information and resources in both of Canada's official languages. This website has numerous resources related to literacy and is supported by the Government of Canada's Office of Literacy and Essential Skills.

Public Health Agency of Canada (PHAC)—Health Literacy

http://www.phac-aspc.gc.ca/cd-mc/hl-ls/index-eng.php

PHAC is developing and sharing tools and products to help Canadians and particularly health care professionals to support and integrate health literacy into their daily practice(s). The information available from this website is intended to help health professionals speak, write, and interact in ways that can be easily understood by Canadians. PHAC also offers subscribers a "health literacy" e-alert notification when new health literacy content is added to the online site.

The Centre for Literacy

http://www.centreforliteracy.qc.ca/

The Centre for Literacy is a centre of expertise that supports best practices and informed policy development in literacy/health literacy and essential skills by creating bridges between research, policy, and practice. The website provides information about upcoming learning events (including institutes and workshops), action research projects and publications, and library services.

CHAPTER 3

POPULATION MEASURES OF LITERACY AND HEALTH LITERACY

Literacy is a bridge from misery to hope. It is a tool for daily life in modern society. It is a bulwark against poverty and a building block of development, an essential complement to investments in roads, dams, clinics and factories. Literacy is a platform for democratization, and a vehicle for the promotion of cultural and national identity. Especially for girls and women, it is an agent of family health and nutrition. For everyone, everywhere, literacy is … a basic human right.… Literacy is, finally, the road to human progress and the means through which every man, woman and child can realize his or her full potential.

—KOFI ANNAN, "MESSAGE ON OCCASION OF INTERNATIONAL LITERACY DAY," 1997

CHAPTER LEARNING OBJECTIVES
- Introduce population level measurement of literacy and health literacy
- Introduce national and provincial findings from literacy and health literacy surveys of Canadians
- Situate population literacy and health literacy results from Canada with other countries

INTRODUCTION

We begin this chapter with a brief review of the concepts—literacy and health literacy—introduced in Chapter 2. We then consider how literacy and health literacy have been measured at the population level, and using these population measures, we present an overall profile of Canadian literacy and health literacy findings. The findings indicate that literacy and health literacy skills of Canadians vary considerably by province and by official language. We describe the literacy and health literacy proficiencies of vulnerable subpopulations—including seniors, immigrants, Aboriginal peoples, and those with limited education—and identify factors that contribute to variations in these proficiencies across the different subgroups. Finally, we conclude with a description of Canada's ranking on literacy and health literacy relative to other economically advantaged countries.

NATIONAL AND INTERNATIONAL MEASUREMENT OF LITERACY AND HEALTH LITERACY

In Chapter 2, a number of literacy tools were introduced. These tools included formulas, such as the SMOG (Simplified Measure of Gobbledygook), which are used to determine the readability of printed information (sometimes known as reading grade levels). There are also instruments and scales to measure health literacy, although most have been developed specifically for use in the United States. Among these instruments are the Test of Functional Health Literacy in Adults (TOFHLA), a measure of comprehension of health information; the Rapid Assessment of Literacy in Medicine (REALM), a test of health literacy in clinical settings; and the Newest Vital Sign (NVS), a measure of health literacy and numeracy. As discussed in the previous chapter, what these instruments and formulas have in common is that they are used to determine the literacy or health literacy proficiency of individuals.

In this chapter, we will focus on the measurement of literacy and health literacy at the population level. These measures involve national and international surveys, with large population samples. One of the most widely used surveys of literacy is the International Adult Literacy Survey (IALS), a multinational assessment that has been administered several times since 1994. The 2003 version of IALS was also known as the Adult Literacy and Life Skills Survey (ALLS or IALSS). For consistency and simplicity throughout this book, the term "IALS" will be used and the specific version indicated by date. A major change from IALS 1994 to IALS 2003 was the inclusion of test items designed to measure health literacy (or, more accurately, self-reported health indicators, which were then correlated with literacy measures) and problem-solving skills.

There have been several rounds of IALS surveys, and Canada has participated twice, in 1994 and again in 2003. To measure population literacy, the initial IALS survey focused on three different domains: prose, document, and quantitative. *Prose* literacy measures a person's ability to read, understand, and use textual information, such as a newspaper editorial, an information brochure, or a story or poem. *Document* literacy measures an individual's ability to find, understand, and use information in items such as maps and job applications. *Quantitative* literacy (also known as numeracy) measures a person's ability to read, understand, and use information that requires the application of arithmetic operations to numbers embedded in printed materials. This could involve calculating how much of a tip to include at a restaurant, determining the amount of interest on a car loan using a chart, balancing a chequebook, or figuring out how many cans of paint are needed to paint a kitchen (Krahn & Lowe, 1999; Sloat & Willms, 2000). The results in each domain were reported as five levels of increasing complexity (sometimes called benchmarks), and on a 0–500 point scale (see Table 3.1). An additional domain—that of problem solving—was added in the IALS 2003 survey. This component was designed to assess knowledge and skills integration reflected in prose and document literacy and numeracy. We will not consider the problem-solving domain of literacy in this chapter for two reasons. First, performance in this literacy component mirrors performance on the prose, document, and numeracy domains. Second, since the problem-solving skill domain was not measured in the first IALS survey (1994), it is difficult to draw solid conclusions as to whether the percentage of Canadians with adequate proficiency in this domain has changed over time. Students are encouraged to review the problem-solving literacy results in the IALS 2003 report (Human Resources and Skills Development Canada [HRSDC] and Statistics Canada, 2005).

TABLE 3.1: IALS 500-POINT SCALE AND CORRESPONDING LEVEL OF DIFFICULTY OF PROSE TEXT

Level	Score (range)
1 (lowest)	0–225
2	226–275
3	276–325
4	326–376
5 (highest)	376–500

Source: Modified from Literacy Basics. (n.d.). Measuring complexity using IALS 500 point scale and HRSDC five-point scale. *Community Literacy of Ontario*. Retrieved from http://www.nald.ca/literacybasics/essentl/history/01.htm [accessed: 15 June 2013].

What do these levels on the IALS scale actually mean in terms of prose literacy abilities? At the lowest level (Level 1), individuals have very basic literacy skills. They can read short, simple texts containing a single piece of information. An example of text at this level of difficulty might be: "Jane went to the grocery store." At IALS Level 2, people can read more complex texts that have a single piece of information, or simpler texts with several pieces of information. An example of text at this level of difficulty might be: "When it stopped raining, Jane went to the grocery store to buy milk, eggs, and bread." At IALS Level 3, people can identify and select relevant information from several parts of a text and make low-level inferences about that information. An example of text at this level of difficulty would be: "When it stopped raining, Jane went to the grocery store to buy milk, eggs, and bread. At the checkout, she noticed that she did not have any cash in her wallet. Jane took out her debit card and proceeded to pay for her purchases." Human Resources and Skills Development Canada identifies IALS Level 3 as the minimum level to function effectively in our contemporary knowledge economy (HRSDC, n.d.-a). And, as Canada increasingly moves away from being a resource-based economy to a knowledge-based one, skill at IALS Level 3 (or higher) will become even more important. At the highest levels of literacy skill, people can integrate, synthesize, and interpret information from difficult texts, make complex inferences, and use general background (Level 4) or specialized knowledge (Level 5) in making these inferences (HRSDC, n.d.-a).

REVIEW AND REFLECT

Individuals at IALS Level 1 are able to identify and select relevant information from several parts of a text and make low-level inferences about that information. Is this statement correct? Explain.

Performance at IALS Level 1 is the minimum level needed to function in the Canadian knowledge economy. Is this statement correct? Explain.

Figure 3.1 provides additional examples of text and skills representative of Levels 1 and 2 (Bow Valley College Centre, n.d.). The full impact of these skill levels will be considered in the section on the national profile of literacy of Canadians.

FIGURE 3.1: SAMPLE TEXT AND QUESTIONS ILLUSTRATING SKILL AT IALS LEVELS 1 AND 2

Example question for IALS Level 1:

When was the dog lost?

LOST DOG

WHERE: Clair Hills area in Waterloo

WHEN: August 25th

DESCRIPTION: Dalmatian, five years old

PLEASE CALL 519-765-4321

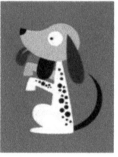

(answers to the name of Randy)

Example question for IALS Level 2:

Who is responsible for backing up files on employee computers?

FROM: Sally Simon
TO: All Employees
CC: Sally Simon
SUBJECT: New Policy on File Management

A new policy on file management has been developed and is effective immediately. Every employee is now required to back up their files on the hard drives of their computer to the company's common network (Z: Drive). Files include letters, statements, data, and other critical documents. With this new policy employees are discouraged from keeping paper files. A program is available to help you in the process.

Source: Adapted from Bow Valley College Centre for Excellence in Foundational Learning. (n.d.). *Read forward.* Retrieved from http://blogs.bowvalleycollegeweb.com/adultreadingassessment/readforward/#tests [accessed: 13 June 2013].

As noted earlier, IALS 2003 included test items to measure the use of information in different health contexts (Canadian Council on Learning, 2007a). Similar to the scoring of prose, document, and quantitative literacy domains, health literacy proficiencies were grouped into five levels, with scores between 0 and 500. Information from IALS (as well as from other surveys) about activities related to health promotion, health protection, disease prevention, health care and maintenance, and health system navigation were collected and used to develop a Health Activity Literacy Scale (Rootman, 2009; Rudd, 2007; Rudd, Kirsch, & Yamamoto, 2004). Unlike the link between IALS scores and necessary workplace and economic skills, the minimum health literacy level needed for informed decision making in personal health care was not established. However, we might expect that Level 3 is also the minimum proficiency needed for a health-literate population.

To summarize the key points thus far, at the population level, literacy has been measured by International Adult Literacy Skills Surveys or IALS (or IALSS, as it was later known). Of importance for students interested in the measurement of health literacy, some of the questions from the IALS 2003 survey of Canada included a health literacy component. While HRSDC suggests that the minimum level to function in the knowledge economy is IALS Level 3, the minimum level of health literacy skill that Canadians require to participate in informed personal health care decision making has not been established.

LITERACY OF CANADIANS

Canada has a long history of adult literacy education that dates to more than a century ago with the establishment of Frontier College (see "A Canadian Milestone" at the end of this chapter). We will not review the history of the adult literacy education movement in Canada; a number of excellent websites and books that focus on this topic are listed at the end of the chapter. However, one important milestone points to a gap in the urgency of the literacy message. That milestone—the October 1, 1986, Speech from the Throne—identified literacy as a priority area for the Government of Canada and led to the establishment of the National Literacy Secretariat (Partnerships in Learning, n.d.). However, it wasn't until almost a decade later, in 1995, that the extent and seriousness of the adult literacy problem in Canada received significant attention with the release of the first IALS survey results. While there had been earlier assessments that indicated a major literacy problem in Canada, these did not provide the necessary momentum to tackle the problem. For example, the Survey of Literacy Used in Daily Activities was conducted in 1987 for the Southam newspaper chain and reported that 24 percent of Canadians were functionally illiterate (i.e., below the level needed for simple reading and writing) (Calamai, 1987). And about 4 percent of Canadians indicated that they needed help in reading product names in stores, and 6 percent that they could not find the expiration date on their driver's license (Darville, 1992). The IALS results, however, revealed the scope of the adult literacy problem and Canada's ranking relative to other countries.

The IALS was cross-sectional in design. It surveyed Canadian adults age 16–65 years, was conducted in the home (rather than by mail), and excluded individuals who were in institutions (such as prisons) or on Aboriginal reserves. The survey coverage was reduced for northern territories and sparsely populated regions of the country (e.g., northern Manitoba). In a later IALS conducted in 2003, the survey population was expanded to include individuals over the age of 65 years. What the IALS data clearly showed was that the literacy level of Canadians was skewed to the lower end of proficiency. Although more than 20 percent of the Canadian adult population scored at Levels 4 and 5, almost half (about 48 percent) scored at or below Level 2 of IALS. Consider the examples in Figure 3.1 of IALS Levels 1 and 2 text. And, of those scoring at Levels 1 and 2, almost 20 percent of adult Canadians scored at the lowest level (Level 1) of proficiency (Rubenson & Walker, 2011). In other words, 1 in 5 adult Canadians had difficulty reading and understanding all but simple text. Did these findings change with the later survey? When results from IALS 1994 and 2003 are compared, the percentage of Canadians at each literacy level remained relatively constant (see Table 3.2). In fact, the percentage of Canadians with low levels of literacy proficiency (Level 2 or less) was slightly more in 2003 (about 48 percent) than the percentage reported almost a decade earlier in 1994 (about 47 percent). Another important finding from the IALS surveys was that literacy skill was not uniformly distributed across the Canadian population. Factors including education, age, language group, Aboriginal status, and province of residence strongly affected literacy scores. The importance of these factors for population literacy has not changed over time.

TABLE 3.2: PERCENTAGE OF CANADIANS AT EACH LEVEL OF PROSE LITERACY, IALS (1994 AND 2003)

Year of survey	IALS Level			
	Level 1 (lowest)	Level 2	Level 3	Levels 4/5 (highest)
1994	21.5%	25.0%	33.9%	19.6%
2003	19.9%	27.8%	35.4%	17.0%

Source: Modified from Human Resources and Skills Development Canada and Statistics Canada. (2005). *Building on our competencies: Canadian results of the International Adult Literacy and Skills Survey 2003*. Table 1.5. Cat. No. 89-617-XIE. Ottawa: Statistics Canada. Retrieved from http://www.statcan.gc.ca/pub/89-617-x/89-617-x2005001-eng.pdf [accessed: 15 June 2013].

One of the strongest predictors of literacy scores was the number of years of formal (or attained) education. As Willms (1997) noted, "[E]ach year of schooling translates to increased literacy scores of about 12% to 13.5% of a standard deviation" (p. 16). On a population basis, individuals with more education scored higher on all domains of literacy relative to those with less education. The impact of education was strong, even after controlling for other background factors—having a first language other than English or French, occupational status, and gender. Table 3.3 shows the summary results from IALS (1994) for Canadian adults age 20–25 years across the three domains of literacy skill (prose, document, and quantitative/numeracy). For young adults who dropped out of high school, the effects on prose and document literacy scores were large and statistically significant. The effects on quantitative literacy were similarly striking (Willms, 1997).

TABLE 3.3: MEAN LITERACY SCORES OUT OF 500 FOR CANADIANS AGE 20–25, BY EDUCATION LEVEL

Young adult group by education	Prose	Document	Quantitative
All Canadians age 20–25 years	286.9	294.1	284.1
Canadians age 20-25 years with less than a secondary school education	231.3	217.8	226.6
Canadians age 20–25 years with some college or university	309.9	322.6	310.9

Source: Modified from Human Resources and Skills Development Canada and Statistics Canada. (2005). *Building on our competencies: Canadian results of the International Adult Literacy and Skills Survey 2003.* Cat. No. 89-617-XIE. Ottawa: Statistics Canada. Retrieved from www.statcan.gc.ca/pub/89-617-x/89-617-x2005001-eng.pdf; data also available at www.nald.ca/library/research/bnch-nae/33.htm (Table 1), www.nald.ca/library/research/bnch-nae/34.htm (Table 2) and www.nald.ca/library/research/bnch-nae/35.htm (Table 3) [accessed: 15 June 2013].

Age was another key variable affecting population literacy scores. Figure 3.2 shows how the proportion of Canadians with low literacy increases with age. And, this relationship is not unique for Canada as literacy scores also decline with age for two comparison countries—the United States and Switzerland. For adult Canadians 66 years of age and older, 51.5 percent scored at Level 1 prose proficiency, and the decline in literacy was particularly pronounced with increasing age (Rubenson, Desjardins, & Yoon, 2007). There were 14.7 percent, 15.9 percent, 26.9 percent, and 51.5 percent of adult Canadians between the ages of 36–45, 46–55, 56–65, and 66 years and over at Level 1 prose proficiency. At the highest prose skill (Level 4/5), the percentage decreased from 20.3 percent (for adults between 36 and 45 years) to 2.2 percent (for adults 66 years and older). Document literacy skill followed a similar age-related association. The percentage of adults at IALS proficiency Level 1 increased from 15.8 (age 36–48 years) to 57.3 (age 66 and over). Only 2.2 percent of adults age 66 and older were at Level 4/5 for document skill level (we will consider numeracy levels later in this section). Moreover, the highest percentage of individuals at Level 3 or higher for prose and document literacy proficiency was among young Canadians age 16–35 years.

Figure 3.3 shows the proportion of Canadians at Level 3 or higher for prose literacy skill as a function of age. This relationship supports the notion that literacy is a practice-driven skill and that steps to enhance practice over the life course may mitigate some of this population decline in literacy level with age. A key priority arising from the IALS data is that literacy is a lifelong endeavour, and daily reading is an essential strategy for maintaining this skill (Public Health Agency of Canada, 2008).

FIGURE 3.2: DISTRIBUTION OF PROSE LITERACY AND NUMERACY LEVELS AS A
FUNCTION OF AGE—CANADIAN IALS (2003) RESULTS RELATIVE TO LEVELS FOR
UNITED STATES AND SWITZERLAND POPULATIONS

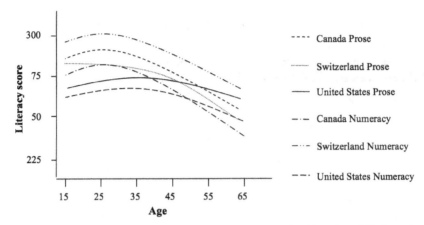

Source: Adapted from Willms, J.D., & Watson, B. (2008). *Literacy, numeracy, and problem-solving skills of Canadian youth.*
Figure 1. Human Resources and Social Development Canada, Learning Policy Directorate, Strategic Policy and Research.
Retrieved from http://publications.gc.ca/collection_2008/hrsdc-rhdsc/HS28-145-2008E.pdf [accessed: 13 June 2013].

FIGURE 3.3: PROPORTION OF CANADIANS AT IALS (2003) PROFICIENCY
LEVEL 3 OR HIGHER FOR PROSE LITERACY AS A FUNCTION OF AGE

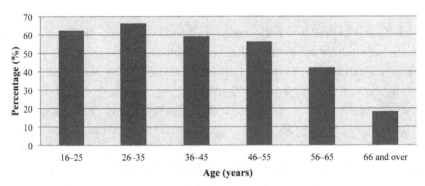

Source: Human Resources and Skills Development Canada and Statistics Canada. (2005). *Building on our competencies:
Canadian results of the International Adult Literacy and Skills Survey 2003.* Table 2. Cat. No. 89-617-XIE. Ottawa: Statistics
Canada. Retrieved from http://www.statcan.gc.ca/pub/89-617-x/89-617-x2005001-eng.pdf [accessed: 13 June 2013].

Not surprisingly, mother tongue (first language) strongly influenced literacy level (Rubenson
et al., 2007). Among francophones (including individuals living in Quebec and those living
elsewhere in Canada), only 45 percent were at or above Level 3 literacy in the IALS 2003 survey
results. This can be compared to 62 percent of anglophones (across Canada, including Quebec)
at Level 3 or higher literacy levels. For individuals whose first language was neither English nor
French, the situation was particularly alarming. Table 3.4 shows the percentage of native-born
and second-language foreign-born Canadians at IALS (1994) levels on prose, document, and

quantitative literacy. These findings were largely unchanged in the 2003 IALS survey: only 40 percent of those age 16–65 had a literacy level of 3 or more compared with age-matched native-born Canadians at 63 percent. Although the total proportion of immigrants with proficiency below IALS Level 3 is expected to decrease from 67 percent in 2001 to 61 percent in 2031, the absolute number of immigrants with low literacy skills will increase to more than 5.7 million by 2031 (Canadian Council on Learning [CCL], 2010c). Persistent disparities in the literacy skills of immigrants are a serious concern for all Canadians, and the findings from the IALS surveys serve as a compelling reminder of the work needed to raise literacy levels.

What accounts for the projected increase in the number of adults with low literacy? The factors vary across the country. Consider the situation in four large urban centres in Canada: Ottawa, Toronto, Vancouver, and Montreal. In Ottawa, the projected increase in adults with low literacy (from about 275,000 in 2001 to almost 500,000 in 2031) is thought to reflect immigration trends (more immigrant adults with low literacy) and demographic changes (a higher percentage of seniors living in the nation's capital region) that are shaped by the current immigration policies (CCL, 2010c). In Toronto, the estimated increase in the number of adults with low literacy is even more striking—from 1.9 million in 2001 to nearly 3.2 million in 2031; the Toronto literacy statistics are thought to reflect a projected increase in the number of immigrants with low literacy. In Vancouver, the projected increase likely reflects the increasing number of senior citizens in that city; adults with low literacy have been projected to increase from approximately 800,000 in 2001 to over 1.3 million by 2031. In contrast, the proportion of adults with low literacy in Montreal is projected to decline, from 54 percent in 2001 to 51 percent in 2031. This trend may reflect steady improvements for the immigrant population in the city (CCL, 2010c). In later chapters, the social and policy implications of Canadian population literacy results for vulnerable subgroups will be considered.

TABLE 3.4: PERCENTAGE OF NATIVE-BORN AND SECOND-LANGUAGE FOREIGN-BORN CANADIANS, AGE 16–65, FOR PROSE, DOCUMENT, AND QUANTITATIVE LITERACY LEVELS, IALS (1994)

Population language group	IALS Level			
	Level 1 (lowest)	Level 2	Level 3	Levels 4/5 (highest)
Native-born				
Prose	12.9%	26.4%	38.9%	21.8%
Document	14.8%	25.6%	35.4%	24.2%
Quantitative	13.8%	28.2%	37.4%	20.6%
Second-language foreign-born				
Prose	50.7%	25.9%	14.4%	(8.9%)
Document	47.5%	27.2%	(9.4%)	(15.9%)
Quantitative	44.7%	24.4%	19.5%	(11.4%)

Note: Values in parenthesis = unreliable estimates.

Source: Modified from Tuijnman, A. (2001). *Benchmarking adult literacy in North America: An international comparative study.* Table 10. Cat. No. 89-572-XIE. International Adult Literacy Survey. Ottawa: Statistics Canada. Retrieved from http://www.statcan.gc.ca/pub/89-572-x/89-572-x1998001-eng.pdf [accessed: 15 June 2013].

REVIEW AND REFLECT

The Canadian Council on Learning developed a tool called PALMM (Projections of Adult Literacy: Measuring Movement) to calculate adult literacy trends between 2001 and 2031.

Using PALMM (www.ccl-cca.ca/PALMM/projection.aspx), how many adult Canadians are projected to be at Level 1 literacy in 2031? How many adults in your province are projected to be at Level 1 literacy in 2031?

Literacy statistics for Canadian Aboriginal peoples are concerning. Overall, the literacy scores for First Nations, Métis, and Inuit people were lower than for non-Aboriginal Canadians. Moreover, the degree of literacy disparities from the IALS 2003 survey varied by province and territory. For example, in the Yukon, 34.5 percent of Aboriginal people had prose literacy at Level 3, whereas in Nunavut, the Northwest Territories, and Manitoba/Saskatchewan, these percentages were 11.1 percent, 28 percent, and 29.8 percent, respectively (Biswal, 2008, Tables A8 and A10). The factors contributing to low literacy among Aboriginal peoples reflect many of the issues that affect the health of other disenfranchised groups and include systematic barriers such as colonialism, racism, poverty, loss of culture, low education, and unemployment. The barriers and disparities faced by Aboriginal peoples relative to non-Aboriginal Canadians underscore the issue of inequity and the importance of social justice (see chapters 1 and 4). Language barriers likely influence the literacy scores of Aboriginal Canadians. According to Government of Canada statistics, there are between 56 and 70 Aboriginal languages (e.g., Eastern Inuktitut, Innu, South Slavey, Ojibwa, Plains Cree, Micmac, and Blackfoot) (Government of Canada, n.d.). According to 2001 Census data, one in four First Nations people speak an Aboriginal language; moreover, some Aboriginal languages are spoken in the home on a "most often" basis, such as Inuktitut at 82 percent and Cree at 69 percent, whereas others, such as Haida (10 percent), are spoken as a home language much less often (Norris, 2007). Since the IALS surveys were conducted in English or French, it is difficult to determine how many people of Aboriginal heritage who participated in the surveys were daily, regular, or (even) infrequent speakers of an Aboriginal language and how many participants were bilingual (an official language and an Aboriginal language). Hence, the low literacy levels may not be representative of actual literacy and should be interpreted cautiously because of the possibility of bias.

Where one lives in Canada influences literacy proficiency. The variation in literacy by province or territory was described in the IALS summary (HRSDC and Statistics Canada, 2005). Using Level 3 prose literacy as the benchmark for adequate skill to participate in the modern knowledge economy, Nunavut fared the worst with only 27 percent of residents 16 years and older scoring at or above Level 3 on the 2003 IALS survey. It is important to point out that this finding was not unique to prose literacy: fewer than 30 percent of adults living in Nunavut performed at or above Level 3 on document literacy and numeracy (26.2 percent and 21.9 percent). By contrast, about 67 percent of residents of the Yukon were at or above Level 3 for prose literacy, well above the Canadian average of 52 percent. The western provinces of Saskatchewan, Alberta, and British Columbia (but not Manitoba) also performed quite well, with 60 percent or more of residents 16 years and older at or above Level 3 prose literacy of IALS. Ontario residents were equivalent to Canada as a whole, with 52 percent of the population at or above Level 3 for prose proficiency. There were proportionally fewer residents of Quebec (45 percent) who were at or above this level. Finally, the results from the Atlantic provinces show relatively poor performance, with the percentage of the population 16 years and older at or above Level 3 IALS for prose skill ranging from 44 in New Brunswick to 55 in Nova Scotia. The provincial and territorial breakdown for prose literacy is shown in Figure 3.4. Similar patterns of provincial and territorial differences in document literacy and numeracy of adult Canadians were also found.

FIGURE 3.4: PERCENTAGE OF POPULATION AT IALS (2003) PROFICIENCY LEVEL 3 OR HIGHER FOR PROSE LITERACY BY PROVINCE AND TERRITORY IN CANADA

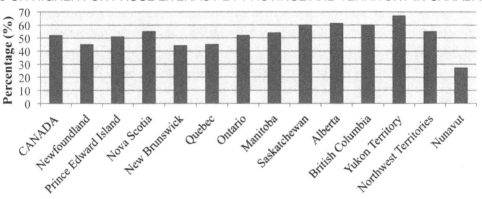

Canada, provinces, and territories

Source: Adapted from Human Resources and Skills Development Canada and Statistics Canada. (2005). *Building on our competencies: Canadian results of the International Adult Literacy and Skills Survey 2003.* Table 1.2. Cat. No. 89-617-XIE. Ottawa: Statistics Canada. Retrieved from www4.hrsdc.gc.ca/.3ndic.1t.4r@-eng.jsp?iid=31#M_1 [accessed: 13 June 2013].

REVIEW AND REFLECT

The percentage of Canadians at each literacy level was relatively constant between IALS 1994 and IALS 2003. Explain.

Language barriers contribute to low literacy levels among Aboriginal people in Canada. Do you agree with this statement?

Before turning our attention to national measures of health literacy, we will address the overall picture with respect to numeracy (the quantitative domain component of the surveys). As described in Chapter 2, numeracy refers to an individual's ability to understand and use mathematical information at school, at work, and in everyday life; as examples, this skill could include handling money, making a household budget, using measurements for cooking, calculating the HST on a purchase, or reading a map (Human Resources and Skills Development Canada [HRSDC], n.d.-b). Numeracy is an important component of health literacy. It is the skill needed to understand a prescription dose or to determine the difference in meaning between good and bad cholesterol levels; it is important for making sense of nutrition labels on food packaging or for calculating and understanding one's risk of developing colon cancer over the lifetime, given family history and other factors. From the IALS 2003 survey data, the national picture of numeracy raises concerns. The percentage of the population below Level 3 numeracy was 55 percent, and in fact, 26 percent of adult Canadians achieved only Level 1 numeracy levels (HRSDC and Statistics Canada, 2005). Not surprisingly, higher levels of attained education were strongly associated with higher levels of numeracy. Consider the following findings: 73.3 percent of individuals with a university degree performed at or above numeracy scores at Level 3 compared with only 17.7 percent of individuals with less than a high school education. In contrast, only 6.3 percent of adult Canadians with a university education were at the lowest numeracy skill level (Level 1) compared with 53.8 percent of the population who did not complete high school. Age had an enormous effect on numeracy skill. The percentage of Canadians with adequate or high numeracy skills (at Level 3 or greater) was more than half (52.5 percent) for younger persons between 26 and 35 years compared to only 12.2 percent of adults 66 years and older.

Aboriginal peoples had low numeracy scores irrespective of province or territory of residence. And, similar to the prose literacy findings, there was some provincial and territorial variation in scores. In the Yukon, for example, the mean numeracy scores among First Nations peoples were marginally higher (244 out of 500) compared with average scores of Aboriginal peoples in Saskatchewan (241 out of 500) and markedly higher than scores reported for Nunavut (194 out of 500) and the Northwest Territories (229 out of 500) (HRSDC and Statistics Canada, 2005). To put these scores into a national perspective, non-Aboriginal residents of the Yukon and Nunavut scored at 287 and 290, respectively.

Do new immigrants fare better or worse on numeracy scores compared with non-immigrants or those individuals who have lived in Canada for many years? Almost 40 percent (39.9 percent) of recent immigrants to Canada, defined as those who have been in the country 10 or fewer years, had numeracy proficiency at or above Level 3, greater than for established immigrants (36.2 percent) (HRSDC and Statistics Canada, 2005). The percentage of both recent and established immigrant populations at Level 3 or higher numeracy skill was significantly less than Canadian-born individuals (53.6 percent). These results suggest ongoing disparities in numeracy skill even for immigrants who have lived for many years in Canada compared with native-born Canadians. Factors in numeracy and literacy skill disparities will be considered in detail in Chapter 4.

Similar to prose literacy, the percentage of Canadians ages 16–65 with Level 3 or higher numeracy proficiency varied across the country: the highest was in the Yukon and the western provinces, and the lowest in Nunavut and the Atlantic provinces. Ontario and Quebec had percentages that were just below the proportion for Canada. Of note was that the average numeracy score for men was higher than for women (HRSDC and Statistics Canada, 2005, Tables 1.2, 3.5C, 3.14A-D, 2.8 for the complete statistics).

To summarize the key points of this section, the IALS surveys of 1994 and 2003 indicate that literacy is a continuing (and alarming) issue in Canada. The literacy skill to function at home, at work, at school, and in civil society varies widely across the country and by subpopulation. Groups at risk for low prose literacy levels include those with less than a high school education, immigrants whose first language is neither English nor French, and Aboriginal peoples. Literacy scores show a strong age-associated decline, and this is most evident in seniors 66 years and older. The percentage of francophones attaining a literacy level of 3 or higher is less than for anglophones. Numeracy skill follows similar subpopulation patterns as those seen with prose literacy. Regionally, the proportion of Canadians with adequate prose literacy and numeracy is higher in the western provinces than in the east; Nunavut has the smallest percentage of individuals at or above Level 3 literacy and numeracy.

HEALTH LITERACY OF CANADIANS

As the Canadian Council on Learning (CCL, 2008a, 2008b) observed, Canada has one of the most highly educated populations in the world, a respected (even if chronically underfunded) public health care system, and recognition at all levels of government that education and learning are essential determinants of economic success. Canada should therefore score very highly on population measures of health literacy. Sadly, this is not the case. There are more people with low health literacy skill (60 percent of Canadians) than with low literacy skill (48 percent of Canadians) (CCL, 2008a). In this section, we will consider population level measurement of Canadians' health literacy. The national profile of health literacy is based on the 2003 IALS survey using participant responses to 12 questions about physical and mental health—the SF-12 (a shortened version of a much longer questionnaire known as the Physical Component Summary and the Mental Component Summary). In the SF-12, participants were asked, for example, questions such as "In general, would you say your health is …?" (response options ranged from excellent to poor) or "During the past 4 weeks, how much of the time has your physical health or emotional problems interfered with your social activities (like visiting friends, relatives, etc.)? Was it …" (response options ranged from all of the time to none of the time) (Statistics Canada, 2002, pp. 53, 55). Participant responses to health status questions were correlated with demographic variables, place of residence, education, linguistic abilities, reading skill, general literacy and numeracy practice, employment, and information and technological literacy items. These associations were used to develop a health literacy scale. The analysis of health and literacy focused on document literacy: this literacy domain corresponds to the skills needed to follow instructions and directions about health care and medications (HRSDC and Statistics Canada, 2005, p. 92).

Analysis of document literacy scores by mental health questions found little support for a link between the mental health component questions and document literacy of Canadians, irrespective of province or territory of residence (HRSDC and Statistics Canada, 2005). Why there was little association between the mental health results and document literacy in IALS is not clear. Many factors could have influenced these findings, including the types of questions asked, the psychometric properties of the questions, the reluctance that people have to discuss mental health issues, the stigma associated with mental health issues, and a general lack of knowledge about mental health. However, document literacy scores for adult Canadians reporting poor physical health were at Level 2, whereas those reporting fair, good, or excellent physical health had Level 3 document literacy. About 50 percent of seniors who scored at Level 1 of document literacy also reported poor physical health (HRSDC and Statistics Canada, 2005, Table 5.1).

The next step in evaluating health literacy involved the development of health-related activity tasks and a health-related literacy scale, using the IALS 2003 physical health component–document literacy links. For the version developed for the United States, at the easiest level, readers were asked to underline the sentence indicating how often the medication should be given. The next difficulty level required readers to identify how much of the medication should be given to a child of a specific age and weight (e.g., 10 years old and 50 lbs.). At the highest level of difficulty, readers were asked to determine the maximum amount of medication that could be given to a child of a specific age and weight over a 24-hour period (Rudd et al., 2004). The Canadian version presented tasks with increasing difficulty levels for the reader. For example, one of the easiest tasks in terms of difficulty (Level 1) asked respondents to look at a medicine label and to determine "the maximum number of days you should take this medicine" (Statistics Canada and OECD, 2005, p. 284). Examples of materials used in health-related tasks are shown in Figures 3.5A and 3.5B. Other tasks in the IALS 2003 survey were designed to assess numeracy skill, a domain highly relevant to health literacy. In Figure 3.5B, for example, a Level 3 difficulty activity requires participants to describe how much Dioxin levels in breast milk had changed from 1975 to 1995.

FIGURES 3.5A AND 3.5B: EXAMPLES OF MATERIALS USED IN HEALTH LITERACY AND HEALTH NUMERACY TASKS, CANADA

MEDCO ASPIRIN   500

INDICATIONS: Headaches, muscle pains, rheumatic pains, toothaches, earaches. RELIEVES COMMON COLD SYMPTOMS.

DOSAGE: ORAL. 1 or 2 tablets every 6 hours, preferably accompanied by food, for not longer than 7 days. Store in a cool, dry place.

CAUTION: Do not use for gastritis or peptic ulcer. Do not use if taking anticoagulant drugs. Do not use for serious liver illness or bronchial asthma. If taken in large doses and for an extended period, may cause harm to kidneys. Before using this medication for chicken pox or influenza in children, consult with a doctor about Reyes syndrome, a rare but serious illness. During lactation and pregnancy, consult with a doctor before using this product, especially in the last trimester of pregnancy. If symptoms persist, or in case of an accidental overdose, consult a doctor. Keep out of reach of children.

INGREDIENTS: Each tablet contains 500mg acetylsalicylic acid.
Excipient c.b.p.   1 tablet.
Reg. No. 88246

Made in Canada by STERLING PRODUCTS, INC.
1600 Industrial Blvd., Montreal, Quebec H9J 3P1

0   67736 11079

Is breast milk safe?

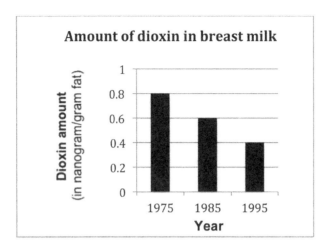

Since the 1970s, scientists have been worried about the amount of dioxin, a toxin in fish caught in the Baltic Sea. Dioxin tends to accumulate in breast milk and can harm newborn babies.

The chart shows the amount of dioxin in the breast milk of Northern European women, as found in studies done from 1975 to 1995.

Source: Statistics Canada and OECD. (2005, pp. 284, 300). *Learning a living: First results of the Adult Literacy and Life Skills Survey. Annex A: A construct-centered approach to understanding what was measured in the International Adult Literacy and Life Skills (ALL) Survey.* Retrieved from http://www.oecd.org/education/country-studies/34867438.pdf [accessed: 13 June 2013].

However competencies are assessed, the health literacy results for Canada raise major concerns (CCL 2007a; 2008a; 2008b). The average health literacy score is only 258, which puts a large proportion of Canadian adults (about 60 percent) at a proficiency level that is simply not adequate to participate in a meaningful way in health decision making. Despite the increasing emphasis on patient- and consumer-centred care, low health literacy presents a significant barrier to people participating in their health care decisions.

There are also striking differences in average health literacy by region. Much of our knowledge about the provincial variation in health literacy can be monitored using an important interactive map tool developed by the Canadian Council on Learning (2010b) (students are encouraged to visit the CCL website for the health literacy map tool at www.ccl-cca.ca/cclflash/healthliteracy/map_health_regions_e.html). This map profiles more than 49,000 communities and neighbourhoods, and allows specificity of health literacy levels to be described by and within regions. To illustrate the usefulness of this interactive mapping tool, we will consider the health literacy assessment of Newfoundland and Labrador (only Nunavut had a greater percentage of adults who were at or below Level 2). The IALS 2003 results indicated that Newfoundland and Labrador had the second largest proportion of adult Canadians with health literacy scores at or below Level 2. However, the scope of the health literacy problem varied across the province. In the Labrador-Grenfell Regional Integrated Health Authority catchment (which includes communities north of Bartlett's Harbour and all of Labrador), 76 percent of the population was at or below Level 2. This contrasts with the Eastern Regional Integrated Health Authority catchment (which includes St. John's), with 52 percent of the population at or below this level.

Another set of indicators developed by the Canadian Council on Learning that is relevant to population health literacy is the Composite Learning Index (CLI). The CLI is a combination of statistical indicators on lifelong learning in the multiple ways and places Canadians learn (e.g., formally, informally; at home, at work, in school, in community settings). The CLI uses a four pillars of learning framework: learning to know, learning to do, learning to live together, and learning to be. What the CLI basically captures are economic (income, unemployment rate) and social (adult literacy, early childhood development, population health, environmental responsibility, voter participation) effects of lifelong learning over time for Canada and for individual communities. The higher the score on the CLI, the greater the state of learning in that community (including the learning conditions needed to succeed economically and socially) (CCL, 2010a). For 2010 the CLI score for Canada was 75 out of 100. Continuing with our Newfoundland and Labrador example, community differences are large: Happy Valley-Goose Bay had a CLI score in 2010 of 43, whereas St. John's had a CLI score of 80 and Corner Brook, 48. The importance of the health literacy map and CLI indicators cannot be overstated. This specificity is a necessary first step in the design and implementation of region-specific interventions to address health literacy problems across Canada. What is clear from the CLI is that greater population health is positively related to increased learning, and higher levels of education correspond to better general health and increased life expectancy (Saisana & Cartwright, 2007; Wolfe & Haveman, 2001).

REVIEW AND REFLECT

What percentage of adults in your province and community are at or below Level 2 health literacy proficiency? (Hint: Go to the Canadian Council on Learning website at www.ccl-cca.ca/ccl/home/ to check out the Composite Learning Index and the health literacy map.)

The health literacy reports by the Canadian Council on Learning (e.g., CCL, 2010a) pointed to a growing problem for a number of vulnerable groups. There is a large gap in the health literacy scores between those over 65 years of age and younger persons, between the employed and unemployed, immigrants and native-born Canadians, off-reserve Aboriginal people and non-Aboriginal Canadians, and those whose mother tongue is neither English or French. Certain factors (being employed, educational attainment, speaking one of the official languages, being born in Canada, and being young) are associated with Level 3 or higher scores on health literacy. In fact, roughly 60 percent of the observed variation in health literacy skill of Canadians can be explained by these determinants (CCL, 2007a). Other factors, including cultural beliefs and living with a disability, affect health literacy outcomes, as do systemic barriers, such as regional differences in educational system funding and philosophy, Internet access, and health system access (more about these systemic factors in later chapters). Table 3.5 shows some key factors influencing health literacy skill for Canadian adults, age 16–65 years. Some of these factors are positively associated with greater health literacy: for example, greater health literacy skill is predicated on higher household income because literacy resources and opportunities are usually more available with greater discretionary income. Other factors tend to influence poor health literacy skill. For example, being an immigrant to Canada is negatively associated with health literacy. This association may reflect fewer employment opportunities for immigrants where literacy skills can be enhanced. Overall, what the factors in Table 3.5 show is that social determinants influence health literacy skill (see Chapter 4). Especially noteworthy about these predictive factors is that Canadians who engage in daily reading practices can enhance, or least maintain, their general literacy and health literacy skills. And, reading practice is not restricted to traditional newspapers, books, or magazines. Participation in any activity (ranging from computer use to volunteering to visits to the library to physical activity programs in community centres) that fosters lifelong learning enhances health literacy in a rapidly changing and complex society (Wister, Malloy-Weir, Rootman, & Desjardins, 2010).

TABLE 3.5: FACTORS INFLUENCING HEALTH LITERACY OF ADULT CANADIANS, AGE 16–65

Factor	Impact on health literacy
Literacy practices at home	+++
Educational attainment	++
Informal learning by self-study	+
Adult education and training	+
Household income	+
Labour-force participation	+
Aboriginal status	-
Community size	-
Being foreign-born	---

Note: +++ = very strong positive effect; ++ = moderate positive effect; + = weak positive effect; --- = very strong negative effect; - = weak negative effect

Source: Modified from Canadian Council on Learning. (2008). *Health literacy in Canada: A healthy understanding.* Figure 5.1. Ottawa. Retrieved from http://www.ccl-cca.ca/pdfs/HealthLiteracy/HealthLiteracyReportFeb2008E.pdf [accessed: 15 June 2013].

To summarize, the health literacy skill of Canadians is cause for concern. Results of the IALS 2003 survey indicate that about 60 percent of the population over the age of 16 years has low health literacy, with a proficiency less than Level 3. This is the minimum level that people need to acquire, make sense of, and evaluate health information (including being able to determine what is based on credible evidence and what is pseudoscience). It is also the skill level that allows individuals to participate in informed personal health care decision making. Many of the provincial variations observed for prose, document, and quantitative literacy skill level also characterize health literacy skill level across the country. Subpopulations—including seniors, Aboriginal people, those with low attained education, and English- or French-as-a-Second-Language immigrants—are at higher risk for low health literacy proficiency. Factors that positively influence health literacy include literacy practices at home, educational attainment, and continued learning throughout the life course (either by informal self-study or by formal adult education). Factors that are negatively associated with health literacy proficiency include not being employed, speaking a first language other than English or French, and not being born in Canada. Nevertheless, regardless of age, background, or mother tongue, Canadians can enhance health literacy proficiency by engaging in daily reading and learning activities.

LITERACY AND HEALTH LITERACY OF CANADIANS RELATIVE TO OTHER COUNTRIES

As Canadians, we often compare ourselves with other countries on many indicators—quality of life, economic well-being, housing starts, hospital waiting times, cost of post-secondary education, demographic trends, obesity levels, happiness, and so on. As noted throughout this chapter, the IALS surveys were international in scope, and therefore it is not surprising that comparisons about the literacy and numeracy skills of adult Canadians are made relative to the performance of adults in other countries around the world. In 1994, eight countries (Canada, Germany, Ireland, the Netherlands, Poland, Sweden, Switzerland, and the United States) participated in the survey. In 1995, five additional countries agreed to participate in the IALS survey (Australia, Belgium, Great Britain, New Zealand, and Northern Ireland). Finally, in 1998, nine more countries, including one from South America (Chile), took part. How did Canada perform compared to other countries participating in IALS? Essentially, Canada was in the middle compared to other countries. Using Level 1 prose literacy of native-born adults age 16–65 years to illustrate, Canada performed much better than Chile (12.9 percent of adults versus 50.3 percent of adults), slightly better than the United States (14.0 percent of adults), slightly worse than Australia (11.7 percent of adults), and much worse than Sweden (5.1 percent of adults) (Tuijnman, 2001). Document and quantitative literacies followed similar patterns for international comparisons of the percentage of adults at the lowest literacy level (Level 1). Did the same middle-of-the-range placement of Canada also occur at Level 3 prose literacy (i.e., able to function well in the knowledge economy)? Table 3.6 shows that more than one-third of adults born in Canada function at Level 3 for prose, document, and quantitative domains.

However, this percentage is still less than that reported for Australia and Sweden (Tuijnman, 2001, Table 10).

There are many factors that contribute to these national differences in the percentage of adults at the various literacy levels. These factors include population composition, geography of the country, linguistic diversity, resources and delivery of education, and even when and which version of the IALS survey was used. Consider, for example, Australia and Sweden, which performed better than Canada on the percentage of adults at proficiency Level 3 literacy. There are a number of differences between the three countries that could affect the literacy performances. Australia and Sweden have smaller populations than Canada (both at the time of the surveys and currently). Using 2011 Census data, Canada had an estimated population of just over 34 million, Australia, just under 21.8 million, and Sweden, 9.1 million (World Factbook, 2011). Australia and Sweden are officially monolingual, whereas Canada is a bilingual nation. Sweden had a much lower immigration rate than either Australia or Canada—for 2011, 1.65 migrants/1,000 of the population compared with Canada at 5.65 and Australia at 6.03 (Central Intelligence Agency, 2012). Nevertheless, the Conference Board of Canada (2012) summed up what these international comparisons to peer countries mean for Canada: we are an average performer and rank 8th out of 13 countries on the percentage of adults scoring low on adult literacy rate tests. Action is needed to improve adult literacy in Canada and narrow the gap between the "best" performers and where we stand internationally.

TABLE 3.6: PERCENTAGE OF NATIVE-BORN POPULATION, AGE 16–65, AT LEVEL 3 OF PROSE, DOCUMENT, AND QUANTITATIVE LITERACY, IALS (1994–1998)

Country	Prose	Document	Quantitative
Canada	38.9%	35.4%	37.4%
Chile	13.1%	11.6%	14.1%
United States	35.0%	34.0%	33.4%
Australia	39.9%	39.9%	39.4%
Sweden	40.4%	40.3%	39.9%

Source: Data taken from Tuijnman, A. (2001). *Benchmarking adult literacy in North America: An international comparative study.* Table 10. Cat. No. 89-572-XIE. International Adult Literacy Survey. Ottawa: Statistics Canada. Retrieved from http://www.statcan.gc.ca/pub/89-572-x/89-572-x1998001-eng.pdf [accessed: 15 June 2013].

How does Canada compare to other countries in terms of health literacy? Earlier in this chapter, it was pointed out that about 60 percent of adult Canadians lack the skills necessary to manage their health literacy needs effectively (scoring below Level 3, which ranges from 276–325) (CCL, 2007a). The average health literacy score for Canadian adults was 258 and was considerably lower for a number of vulnerable subgroups in Canada: seniors over 65 years (between 190–215; Level 1 scores range from 0–225) and immigrants for whom English or French was not their first language (between 215–240; Level 2 scores range from 226–275) (Rootman & Gordon-El-Bihbety, 2008). Although health literacy results for many of the

IALS participating countries are still forthcoming, data for the United States are available. For U.S. adults between the ages of 16 and 65 years, about 53 percent had Level 3 health literacy scores (termed intermediate health literacy, between 206–309 on the health literacy scale) (Kutner, Greenberg, Jin, Paulsen, & White, 2006). Adult men in the U.S. tended to have slightly lower health literacy scores (average of 242) compared with women (average score of 248). Thus, while Canadian adults performed marginally better on health literacy measures than adults in the U.S., the size and extent of the low health literacy problem in both populations is considerable and remains especially concerning for older adults.

KEY LEARNING POINTS

Profiles of literacy and health literacy of Canadians have been based on a series of international assessments, known as the International Adult Literacy Skills (IALS) Survey, administered in 1994 and 2003. The 2003 version included items designed to measure general health status and that led to the development of a health literacy instrument and scale. What the first IALS survey revealed was that about 48 percent of adult Canadians between 16 and 65 years of age did not meet the minimum prose, document, and quantitative literacy proficiency level (Level 3) necessary to function in a knowledge-based economy. Moreover, the proportion of the adult population with low literacy did not change fundamentally between 1994 and 2003. The surveys also pointed to some disturbing patterns for vulnerable subgroups. Educational level, not speaking English or French as one's first language, being of Aboriginal heritage, and immigrant status were key determinants influencing adult literacy. Seniors were at high risk for low literacy level, especially adults over the age of 65 years. Across the country literacy levels varied considerably, with a higher percentage of adults with low literacy levels in the Atlantic provinces compared with the western provinces and the Yukon. Even more alarming was the profile of health literacy levels of Canadians. An estimated 60 percent of adult Canadians have low health literacy skill, which indicates an even larger problem than that of low literacy in general. Low health literacy has profound consequences for informed health decision making at the individual level, for the cost of the national health care system, and for promoting equity for all Canadians. Internationally, Canada ranks about the "middle of the road" in literacy proficiency, performing somewhat better than the United States and much worse than Sweden. There are few international comparisons of health literacy performance. Given the current high prevalence of low health literacy and the projected trends of population aging and increased immigration, the magnitude of the problem will likely become more dire in the future for Canada and other member countries of the Organisation for Economic Co-operation and Development.

In October 2013, the Canadian results of the Programme for the International Assessment of Adult Competencies (PIAAC) were released. This 2012 survey of over 27,000 adult Canadians age 16–65 years built on earlier IALS assessments. Among the key findings are that Canada has a higher proportion of its population at the top and bottom ends of literacy proficiency relative to other OECD countries: 14 percent at Level 4 or 5 and 17 percent at Level 1 or below. The results for numeracy proficiency are also striking: 13 percent of adult Canadians scored at Level 4 or 5 and 23 percent were at Level 1 or below (Statistics Canada, 2013).

A CANADIAN MILESTONE

The literacy movement in Canada has a long and rich history. An important milestone was the founding of Frontier College in 1899 by Alfred Fitzpatrick. Fitzpatrick, a Nova Scotian by birth, was a leader in adult education who passionately believed that education should be available for all adults, regardless of background and where they lived. He developed the idea of the Labourer–Teacher, an instructor who would labour alongside of workers (miners, those on the railroads, farmers, lumberjacks, factory workers, and so on) during the day and teach them at night when the work was done. Frontier College Labourer–Teachers travelled across Canada, from remote areas in the northern bush to farming communities on the prairies. The spirit of "have book will travel" was a guiding principle. Today Frontier College continues to work with adults—in the workplace, with homeless street youth, prison inmates, persons with disabilities, seniors, and immigrants—drawing on the philosophy that literacy is a right of all Canadians.

The information about Alfred Fitzpatrick and the history of Frontier College is taken directly from www.frontiercollege.ca/english/learn/alfred_fitzpatrick. html and www.frontiercollege.ca/english_literacy.html. There are also a number of excellent books about Alfred Fitzpatrick and the founding and development of Frontier College. You may want to read *Frontier College Letters: One Hundred Years of Teaching, Learning and Nation Building* by Larry Krotz, Erica Martin, and Philip Fernandez (1999), available at nald. ca (www.nald.ca/library/learning/frontier/letters/letters.pdf), and *University in Overalls: A Plea for Part-Time Study* by Alfred Fitzpatrick (Thompson Educational Publishing, 1999).

ADDITIONAL RESOURCES OF INTEREST

Educational Testing Service (ETS)—ETS Literacy Services
http://litdata.ets.org/ialdata/search.asp
This searchable database allows users to select a scale (such as numeracy), country (including Canada), and category (such as health) to identify the responses from the International Adult Literacy Survey (IALS) (1994) and the IALS/Adult Literacy and Skills Survey (ALSS) (2003).

Murray, T.S., McCracken, M., Willms, D., Jones, S., Shillington, R., & Stucker, J. (2009).
Addressing Canada's Literacy Challenge: A Cost/Benefit Analysis.
http://www.en.copian.ca/library/research/cost_benefit/cover.htm
This excellent position paper describes Canada's literacy problem as an economic one, with recommendations about unique literacy markets and best practice program responses.

Quigley, B.A. (2007). Literacy's Heroes and Heroines: Reclaiming Our Forgotten Past. *Literacies, 7,* **411.**
http://www.literacyjournal.ca/literacies/7-2007/htm/quigley.htm
This paper discusses a number of pioneers in the literacy movement in the United Kingdom, Canada, and the United States, including Alfred Fitzpatrick and Frontier College.

Quigley, B.A., Folinsbee, S., & Kraglund-Gauthier, W.L. (2006). *State of the Field Review: Adult Literacy.* **Ottawa: Canadian Council on Learning**
http://www.ccl-cca.ca/pdfs/AdLKC/stateofthefieldreports/AdultLiteracy2008.pdf
This comprehensive report on adult literacy in Canada includes a brief section on the history of literacy education.

Willms, J.D., & Murray, T.S. (2007). *International Adult Literacy Survey: Gaining and Losing Literacy Skills over the Lifecourse.*
http://www.en.copian.ca/library/research/gaining/cover.htm
This important paper describes the changes between the 1994 and 2003 Canadian findings from the International Adult Literacy Surveys (IALS). Factors that might explain why some subgroups gained and others lost literacy skills and what policy-makers need to do reduce the future literacy skill loss of Canadians are discussed.

CHAPTER 4

HEALTH LITERACY AS A SOCIAL DETERMINANT OF HEALTH

> When people are illiterate, their ability to understand and invoke their legal rights can be very limited. This can be a severe handicap for those whose rights are violated by others, and it tends to be a persistent problem for people at the bottom of the ladder, whose rights are often effectively alienated because of their inability to read and see what they are entitled to demand and how.
>
> —AMARTYA SEN, *LITERACY AS FREEDOM*, 2003

CHAPTER LEARNING OBJECTIVES

- Provide an overview of the concepts of determinants of health, health equity, and social justice
- Discuss the relationship between health literacy and the determinants of health as defined by the Public Health Agency of Canada
- Describe the relationship between health literacy and health promotion, empowerment, and equity

INTRODUCTION

In this chapter we will consider societal factors that contribute to health and health promotion within Canada and globally. We will provide a brief historical review of the development of health promotion to set the context for the remainder of the chapter. You will be asked to consider "health" (and access to health care) as a human right rather than as the absence of disease. A number of frameworks that consider broad societal factors as influential in shaping one's health are presented, and you will have the chance to look at the more commonly used "determinant of health" (DOH) frameworks.

Using intersectionality theory (Hankivsky & Christoffersen, 2008; Hankivsky & Cormier, 2010), we look at how certain health determinants influence other health determinants in the construction of individuals' experiences of health. We will challenge you to consider how the same factors or determinants that promote health can also create disparate and inequitable health experiences and outcomes among Canadians, such as the following:

- The homes of Aboriginal individuals/families relative to non-Aboriginals are:
    - 2 times more likely to be in need of major repair
    - 90 times more likely to have no piped water supply
    - 5 times more likely to have no bathroom facilities
    - 10 times more likely to have no flush toilet
- Men in Canada (as a whole) live seven years longer than Aboriginal men and non-Aboriginal females live five years longer than Aboriginal women;
- Injury-related mortality among Aboriginal infants is four times greater than non-Aboriginal infants;
- Ten percent of Canadian households, approximately three million people, experience food insecurity (lack of safe food and potable water) each year, mostly those who rely on social assistance, single mothers with children, Aboriginal people, and those living in rural and remote communities (food insecurity is associated with poorly perceived health, chronic health conditions, distress and depression);
- The availability of health and medical services (and no-cost additional services for individuals of Indian status or otherwise subsidized) has not eliminated major health disparities; and
- Increases in health care spending—up 55 percent between 1997 and 2003—have not eliminated health disparities (Adelson, 2005; Health Disparities Task Group, 2005).

We will focus in this chapter on how literacy and health literacy contribute to these health disparities and discuss how health promotion, in its most fundamental form, can serve as a means to promote health equity. An exploration of the nuanced difference between health equity and health equality will help us to understand why the disparities listed above continue to persist in Canada. More importantly, this chapter will begin to sketch out the intersection between literacy and health literacy abilities and other determinants of health (e.g., employment, education, culture) that have a powerful impact on determining the health of Canadians.

HEALTH PROMOTION AND THE DETERMINANTS OF HEALTH

On November 21, 1986, attendees at the first International Conference on Health Promotion, held in Ottawa, created a charter for action to achieve "health for all" by the year 2000 and beyond. This important meeting of international health promotion scholars and health care providers resulted in the document now known as the Ottawa Charter (World Health Organization [WHO] et al., 1986). This landmark policy paper built on previous discussions and developments documented in the *Declaration at Alma-Ata* (WHO, 1978) and *Health for All* (WHO, 1981). Importantly, the Ottawa Charter defined "health" as more than an experience of illness; it posited health as a positive (e.g., supportive resource for everyday living) rather than as a negative (e.g., illness) concept. In this sense, health pertains to individuals' physical, social, and personal capacities and resources. The prerequisites for health identified in the Ottawa Charter reiterated and reinforced the seminal work introduced by Marc Lalonde (1974) in *A New Perspective on the Health of Canadians* (known as the Lalonde report). This working document challenged commonly held assumptions about health and advised Canadians to consider the health care system(s), the physical and social environment, and lifestyle, and not just human biology, as influential in determining one's health.

The authors of the 1986 Ottawa Charter emphasized that health is determined by diverse prerequisite conditions and resources. Some of these prerequisites were "obvious" in their relation to health, such as food, shelter, income, and education; others were less "obvious" but also of importance, including peace, a stable ecosystem, sustainable resources, social justice, and equity. Health promotion is defined as the process of enabling people to increase control over, and to improve, their health (WHO et al., 1986). Empowerment, a proposed outcome of health promotion activity and enhanced literacy and health literacy, is defined as the means to attain power, whereby individuals with relatively little power are able to increase control over resources and decision making related to the events that shape their lives and health. Empowerment is not something one person can provide for another person. Rather, empowerment must be gained by those who seek it (Laverack, 2006). The participants of the first International Conference on Health Promotion highlighted equity and social justice as the principles guiding health promotion strategies for action (WHO et al., 1986). In essence, the goal of health promotion is to minimize existing health disparities while working toward the creation of conditions (i.e., DOH) that promote equity and social justice (Potvin, Mantoura, & Ridde, 2007; WHO et al., 1986). Excellent resources to further extend your understanding of the determinants of health include *Closing the Gap in a Generation: Health Equity through Action on the Social Determinants of Health* (Commission on the Social Determinants of Health, 2008), and the *Social Determinants of Health: The Canadian Facts* (Mikkonen & Raphael, 2010).

Other DOH frameworks include the Toronto Charter for a Healthy Canada (Raphael, Bryant, & Curry-Stevens, 2004) (see Box 4.1 for a summary of this framework) and the widely recognized DOH framework by the Public Health Agency of Canada (PHAC, 2011).

BOX 4.1: THE TORONTO CHARTER FOR A HEALTHY CANADA

In collecting and providing the evidence and, in part, drawing on Canada's obligation to honour the UN Human Rights treaty, the Toronto Charter for a Healthy Canada identifies the following as those that determine health:

- early childhood development
- education
- employment and working conditions
- food security
- health care services
- housing (shortages)
- income and its equitable distribution

- social exclusion
- social safety nets
- employment security

Source: Raphael, D., Bryant, T., & Curry-Stevens, A. (2004). Toronto charter outlines future health policy directions for Canada and elsewhere. *Health Promotion International, 19*(2), 269–273.

PHAC scientists and researchers have further refined the DOH list with a resultant 12 health determinants (see Table 4.1) (PHAC, 2011). PHAC emphasizes the interactive nature of the social and economic factors, the physical environment, and the individual behavioural factors that "determine" health. The challenge for health care providers, researchers, educators, and individuals in creating effective health promotion strategies or plans is that the DOH do not exist in isolation from each other; rather, it is the combined influence of these factors that determines health status (PHAC, 2011).

TABLE 4.1: PUBLIC HEALTH AGENCY OF CANADA DETERMINANTS OF HEALTH

1. Income and social status	2. Social support networks
3. Education and literacy	4. Employment/working conditions
5. Social environments	6. Physical environments
7. Personal health practices and coping skills	8. Healthy child development
9. Biology and genetic endowment	10. Health services
11. Gender	12. Culture

Source: Modified from Public Health Agency of Canada. (2011). *What determines health?* Retrieved from http://www.phac-aspc.gc.ca/ph-sp/determinants/index-eng.php#What [accessed: 15 June 2013].

Proposed additional refinements to the PHAC list of health determinants include incorporating concepts of "power" (decision making) and social inclusion or exclusion (Hankivsky & Christoffersen, 2008; Potvin et al., 2007; Raphael et al., 2004). Hankivsky and Christoffersen (2008) state that having "power" (a foundational concept to intersectionality theory, discussed later in this chapter) contributes to the development of health equity through the opportunity to determine issues of importance, set policy, and allocate resources. Examples of a lack of "power" include the persistent social stigma experienced by, and lack of resources available for, those with mental health problems or people who are transgendered in their sexuality. Similarly, Raphael and colleagues (2004) persuasively argue that those who are socially excluded, who are marginalized in society (e.g., individuals with low socio-economic status, living homeless, managing mental health issues), are without "voice" and have little opportunity to set health priorities and determine resource allocation (Raphael, Curry-Stevens, & Bryant, 2008). These researchers define social exclusion as the processes that deny Canadians—mostly those who are poor, of Aboriginal heritage, immigrants, and in the non-dominant race, ethnicity, or religious affiliation—opportunities to participate in many aspects of cultural, economic, social, and political life.

REVIEW AND REFLECT

Using the listed determinants of health (DOH) from the Public Health Agency of Canada in Table 4.1, consider how these factors influence your own health. How might the DOH influence your own family, neighbourhood, and community? Then have a look on the PHAC website (see "Additional Resources of Interest" at the end of the chapter) for further evidence of factors that determine health.

A number of Canadian educators and scholars have studied and written about the DOH and more specifically on the social determinants of health (SDOH). The SDOH, also referred to as the non-medical, non-biological DOH, encompass the conditions or the contexts that shape people's everyday lives. The World Health Organization states that the life context of people (e.g., the homes they live in, where they live, their level of education, literacy skill, income, gender, and culture) are shaped by the distribution of money, power, and resources at global, national, and local levels. (You may want to explore additional information on social determinants of health from the WHO [2012], available at http://www.who.int/social_determinants/en/). Similar to the messages from the Ottawa Charter and PHAC, the WHO states that the SDOH are the factors mostly responsible for existing health inequities within countries and among countries around the world—including Canada.

Responding to increased concerns about persistent and widening inequities within health, the WHO established the Commission on Social Determinants of Health in 2005 to provide evidence and recommendations for reducing inequities. Powerful SDOH include income (particularly income-based inequality), unequal distribution of wealth, and political power (decision-making power) (Subramanian & Kawachi, 2004). An "endless circle of disadvantage" is created among those who are the poorest, the most disempowered, the sickest, and the least likely to be able to change their circumstances (Adelson, 2005). A leading Canadian researcher at York University, Dr. Naomi Adelson, investigated the health circumstances of Aboriginal peoples in Canada and believes the "endless circle of disadvantage" describes the circumstance of many Aboriginal people who are caught in a cycle of poverty, violence, limited education, and chronic health concerns (Adelson, 2005).

The work of other Canadian scholars and practitioners (see Box 4.2) reflects the lesser known or understood SDOH.

BOX 4.2: ONTARIO MEDICAL ASSOCIATION PRESS RELEASE
DOCTORS POINT TO POVERTY AS MAJOR CAUSE OF ILLNESS

Toronto, July 29, 2008—A new report by a group of Ontario doctors highlights the ways in which poverty affects the health outcomes of adults and children and the role health-care professionals can play in reducing the impact of poverty on people's health. The report, "Why poverty makes us sick," authored by The Ontario Physicians Poverty Work Group, reveals that poverty substantially raises the rate of chronic illness, infant mortality and lowers life expectancy.

"As doctors, we are concerned with the widespread impact that poverty has on people's health," said Dr. Gary Bloch, a family doctor and member of the Ontario Physicians Poverty Work Group. "Demographic trends show that poverty is now a key indicator for health status when we treat our patients, which is why doctors are highlighting how poverty can affect us and what patients need to do to minimize the negative impact."

The Ontario Physicians Poverty Work Group, which is made up of Medical Officers of Health and physicians who specialize in family medicine, is raising awareness about the role health care providers can play in treating patients from lower socio-economic backgrounds and the need to have a province-wide plan to address poverty.

"The faces of poverty are often hidden to physicians, but there are ways to understand how patients are living and their level of risk for illnesses associated with poverty," said Dr. Itamar Tamari, member of the Ontario Physicians Poverty Work Group. "Doctors are working hard to ensure this part of the patient population does not go untreated, but tackling poverty must be a coordinated effort including governments and communities."

In 2007, the Ontario provincial government pledged to tackle poverty in their election platform. According to the Ontario Physicians Poverty Work Group, health care professionals look forward to working with the government to address the negative impact of poverty on health.

The report provides practical clinical advice to physicians such as becoming aware of different population groups in the community so that appropriate preventative steps and education are provided to patients. The report also suggests that doctors can encourage patients to apply for government support programs and advocate for their patients by preparing letters of support.

"In order to address the problem of poverty we need strong leaders. Doctors can fulfill that role by advocating for better care for their patients," said Dr. Michael Rachlis, member of the Ontario Physicians Poverty Work Group. "It is our hope that the provincial government will work with health-care providers in the fight against poverty and the preventable illnesses that it is responsible for."

Source: Ontario Medical Association Press Release. (2008, July 29). *Doctors point to poverty as major cause of illness* [Press release]. Retrieved from www.newswire.ca/en/story/300711/doctors-point-to-poverty-as-major-cause-of-illness.

One of the most dramatic conclusions in the report is that poverty is likely the most important determinant of illness and early mortality. Research shows the startling impact that low income can have on a person's health status. For example, low-income Ontario women are nearly four times more likely to suffer from diabetes than high-income women, and the prevalence of depression among low-income individuals is 60 percent higher than the Canadian average.

Unfortunately, public awareness of the SDOH influence on health has not yet attained "mainstream" status (Daghofer, 2011). Different from the health promotion messages encouraging Canadians to change habits and take "ownership" of their individual lifestyle choices (e.g., to increase their intake of fruits and vegetables, increase physical activity, stop smoking, drink alcohol in moderation), the impact of the SDOH are not well understood by the average Canadian (Daghofer, 2011; Gasher, Hayes, Hackett, Gutstein, & Dunn, 2007; Hayes et al., 2007). In fact, Hayes and colleagues (2007) analyzed the content of 4,732 news stories from 13 Canadian daily newspapers (10 English, 3 French) for the years 1993, 1995, 1997, and 2001 and concluded that topics related to health care (e.g., issues of service provision, delivery, management, regulation) were prominent. Knowing that the mass media are very influential in shaping public ideas about health, it was troubling that socio-economic issues, frequently cited in the research literature as being most influential in shaping population health outcomes, were rarely reported on (Hayes et al., 2007). Yet, the majority of Canadians claim they have good to excellent understanding of health issues, identifying the most important health factors as diet and physical activity. When asked, only one in three Canadians recognized that social and economic conditions (e.g., income and housing) and community characteristics (e.g., supportive services) influence health. Moreover, research shows that mass media coverage of the SDOH is extremely limited (Daghofer, 2011; Gasher et al., 2007; Hayes et al., 2007). And, of the SDOH, employment and education were most likely to be linked to health outcomes. Literacy and health literacy (which are necessary for and related to employment and income) were not recognized within the public sphere as DOH (Daghofer, 2011).

HEALTH AS A HUMAN RIGHT

Taking action to promote health involves strategies that advocate for favourable political, economic, social, cultural, environmental, behavioural, and biological conditions. The Ottawa Charter frames health and health promotion from a human rights perspective, calling for equity in health achievable through actions that reduce differences in health status and ensure equal opportunities and resources to enable all people to achieve their fullest health potential. Essentially, these prerequisites for health assert the need for access to supportive environments, access to information, developed life skills, and opportunities for making healthy choices. Given the multiplicity of factors influencing health, "health promotion demands coordinated action by all concerned: by governments, by health and other social and economic sectors, by non-governmental and voluntary organizations, by local authorities, by industry and by the media" (WHO et al., 1986). The suggested health-promoting strategies of building healthy public policy, creating supportive environments, strengthening community action, developing personal skills, and reorienting health services proposed within the Ottawa Charter are intended to promote health among individuals, families, and communities and "to tackle the inequities in health" (WHO et al., 1986).

Furthermore, the United Nations (UN) Universal Declaration of Human Rights (1948) states: "Everyone has the right to a standard of living adequate for the health and well-being of [the individual] and of [their] family, including food, clothing, housing and medical care ... [and] the right to security in the event of ... sickness, disability" (UN, 1948) (see Figure 4.1 for a summary of the links between health and human rights). While Canada played a key role in the development of the UN Human Rights Declaration, it is interesting to note that the Canadian government uses the term "values" rather than "rights" in documents describing the principles underlying the Canadian health system. What is meant by "values" as opposed to "rights"? The values we hold guide our thinking and behaviour. For example, MacDonald (2002) argues for a values-based approach to health promotion. She contends that all health promotion activity—program development, implementation, and evaluation—should be guided by the values of empowerment, equity, collaboration, partnering, and a bottom-up approach (MacDonald, 2002). A rights-based approach, in contrast, would expect all health promotion activity to be based on ensuring equity, collaboration, partnerships, and empowerment. We will consider values-based and rights-based approaches again in Chapter 5 when the focus turns to culture and health literacy.

REVIEW AND REFLECT

Do you think that our health care system operates from a values-based approach to promoting health? Why or why not?

Should we as Canadians be concerned that the "right to health" is not in the Canadian Charter of Rights and Freedoms? (Review the Canadian Charter of Rights and Freedoms found on the Government of Canada website at http://laws-lois.justice.gc.ca/eng/Const/page-15.html)

Leary (2009) found that the values of equity and fairness were evident in the Canadian health care system and were reflected in the Romanow report (2002) that advocated for health care universality, portability, comprehensiveness, accessibility. and public administration. She states that "the phrase 'right to health' is not used in the Canadian Charter of Rights and Freedoms and to date there has been an apparent reluctance to give legal recognition to health as a human right in Canada" (Leary, 2009, p. 473). Yet, the recommendations of the Romanow report also called for equitable access to and enhanced quality of health care, greater attention to the social determinants of health, greater system transparency and accountability, and a focused attention on the health needs of marginalized populations (Leary, 2009). The right to health is not separate from other rights, including the right to a decent standard of living and education, as well as to freedom from discrimination, and so forth. From a human rights perspective, health promotion is built on the right to have equal opportunities to be healthy, not only in terms of health status, but with respect to all of the SDOH (Braveman & Gruskin, 2003).

FIGURE 4.1: LINKS BETWEEN HUMAN RIGHTS AND HEALTH

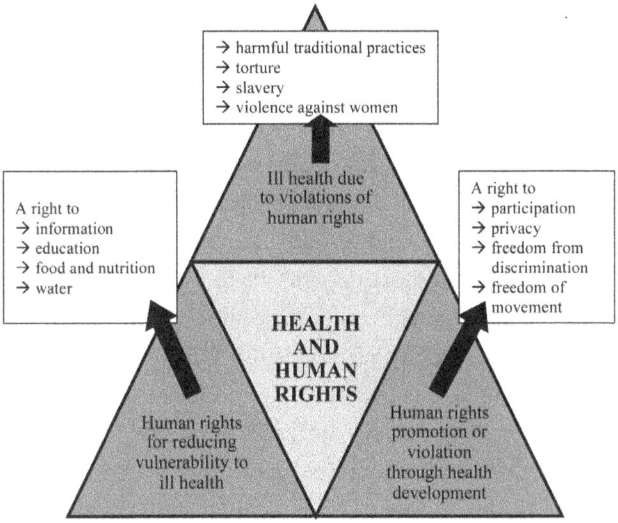

→ harmful traditional practices
→ torture
→ slavery
→ violence against women

Ill health due to violations of human rights

A right to
→ information
→ education
→ food and nutrition
→ water

A right to
→ participation
→ privacy
→ freedom from discrimination
→ freedom of movement

HEALTH AND HUMAN RIGHTS

Human rights for reducing vulnerability to ill health

Human rights promotion or violation through health development

Source: Figure modified from World Health Organization. (2012). *Linkages between health and human rights*. Retrieved from www.who.int/hhr/HHRlinkages.pdf

Framing health as a human right (rather than a value) holds governments and organizations accountable for creating the conditions, policies, processes, and procedures that determine the health of individuals. For example, Leary (2009) credits Canada with a model health care system but also points to persistent health disparities that exist among Aboriginal peoples relative to non-Aboriginal Canadians as a violation of the perspective of health as a human right. Leary (2009) states:

> Recognizing health as a human right can help to underscore the importance of human health as more than access to health care, to include socio-economic determinants such as the environment, access to clean drinking water and food, and adequate housing, as well as health promotion. The right to health also ... highlights the disparate health status of marginalized populations and ultimately ensures that health systems ... meet the health needs of all. (p. 478)

To summarize the chapter so far, we consider health as being influenced by social, economic, policy, and physical factors and conditions, and as much more than the simple absence of disease; health is a fundamental resource for everyday living (Public Health Agency of Canada, 2011; WHO et al., 1986). We have discussed health and the promotion of optimal health as a human right. The factors and conditions that influence health, referred to as the "determinants of health" (DOH), consist of multiple and intersecting personal, social, economic, and environmental factors that determine the *health status* of individuals or populations throughout the lifespan. The SDOH, factors with a powerful impact on health, are not widely understood and tend to be underappreciated as important to health by the general public. The Ottawa Charter, the health promotion "road map," lists strategies for action on all DOH to reduce inequities and to enhance the health of all Canadians. The principles established for the practice and promotion of health are founded on the concepts of social justice and equity (a more detailed explanation of these concepts are provided later in this chapter); through this lens, differences in health status, opportunity, and access to resources are minimized through supportive environments, access to information and services, the development of effective life skills, and the opportunity to control choices.

Health promotion and health communication experts point to the limited attention within health promotion research, education, and practice to issues that create health inequities (Dutta, 2010; Potvin et al., 2007). This lack of attention to the conditions that create health inequities is despite the fact that the Ottawa Charter highlights inequities as a focus of health promotion activity. The following section will provide a brief overview of the concepts of equity and social justice. For an in-depth exploration of the concepts of equity and social justice, students are encouraged to read the works of Margaret Whitehead (Whitehead, 1991; 1996) and Paula Braveman (Braveman, 2006; Braveman & Gruskin, 2003; Braveman et al., 2011), among others.

EQUITY, EQUALITY, AND SOCIAL JUSTICE

"Equity means social justice or fairness; it is an ethical concept, grounded in principles of distributive justice" (Braveman & Gruskin, 2003, p. 254). Social justice is defined as the *socially defined* view in society about what is fair, just, and right; these views or judgments are dictated by the current moral beliefs and values of the society (Whitehead, 1991; 1996). It is also the case that whoever determines how these judgments, morals, and beliefs are put into action (e.g., setting policy or creating laws) also tends to have greater privilege, status, and power—a greater voice in making decisions that affect the population at large.

Health equity implies that all people have an equal opportunity to develop and maintain their health through fair and just access to resources for health. Whitehead (1991) argues that the goal of health equity is "not to eliminate all health differences so that everyone has the same level and quality of health, but rather to reduce or eliminate those [differences] which result from factors which are considered to be both avoidable and unfair" (p. 220). Equity does not guarantee that all Canadians enjoy the same or equal level of health but that there should be *equal opportunity* for individuals to attain optimal health potential. Alternatively, inequities in health "systematically put groups of people who are already socially disadvantaged (for example, by virtue of being poor, female, and/or members of a disenfranchised racial, ethnic, or religious group) at further disadvantage with respect to their health" (Braveman & Gruskin, 2003, p. 254).

> **REVIEW AND REFLECT**
>
> Look at the differences in health care within your family, community, and province, and ask yourself whether the differences you witness are in fact inequitable or unequal. Explain the difference between health inequity and health inequality.

Braveman and Gruskin (2003) make an important distinction between disparities within health that are labelled as inequitable (lacking fairness) rather than as unequal. Health inequities are created from a systematic lack of fairness of the distribution of resources and processes (determinants of health) that influence health care and status. The apparent disparity of the general health status of younger Canadians relative to senior Canadians constitutes an inequality but is not viewed as inequitable. The inequality (not inequity) in health status is illustrated by the prevalence of coronary heart disease, which is more prevalent in older men compared to young men. This difference in prevalence is not unexpected, and despite the greater number of older men with heart disease, this disparity would not be considered inequitable. Alternatively, the higher rates of ill health resulting from a lack of resources, low education, and income that limits choices related to food security, housing, safe working conditions, or stable and secure employment are inequitable. Inequitable access to health services occurs when people are either denied health services or cannot access these services because of income, race, sex, age, religion, literacy/health literacy, or other factors not directly related to the need for care (Whitehead, 1990).

Equal quality of care for everyone also implies that health care providers will strive to put the same commitment into the quality of services they deliver for all population segments of a community. Inequities in care can arise from the manner in which certain groups (for instance, those with low literacy or who are homeless) are treated by health care providers and health care systems who do not put the same effort into their work and offer less of their time or professional expertise (Institute of Medicine, 2012; Whitehead, 1990; Zrinyi & Balogh, 2004).

From a health systems perspective, the health inequities experienced by Canadians who are First Nations stem from a fundamental difference in an understanding of "health." Broadly speaking (and admittedly a generalization), First Nations people have traditionally framed health around the physical, emotional, mental, and spiritual wellness of a person, family, and community. This understanding of health contrasts with the biomedical model of health care that tends to dominate the Canadian health care system. Disparate or inequitable health care results when non-Aboriginal health care workers are disadvantaged in attending to and communicating about health (disease) using the language and the culture of biomedicine (Adelson, 2005). A study by the Montreal Native Friendship Centre found that HIV-positive Aboriginal people often do not access the available services because of the multiple stigmas associated with HIV and AIDS; many living with HIV/AIDS prefer to remain anonymous and refuse to seek care or support until the later stages of the disease (Adelson, 2005). These examples of inequities are inconsistent with Canadian values, are avoidable, and can be successfully addressed. Nevertheless, these inequities persist and, in some cases, are increasing across the country (Health Disparities Task Group, 2005). Earlier we commented that the DOH can either enhance or negatively influence health status. What follows is a more detailed discussion of how the DOH of education and literacy and health literacy contribute to health.

LITERACY AND HEALTH LITERACY AS DETERMINANTS OF HEALTH (DOH)

The United Nations Economic and Social Council Ministers identified health literacy as an important health determinant and set forth a number of recommendations to guide the development of health literacy best practices within the countries represented at the meeting:

> [E]ffective health literacy interventions; demonstrating how improved health literacy can enhance the effectiveness of primary health care; developing culturally appropriate measures for reporting progress; strengthening joint action within and beyond the health sectors; promoting use of modern information and communications technology (ICT) and encouraging the media to ensure information accuracy; and building community capacity through empowerment and institutional capacity for sustainable action, including the use by practitioners of the evidence-based approach. (United Nations Economic and Social Council, 2009, p. 2)

We will use intersectionality theory to focus on the multiple and intersecting factors that influence health, such as issues of education, literacy, and health literacy. Intersectionality theory holds that no one factor is more important than another. Rather, it is at the intersection of many factors (e.g., race/ethnicity, religion, culture, socio-economic status, sexuality, gender) where an individual's health experience is defined and created (Hankivsky & Christoffersen, 2008). In using an intersectional approach to understanding health and health promotion, you would not

> simply add social categories to one another in an attempt to understand diverse experiences. Instead, ... an intersectional paradigm seeks to uncover the convergence of experiences, including multiple forms of discrimination and oppression. In terms of a health determinants framework, examinations of health inequities that are reduced to any one single determinant or marker of difference would be viewed as inadequate for understanding the various dimensions that are always at play in shaping and influencing social positions and power relations. (Hankivsky & Christoffersen, 2008, p. 276)

Working from an intersectionality framework helps us to understand the complex interplay of all determinants of health (DOH) on an individual and population level (Hankivsky & Christoffersen, 2008).

For example, an intersectionality perspective helps us to understand the DOH impact on Aboriginal populations within Canada. Intersectionality emphasizes the "construction" of health by the cultural, language, and social differences between and among the diverse Canadian Aboriginal populations (e.g., Inuit, Haida, Annishnabe, Cree). Understanding the impact on health from an intersectionality perspective accounts for differences related to Aboriginal ancestry, gender, age, residence (urban, rural, and remote locations), (un)employment, level of income, (non)education, differences in treaty-related rights, and power(lessness)— creating in a unique way the experiences of health among Aboriginal populations within Canada (Adelson, 2005). The concepts of culture, cultural mosaic, and multiculturalism and how these are influenced by language, history, and literacy are considered in more detail in Chapter 5.

We know from our discussion above that health status is influenced by multiple and intersecting factors. While we will discuss select DOH, focusing on the social determinants of health (SDOH) that align with literacy and health literacy, it is beyond the scope of this chapter to discuss all 12 of the DOH in detail (see the Public Health Agency of Canada's website at www.phac-aspc.gc.ca/ph-sp/determinants/index-eng.php for a full discussion and additional DOH resources). An interesting "conversation" emerging among researchers and practitioners in the health promotion area points to health literacy as an indicator of health disparities. Patterns of health disparities mirror observed differences in health literacy skill (Dutta-Bergman, 2004a, 2004b). In many ways, addressing the development of literacy and health literacy skills supports health and minimizes inequities in health, particularly as they pertain to certain groups of populations, such as Aboriginal peoples, older Canadians, women, those living in rural areas, and immigrants, who are vulnerable to serious health disparities (Health Disparities Task Group, 2005; Murthy, 2009). Older Canadians, First Nations/Inuit peoples, newcomers to Canada, and individuals with limited education, income, and language skill all show evidence of low health literacy skills. This composition of little education, literacy, and health literacy skills limits individuals' access to health information, resources, and services, and sets the stage for inequities within health that arise when health resources and services are unevenly distributed (Health Disparities Task Group, 2005; Whitehead, 1991; 1992). These population segments also tend to experience significantly worse health outcomes, including higher rates of ill health and disability (e.g., higher incidence of cancer, diabetes, high blood pressure, and HIV/AIDS), that align with inadequate health literacy skills (Murthy, 2009). Effective communication and access to timely and relevant information are necessary for chronic disease management. Despite the need for effective communication, a number of SDOH pose challenges to health care providers and public health and health promotion educators to effectively accommodate the information and services needs associated with chronic health issues for disenfranchised groups (Murthy, 2009). Chief among these SDOH are language, cultural barriers, and time constraints.

Similarly, the population level measures of literacy skill discussed in detail in Chapter 3 reflect a basic disparity in information access among Canadian adults. Those who scored at Level 3 literacy skill and above on the International Adult Literacy and Skills Survey prose literacy scale have a reading skill level that enables them to use their reading skill in order *to learn*. This means that Canadians with a Level 3 to 5 skill have greater comprehension abilities and are able to determine the meaning of unfamiliar words or context that supports problem solving, allowing them to seek and understand new and unknown topics. Canadians with Level 3 to 5 skill have reached the level of "reading to learn" (Canadian Council on Learning [CCL], 2008b). In contrast, adults scoring at Levels 1 and 2 on the IALS do not have the same fluency in reading skills and, as a result, much of their reading effort is geared to "learning to read," limiting access to and comprehension of a large proportion of health information (CCL, 2008b).

Research exploring different channels and outlets for obtaining information—such as newspapers, magazines, the Internet, television—extends our understanding of inequitable access to (health) information. Differences in how people attend to, understand, and make use of health information depends more on their literacy level and less on their level of formal education (Viswanath & Ackerson, 2011). Education provides individuals with the skills, knowledge, and confidence to seek specific health information, whereas literacy skill determines the source of health information that individuals specifically seek out. For example, newspapers, magazines, and the Internet are health information sources that require well-developed literacy skills; in contrast, information seekers with fewer literacy skills depend on television and radio to learn about health issues. An interesting question that arises is whether the quality of the health information (e.g., the accuracy, detail, and clarity) from the various sources also differs and, if so, does this difference contribute to inequities in health? We might ask whether the clarity, accuracy, and detail of information about a potential health threat (e.g., the occurrence of West Nile Virus in a specific area) differ between television and newspapers, and if so, how this difference in information characteristics affects individual health behaviour and action.

REVIEW AND REFLECT

Choose a current health issue of interest to you and compare the information about this issue gathered from your local newspaper, televised news broadcasts, and the Internet. Do you notice a difference in the amount, type, and difficulty of the content of information across these media sources?

A lack of community participation also creates a context of isolation and exclusion and eliminates potentially important channels of health information and social support from peer networks (Basu & Dutta, 2008; Eysenbach, 2008). Changing patterns of information access highlight the community as an important and sometimes preferred repository of health information. Because of the increased reliance on social network health information sources, individuals with low levels of participation in their communities lack the benefit of this increasingly important health information resource. Individuals who actively participate in their local communities tend to have greater confidence in their ability to find information and to search for health information (Basu & Dutta, 2008). This information supports the addition of "social exclusion" as an important DOH (Raphael et al., 2004). The "condition" of low literacy and low health literacy creates situations of health inequity with respect to limitations in health information sources and resource access (Rootman & Gordon-El-Bihbety, 2008).

Health communication researchers have determined that communication channel type—active or passive—also influences access to information (Dutta-Bergman, 2004a, 2004b). Active channels (e.g., the Internet) require greater cognitive effort and engagement by individuals to seek out, understand, and ultimately make use of the information. Alternatively, passive information channels (e.g., television) require less personal effort. In addition, individuals using active channels tend to require greater motivation for use in contrast to using passive channels that are typically categorized as "low involvement." Not surprisingly, there is a notable and systematic difference in health literacy skill with respect to the use of active and passive channels of health information. Individuals with low health literacy prefer passive sources of information such as television, spend little time gathering information from active sources such as the Internet, and are less likely to put much trust in online health information (Dutta-Bergman, 2004a, 2004b; Rudd et al., 2004; Viswanath & Ackerson, 2011). "Motivated" health information seekers (those with higher literacy skill) are more likely to learn health information from active communication channels such as the Internet (Dutta-Bergman, 2004a, 2004b, 2004c). Individuals identified as non-information seekers, but who had active chronic health concerns (such as cancer or diabetes), tended to have low income and education, paid little attention to health in the media, and had little trust in mass media health information; they also scored lower on preventive health behaviours (Ramanadhan & Viswanath, 2009).

EQUITABLE ACCESS TO INFORMATION

It seems counterintuitive to think that increased information may actually lead to a widening of the gaps in knowledge between different population groups. Yet, we are beginning to learn that the benefits from increased availability of information are not equally distributed among all Canadians (Viswanath et al., 2006). Advantaged groups are able to acquire new information at a faster rate than disadvantaged groups, and this widening of the information/knowledge gap may account for some of the differential lifestyle behaviours among groups of people. This in turn creates great potential for information disparities that contribute to health disparities (Beacom & Newman, 2010; Viswanath et al., 2006).

Viswanath and Krueter (2007) provide a more critical look at the processes that support the knowledge gap hypothesis, which challenges the assumption that increasingly accessible information (e.g., Internet-based information) is equally accessible to all social classes of people. Their research found that current communication and health policies perpetuate information inequities and contribute to the construction of the "information-haves" and "information have-nots." Part of the digital divide (see Box 4.3) is created by the relatively limited demand for broadband Internet services among the geographical areas with concentrated populations of lower socio-economic communities.

BOX 4.3: THE DIGITAL DIVIDE

Differences in Internet access persist among different demographic groups (e.g., seniors, non-white, lesser education), especially when it comes to access to high-speed broadband at home. People's connection to the Internet is much more diverse today than even in 2000. The International Adult Literacy and Life Skill Survey (ALLS) 2003 survey found that people who use computers consistently scored higher on average on the prose literacy scale than those who didn't.

Sources: Statistics Canada and OECD. (2005). *Learning a living: First results of the Adult Literacy and Life Skills Survey* (p. 276). Ottawa and Paris. Retrieved from http://www.oecd.org/education/country-studies/34867438.pdf [accessed: 19 August 2013]; and Zickuhr, K., & Smith, A. (2012). *Digital differences* (p. 41). Washington, DC: Pew Internet & American Life Project. Retrieved from http://pewinternet.org/Reports/2012/Digital-differences.aspx [accessed: 19 August 2013].

The digital divide is evident among Aboriginal populations and others living in remote areas of Canada who do not have access to the Internet (or only limited access). Challenges remain for many northern and rural communities to gain Internet services that are efficient (high speed) and of comparable quality and cost to those enjoyed by highly populated, urban communities (Government of Canada, 2004). We will consider the impact of the Internet and new media technologies, and the consequences of the digital divide on health in greater detail in Chapter 6.

REVIEW AND REFLECT

Ask your family and friends about their preferred health information sources. Compare the preferred sources of information relative to each individual's age, gender, ethnicity, and geographical location.

KEY LEARNING POINTS

As we stressed in this chapter (and earlier chapters), the development of health literacy allows individuals to gain access to, understand, and use information in ways that promote good health. Health literacy allows people to engage with others and to influence change and exert greater control over their lives. In this chapter we have discussed how determinants of health intersect and influence (both positively and negatively) the health of individuals and populations. We have focused specifically on literacy and health literacy as increasingly important factors in improving health status and in reducing health inequities that exist within Canada. We have considered a "values-based" approach and a "rights-based" approach in access to the intersecting factors that influence health. Finally, we looked at health literacy development among some of the most marginalized Canadians through the lens of intersectionality theory and the social determinants of health.

A CANADIAN MILESTONE

THE CANADIAN PUBLIC HEALTH ASSOCIATION—HEALTH LITERACY PORTAL

The Canadian Public Health Association (CPHA) is a national, independent, not-for-profit, voluntary association representing public health in Canada. This organization, with the support of the Expert Panel on Health Literacy, and many health literacy scholars since, created an online information access portal for information and resources specific to the health literacy of Canadians. The portal reports on ongoing health literacy research between the CPHA and Canadian researchers. CPHA's National Literacy and Health Program (NLHP), in existence since 1994, was created to promote and educate health professionals about the relationship between literacy and health. The program advocates for health information in plain language and clear verbal communication within health care encounters.

The CPHA health literacy portal can be found at www.cpha.ca/en/portals/h-l.aspx.

ADDITIONAL RESOURCES OF INTEREST

The United Nations
http://www.un.org
The United Nations is an international organization founded in 1945 after the Second World War by 51 countries committed to maintaining international peace and security, developing friendly relations among nations, and promoting social progress, better living standards, and human rights. This website provides additional resources related to human rights issues that addresses all of the determinants of health. See also the United Nations Universal Declaration of Human Rights, available at www.un.org/en/documents/udhr/.

The Public Health Agency of Canada
http://www.phac-aspc.gc.ca/
For information regarding the PHAC determinant of health framework, see www.phac-aspc.gc.ca/ph-sp/determinants/determinants-eng.php. Another useful resource is "How Does Literacy Affect the Health of Canadians?" available at http://en.copian.ca/library/research/howdoes/howdoes.pdf.

**United Nations Educational, Scientific and Cultural Organization (UNESCO)—
Literacy Portal**

http://www.unesco.org/new/en/education/themes/education-building-blocks/literacy/

The United Nations Educational, Scientific and Cultural Organization provides a Web portal with numerous resources on literacy from a global perspective.

CHAPTER 5

CULTURE AND HEALTH LITERACY

It is hereby declared to be the policy of the Government of Canada to: (a) recognize and promote the understanding that multiculturalism reflects the cultural and racial diversity of Canadian society and acknowledges the freedom of all members of Canadian society to preserve, enhance and share their cultural heritage; (b) recognize and promote the understanding that multiculturalism is a fundamental characteristic of the Canadian heritage and identity and that it provides an invaluable resource in the shaping of Canada's future; [and] (c) promote the full and equitable participation of individuals and communities of all origins in the continuing evolution and shaping of all aspects of Canadian society and assist them in the elimination of any barrier to that participation.

—GOVERNMENT OF CANADA, CANADIAN MULTICULTURALISM ACT, 1985

CHAPTER LEARNING OBJECTIVES
- Introduce the concepts of culture and ethnicity
- Introduce the concepts of acculturation and assimilation and how they are measured
- Introduce the concepts of cultural awareness, competence, and safety
- Introduce the concepts of multiculturalism and the cultural mosaic in Canada
- Describe how culture affects the health literacy of Canadians

INTRODUCTION

People are experts at categorizing, classifying, labelling, sorting, and analyzing information. We find patterns even when they are subtle. Our search for associations extends to health literacy; identifying meaningful differences in health literacy levels within a population is a necessary first step in responding to those differences. In chapters 2 and 3 we considered the relationship between literacy and health: people with low literacy levels have poorer health outcomes compared to those with higher levels of literacy. The health literacy performance of adult Canadians was related to a number of demographic factors, such as education, income, immigration status, age, Aboriginal status, and province of residence. We also learned why low health literacy is an issue of social justice in Canada.

Another key factor that affects health literacy skill is *culture*. How an individual understands and uses health information is strongly influenced by his or her cultural background, beliefs, values, and language. Culture shapes what people believe, what people feel it is important to know, who they feel needs to know it, and what action follows from this knowledge. Culture is an essential component of health literacy.

To introduce the importance of culture for health literacy, consider what health information is provided and to whom. In a study by Feldman, Zhang, and Cummings (1999), 20 Chinese internists in Beijing and 20 U.S. internists in San Francisco were asked whether they would tell their patients about a terminal cancer diagnosis. Almost all of the U.S. doctors, but none of the Chinese doctors, indicated that they would tell their patients about a cancer diagnosis. When the family members' wishes conflicted with the patient's preferences regarding chemotherapy for the cancer, 65 percent of the Chinese doctors followed the family's preferences whereas only 5 percent of U.S. doctors did. Although there are many reasons for these differences in physician–patient communication, and recognizing that this was a small sample, cultural perspective likely plays a role. Underlying decisions about who to inform is the emphasis on individualism, collectivism, or both (Triandis, 1993). Although no culture group (or individual) is exclusively one or the other in orientation, some stress individualism and personal responsibility, freedom of choice, and personal autonomy. Others emphasize collectivism and interdependence, shared responsibility, and group accountability (Neuliep, 2012). For the U.S. (and by extension, Canadian) physicians, ethical, cultural, and legal frames of individual rights and patient autonomy (Kaufert & Putsch, 1997) may contribute to the decision about who to inform of the cancer diagnosis. For the Chinese-trained doctors, cultural values based on social relationships (Surbone, 2006) may influence their decisions about who to inform about diagnosis and treatment.

Language, an essential component of culture, also affects health literacy. This interplay between language and culture is illustrated by a case described by Pottie (2007). "Mrs. A" and her newborn daughter were new refugees to Canada from Sierra Leone. The baby was taken away from the mother and placed in a foster home because of the misinterpretation of Mrs. A's Krio native language as "broken" English, the assessment of Mrs. A as having low literacy and being of low intelligence (because of language barriers), and inaccuracies in the translation of Krio to English.

Consider a situation where individuals speak the same language, but because of cultural perceptions, each person "hears," "interprets," and "processes" different things. Simple words between a health care provider and a patient may not be understood because of differing values, meanings, and associations of words. For the physician, the phrase "this medication for depression may help" might mean that there is no conclusive evidence about the effectiveness of the medication in someone with intractable depression (e.g., a selective serotonin reuptake inhibitor). For the patient with depression, however, this statement might mean "this medication will help me."

What these three examples illustrate is that cultural factors are crucial for health literacy: failure to recognize differences in explanatory models of health and illness, cultural values, perceptual biases, the meaning of words, and language barriers contribute to inequities in health decision making and health outcomes for Canadians. Nevertheless, culture is difficult to define, and there is no homogeneous or single culture for any given group, including Canadians. People move between groups depending on situations and experiences. Culture is a dynamic and fluid concept. We also need to be very careful about our underlying assumptions about "cultural effects" on health and health literacy, since these assumptions can result in stereotyping, stigma, and bias (Kleinman & Benson, 2006a).

In this chapter we will focus on culture and why it is a necessary but challenging component of health literacy. We begin with a brief consideration of the "slippery slope" of defining culture and ethnicity. We introduce the concepts of cultural awareness, cultural competence, and cultural safety, and discuss why these are important for reducing disparities in health literacy. We explore the relationship between culture and language, and ask whether they have different (or similar) effects on health literacy. The chapter concludes with a discussion of multiculturalism, the Canadian "cultural" mosaic, and its implications for addressing health literacy gaps.

DEFINING CULTURE—A SLIPPERY CONCEPT

The concept of culture is notoriously difficult to define. Culture and cultural conversations are always drawn from people's perspectives and are socially constructed (Allen, 1999). In this section we will briefly outline some key definitions of the term *culture*, how these definitions vary across social science and public health disciplines, and why the act of defining the term has been so contentious. Our intent here is to help students understand why culture narratives matter within the context of health literacy, rather than to review the issue of culture in its entirety. It is beyond the scope of this chapter (and this book) to describe the scholarly debates, and the reasons for these debates, about the meaning of culture; nevertheless, our aim is to highlight some of the complexities, difficulties, and ambiguities inherent in this construct.

Multiple social science disciplines have put forward definitions of "culture," including anthropology, psychology, sociology, geography, and public health. Definitions among each discipline differ with respect to scope and research focus. For example, the anthropologist Clifford Geertz (1973) provided the following definition: "Believing, with Max Weber, that man is an animal suspended in webs of significance he himself has spun, I take culture to be those webs, and the analysis of it to be therefore not an experimental science in search of law but interpretative in search of meaning" (p. 5). In anthropology, research methodology is interpretative and the primary interest is on understanding how culture is represented and defined by individuals within a self-defined group (what is known as an "emic" or insider's perspective). Psychology takes a different focus in that the primary goal of studying culture is to identify its effects on human behaviour using experimental methods and the approach is often from an "etic" (or observer's) perspective. Segall, Lonner, and Berry (1998) capture this view of culture with their definition: "Culture is treated as comprising a set of independent or contextual variables affecting various aspects of individual behavior" (p. 1102). Public health definitions of culture fall somewhere in between the anthropological qualitative and interpretive search for meaning and the psychological quantitative search for axioms. In a review of the use of culture in public health research, Kreuter and McClure (2004) provide the following definition: "Culture is learned, shared, transmitted intergenerationally, and reflected in a group's values, beliefs, norms, practices, patterns of communication, familial roles, and other social regularities. Culture is also dynamic and adaptive" (p. 440). It is important to note the reference to culture as being dynamic and adaptive. As we will see later in this chapter, measurement of culture often does not capture its changing, dynamic process. Sociology tends to focus on the interplay of culture and society, as demonstrated by this quote: Culture is "a repertoire of socially transmitted and intra-generationally generated ideas about how to live and make judgments, both in general terms and in regards to specific domains of life" (Patterson, 2000, p. 208). Like public health, geography uses both qualitative and quantitative methodologies. However, the frame through which geography approaches questions of culture is quite different. The primary interest is how culture both influences and is influenced by physical space occupation and use (Jordan-Bychkov, Domosh, Neumann, & Price, 2006). Here the study of culture is secondary; culture is considered important in how it affects human behaviours of interest, whether the motivations to engage in physical activity or elements of neighbourhood design. Table 5.1 provides a brief snapshot of some important discipline-based distinctions of the concept of culture. (For in-depth discussions about culture, see the classic work of Kroeber, Kluckhohn, & Untereiner [1952]; the excellent review by Kreuter & McClure [2004]; and the interesting paper by Segall, Lonner, & Berry [1998], as well as the suggestions at the end of this chapter.)

TABLE 5.1: SOME KEY "GENERAL" FEATURES OF SOCIAL SCIENCE AND PUBLIC HEALTH APPROACHES TO CULTURE

Discipline	Key emphasis behind the study of "culture"
Anthropology	* Method of data analysis tends to be qualitative * Emphasis on the interpretation of material goods and symbols as means of communicating culture or representing membership
Sociology	* Method of data analysis tends to be quantitative * Emphasis on understanding and identifying the components of culture that people share in a particular society
Psychology	* Method of data analysis tends to be quantitative * Emphasis on culture as a set of independent variables or constituent components used to explain human behaviour
Geography	* Method of data analysis tends to be quantitative * Emphasis on the components of culture that shape patterns of land use
Public health	* Method of data analysis tends to be both quantitative and qualitative * Emphasis on identification of components of culture that enable customization of information and services for different groups of people

Definitions of culture reflect the goals, motivations, and knowledge frameworks of the individual, group, or discipline crafting the definition. For this reason, agreeing upon one definition has been challenging. Given such variability, can we define Canadian culture? Canada is a large country with vast differences in terms of geography and language. It is also a nation that enjoys a high rate of immigration. Canadian census data indicate that in 2006 just under 20 percent of the population was born outside of Canada (Statistics

Canada, 2009a). As a diverse nation it is neither easy nor useful to construct one definition of Canadian culture. The Canadian Multiculturalism Act declared that it was government policy to "recognize and promote the understanding that multiculturalism is a fundamental characteristic of the Canadian heritage and identity and that it provides an invaluable resource in the shaping of Canada's future" (Government of Canada, 1985). In regard to another indicator of culture, there are over 80 languages other than French or English spoken at home (Statistics Canada, 2009b). Diversity is what is truly at the heart of a definition of Canadian culture.

REVIEW AND REFLECT

Why has it been difficult to come up with a single definition of culture?

DEFINING ETHNICITY—MORE TRACTION BUT STILL SLIPPERY

Similar to culture, ethnicity is an elusive and complex concept. It is also one that has been fraught with controversy. The political use of the term *ethnicity* (or ethnic groups) to identify "otherness" comes, in part, from the work of anthropologist Fredrik Barth, who described ethnicity as a fluctuating boundary between groups (whether self-proclaimed, ascribed, or both) (Barth, 1969). More recently, Eriksen (2001) defined ethnicity as a socially sanctioned idea of shared ancestry including religion, language, politics, or history. Eriksen suggested that "ethnicity is the enduring and systematic communication of cultural differences between groups considering themselves to be distinct. It appears whenever cultural differences are made relevant in social interaction, and it should thus be studied at the level of social life" (2002, p. 58).

Yet defining ethnicity is as difficult as defining culture. In public health and health literacy studies the term *ethnicity* is often used interchangeably with the terms *race, culture, minority*, or *ethnic minority*. And, the concept of ethnicity, much like the term *race*, carries historical, political, and social baggage (Oppenheimer, 2001). Egede (2006) points out that current definitions of ethnicity that have been applied to health behaviour and health outcomes are poorly conceptualized and ill-defined. For example, "Hispanic" has been used (especially in the United States) to indicate a certain ethnicity; however, this term includes millions of people from many different groups and subgroups and countries who perhaps share only a common language (or language history). Students may want to consider how the term *Indians* (in the Constitution Act of 1867) has been used to exclude specific Aboriginal peoples, and the implications of the January 2013 Federal Court of Canada decision (*Daniels v. Canada*) on Métis and non-status Indians (see http://decisions.fct-cf.gc.ca/site/fc-cf/decisions/en/item/61753/index.do).

The importance of considering ethnicity in health and health literacy is not diminished by the problematic approach to defining and using the concept. Disparities between groups have been identified in access to health services, in exposure to usual or "mainstream" channels of health information dissemination, and in how health information is interpreted and acted on (Viswanath & Bond, 2007). To identify and address the primary drivers of these disparities, a more precise understanding of ethnicity is needed. In his study of health care barriers among

Vietnamese refugees to British Columbia, Stephenson (1995) carefully considered the contextual issues influencing health care for this community. Examination of specific community-based elements shared by members of this ethnic group, such as language, health beliefs, and immigration and settlement experiences, enabled the identification of specific ways in which communication with health care providers could be improved. For example, Vietnamese participants may have practised dermabrasion (*cao gio*), which breaks the capillaries near the surface of the skin and is used to "rid oneself" of fevers, influenza, and colds. Because this practice could be mistaken for abuse, health care practitioners were urged to consider their assumptions and communication about the causes of welts and small bruises, particularly in children.

The terms *culture* and *ethnicity* have proven difficult to define. Culture is taken to mean the material goods, symbols, and other components that embody and influence (and are influenced by) values, beliefs, and behaviours. Ethnicity is used to more specifically differentiate between culture groups engaged in social interactions. While inclusion of ethnicity in public health and health literacy studies is driven by a desire to reduce disparities, its continued use will require more careful definition and recognition of underlying assumptions and biases.

REVIEW AND REFLECT

What is the relationship between culture and ethnicity?

ACCULTURATION AND ASSIMILATION—MEANING AND MEASUREMENT

Globalization has enabled people to migrate at unprecedented rates, stimulating a renewed interest in the study of culture and cultural differences. In order to incorporate and study the effects of "culture" on human behaviours, concepts such as assimilation and acculturation have been used. These concepts are important to distinguish and understand because health literacy may not be uniformly distributed even within a specific ethnocultural, language, or immigrant group; subgroups and individuals experience different rates and degrees of assimilation and acculturation.

Assimilation is defined as a gradual and irreversible change in the values, behaviours, and attitudes of one culture group to that of the "host" culture group (Gordon, 1964). Implicit in the definition of assimilation is an assumption that the changes within the non-dominant culture involve becoming more like the host culture. *Acculturation* is more broadly defined as the process of interaction between cultures whereby aspects of two or more cultures create a hybrid experience containing elements of both the dominant and non-dominant groups (Redfield, 1936). Harmon and colleagues provide the following definition: "Acculturation is a process of cultural adaptation that occurs when groups of individuals from different cultures come into contact, leading to changes in the cultural patterns of either or both groups" (Harmon, Castro, & Coe, 1996, p. 39). Canadian psychologist John Berry (1997) from Queen's University outlined four acculturative strategies (see Table 5.2) that an individual may use depending on their goals for (1) maintaining their culture of origin traditions, and (2) adopting the "host" culture traditions.

TABLE 5.2: FOUR ACCULTURATIVE STRATEGIES

	High culture-of-origin maintenance	Low culture-of-origin maintenance
High participation in host culture	Integration: Cultural patterns from both host and culture of origin are integrated	Assimilation: Host cultural patterns are adopted in place of culture-of-origin patterns
Low participation in host culture	Separation: Culture-of-origin patterns are maintained and host cultural patterns are not adopted	Marginalization: Believed to occur as a result of forced assimilation and segregation; thus, neither cultural group patterns are explicitly adopted or maintained

Source: Modified from Berry, J.W. (1997). Immigration, adaptation, and acculturation. *Applied Psychology: An International Review, 46*(1), 5–34.

Several scales measure an individual's level of acculturation. Three widely used scales are the Suinn-Lew Asian Self-Identity Acculturation Scale (Suinn, Ahuna, & Khoo, 1992), the Bidimensional Acculturation Scale (BAS) for Hispanics (Marin & Gamba, 1996), and the Acculturation Rating Scale for Mexican Americans II (Cuellar, Arnold, & Maldonado, 1995). These scales pose a series of questions to determine the "cultural orientation" of the individual. Essentially, these scales are checklists of items that represent "cultural markers" and indicate one's primary cultural affiliation through elements such as language use, media preferences, and social interaction. Acculturation rating scales have many limitations (Hunt, Schneider, & Comer, 2004; Salant & Lauderdale, 2003; Thomson & Hoffman-Goetz, 2009), which include:

- overreliance on language as a key marker of exposure to cultural norms and information;
- lack of a guiding theoretical orientation; and
- assumptions about the homogeneity of both the original cultural background and the adopted culture.

Although the majority of acculturation research has been conducted in the United States, both the Suinn-Lew Asian Self-Identity Acculturation Scale and the Bidimensional Acculturation Scale for Hispanics have been applied in slightly modified versions to broadly assess the acculturation of Canadian immigrants (Todd & Hoffman-Goetz, 2011; Thomson & Hoffman-Goetz, 2011). Importantly, acculturation scales do not assess the changes that can occur in the "host" culture. For example, British Columbia and Ontario have established Colleges of Traditional Chinese Medicine and Acupuncture (CTCMPAO; CTCMA), which act as professional licensing bodies in those provinces (to learn about Health Canada's creation of an advisory council on traditional Chinese medicine, go to www.hc-sc.gc.ca/ahc-asc/media/nr-cp/_2012/2012-03bk-eng.php). The establishment of these professional bodies is indicative of the dynamic and changing ideas about health and illness within the Canadian health care landscape. The incorporation of alternative medical models will influence how health is conceptualized, how illness is identified, and how decisions are made about which health care services to seek. The lack of inclusion of these alternate care modalities in health literacy research and practice can lead to a failure to recognize the full spectrum of ways in which people interpret and act on health information.

The concepts of acculturation and assimilation can be found historically in Canadian governmental policies regarding First Nations peoples. The consequences of these policies are still relevant to the discussions of health literacy among Canada's First Nations. Beginning in 1857 with "An Act for the Gradual Civilization of the Indian Tribes in the Canadas," the Canadian government implemented several assimilationist policies aimed at making Canada's First Peoples "Canadian" by attempting to change their language, religion, values, and behaviours. These policies mandated child attendance at church-administered residential boarding schools (see "The Indian Residential Schools Truth and Reconciliation Commission" on the role of the Canadian government in the history of the Indian Residential Schools, available at www.parl. gc.ca/Content/LOP/researchpublications/prb0848-e.htm), restrictions on land ownership, and regulations that defined cultural identity and group membership, particularly for women and children (e.g., a woman and her children would lose matrilineal kinship claims if she married outside of her community). Understanding the lasting effects of these policies, which caused the dispossession of land, damage to community and family values, and loss of relationships, languages, and shared cultural histories, is critical when considering the current context of access and use of health information and services among the Aboriginal peoples of Canada.

As an example, consider health care professionals, such as nurses, who are working in First Nations communities. Nurses who are aware of the history and events contributing to some of the current health issues experienced by First Nations communities will be better equipped to understand behaviours such as "non-compliance" with Western biomedical interventions and better positioned to build healthy relationships built on mutual respect and trust (Browne & Fiske, 2001; Foster, 2006). "Non-compliance" would not likely be an issue in authentic and mutually respectful people-centred care.

CULTURAL AWARENESS, CULTURAL COMPETENCE, AND CULTURAL SAFETY: MORE THAN A MATTER OF WORDS

In this section we consider three terms: *cultural awareness, cultural competence,* and *cultural safety.* Although they have been used interchangeably, there are subtle differences in their meaning and in the underlying assumptions. Why is it important to reflect on how these concepts differ? The type of intervention and its effectiveness in addressing low health literacy among communication-vulnerable Canadians will depend on whether its focus is that of cultural awareness, cultural competence, or cultural safety. The American Medical Association identifies individuals at risk of experiencing communication gaps about health as being communication-vulnerable. People who are communication-vulnerable have little or no English proficiency, are part of a culture that may not be understood by health care personnel or the larger health care system, and have limited health literacy (American Medical Association, 2006). A 2011 Alberta Health Services Report identified health-vulnerable populations as including Aboriginal people, people living in poverty, immigrants, refugees, people who are homeless, and people with low literacy skills; in other words, health-vulnerable people were also communication-vulnerable people. As we will describe later in this chapter, most approaches to improving the health literacy skill of communication-vulnerable Canadians have emphasized cultural awareness and cultural competence. There has been much less emphasis on cultural safety.

Cultural awareness is the first step in a process to enhance health literacy and reduce inequities in the health of Canadians. Cultural awareness involves observing how people carry out their daily lives, developing sensitivity toward another ethnocultural group, and not assigning values (i.e., better/worse; right/wrong; good/bad) to cultural differences (Lister, 1999). An example of cultural awareness applied to health literacy would be an information pamphlet that describes the prevalence of obesity in Nunavut but also presents the cultural, economic, and geographical factors that contribute to obesity rates: for example, Inuit communities have very limited access to low-cost, low-fat foods and greater access to low-cost, high-fat foods. However, being culturally aware means paying attention not only to the obvious aspects of another culture (e.g., food preferences) but also to deeper aspects of culture (e.g., facial expression upon seeing a specific food). Figure 5.1 illustrates the many layers of cultural awareness, some of which are obvious and directly visible and others, subtle or hidden.

FIGURE 5.1: EXAMPLES OF LAYERS OF CULTURAL AWARENESS

Primarily in awareness

- dress   - dancing   - music   - games   - art

- literature   - cooking   - drama

- concept of beauty   - concept of justice   - work tempo

- arrangement of space   - eye contact   - theory of disease

- notions of leadership   - conversational patterns   - cosmology

- nature of friendship   - concept of self   - ordering of time

Primarily not in awareness

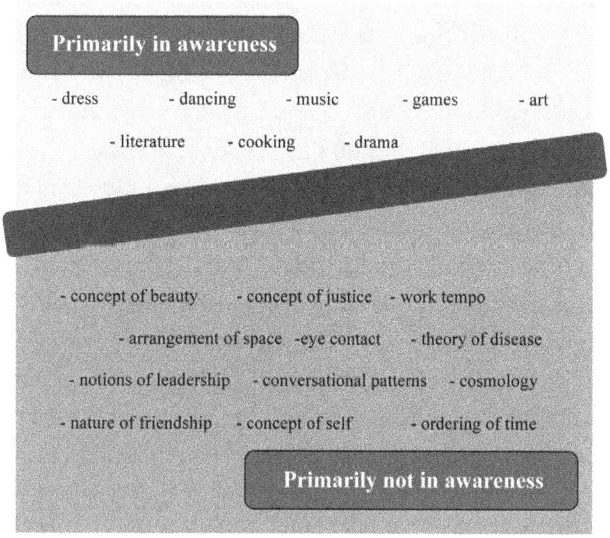

Source: Modified from Nova Scotia Department of Health and Wellness, Primary Health Care. (2011, p. 4). *An introduction to cultural competence in health care—Session I: Culture in health & care participant materials.* Retrieved from http://www.gov.ns.ca/health/primaryhealthcare/documents/bbtt/Culture-Cometence-Participant-Materials-Session-1.pdf. [accessed: 13 June 2013].

Cultural competence is a term that is commonly used in Canadian health care. Researchers, policy-makers, government workers at every level, organizations from hospitals to health charities, individuals engaged in health promotion to practitioners addressing end-of-life care all strive to be culturally competent. But what is cultural competence? The U.S. Office of Minority Health defines cultural competence as "a set of congruent behaviors, attitudes, and policies that come together in a system, agency, or among professionals that enables effective work in cross-cultural situations" (U.S. Department of Health and Human Services, Office of Minority Health, 2005). The Association of Faculties of Medicine of Canada (n.d.) defines cultural competence as "the attitudes, knowledge, and skills of practitioners necessary to become effective health care providers for patients from diverse backgrounds. Competence requires a blend of knowledge and conviction, plus a capacity for action." The Government of Nova Scotia provides the following definition: "Cultural competence refers to the attitudes, knowledge, skills, behaviours, and policies required to better meet the needs of all the people we serve" (Nova Scotia Department of Health and Wellness, 2011, p. 7). Betancourt, Green, Carrillo, and Ananeh-Firempong (2003) concluded that cultural competence in health and health care involves "understanding the importance of social and cultural influences on patients' health beliefs and behaviors, considering how these factors interact at multiple levels of the health care delivery system, and devising interventions that take these issues into account to assure quality health care delivery to diverse patient populations" (p. 297). What these slightly different definitions share is the perspective that cultural competence involves the effective integration and transformation of knowledge found in different cultural settings to improve health care delivery. Cultural competence focuses on the skills of the health care practitioner rather than the consumer or patient. An example of cultural competence applied to health literacy is ensuring that nursing staff receives training about informed consent for diverse cultural communities. For non-native speakers of English or French, the information would be given in a clear fashion, be understood by the patient, and recognize and respect differing cultural perspectives about health, illness, and treatment.

One problem with cultural competence is that it can become a set of stereotyped "do's" and "don'ts" for health care and health literacy delivery. Consumers or patients become defined by a fixed set of ethnic or cultural attributes or traits (Betancourt, 2004). In contrast, *cultural safety*, and similarly cultural humility, shifts the narrative to what matters to the individual. As Kleinman and Benson (2006b) point out, cultural safety is intensive and imaginative empathy for the experience of the person. Cultural safety is not about health care practitioners "knowing" the customs of any given ethno-specific culture and transferring that to clinical situations. Rather, cultural safety involves mutual recognition and shared respect for individual differences and an understanding of differences in power relationships between the health service provider and the individual (Papps & Ramsden, 1996). Cultural safety "assumes that each health care relationship between a professional and a consumer is unique, power-laden and culturally dyadic.... This bicultural component not only involves unequal power and different statuses but it also often involves two cultures with differing colonial histories, ethnicities or levels of material advantage" (Papps & Ramsden, 1996, p. 494). Cultural safety involves creating safety in health care and health services as defined by the people who receive the health service. It recognizes that health care providers, including those involved in health literacy, have their own explanatory models and beliefs that influence person-to-person interactions. Cultural safety is "the outcome of culturally competent care" (National Aboriginal Health Organization, 2008, p. 8).

How do these concepts of cultural awareness, cultural competence, and cultural safety build on each other? Lister (1999) developed a hierarchal framework for planning from cultural awareness, to cultural knowledge, to cultural understanding, to cultural competence. Lister's model encourages thinking about complex health inequities and how people negotiate their identities in light of their particular circumstances and the role expectations of others both within and outside of the health care system. Another way of thinking about the relationship between cultural awareness, competence, and safety as applied to health literacy is to consider the level of cultural reflection that each of these concepts entails. Table 5.3 shows how each level of cultural reflection can be applied to health literacy practice.

TABLE 5.3: CULTURAL REFLECTION CONCEPTS APPLIED TO HEALTH LITERACY

Cultural reflection	Application to health literacy	Example of what this may mean in practice
Cultural awareness	Health information provider realizes importance of culture in information exchange	Creation of language-appropriate written materials
Cultural competence	Health information provider realizes importance of culturally supportive environment	Involvement of linguistically and culturally congruent navigators/interpreters in health information exchange
Cultural safety	Health information provider actively creates environment where individual feels culturally safe and without risk	Provision of safe physical, emotional, and spiritual space where health and cultural conversations are not compromised; traditions are valued and encouraged

It is important to briefly mention tools for assessment. There are no specific evaluation instruments for cultural awareness, competence, or safety for health literacy. As an alternative, the "cultural sensitivity" (also called "cultural appropriateness") of printed health information for health literacy research has been measured using specific tools, instruments, and checklists. Cultural sensitivity refers to the attempt to craft communication using characteristics that are familiar to or preferred among members of the target population (Resnicow, Baranowski, Ahluwalia, & Braithwaite, 1999). Two measurement instruments are the Suitability Assessment of Materials (SAM) (Doak, Doak, & Root, 1996) and the Cultural Sensitivity Assessment Tool (CSAT) (Friedman & Hoffman-Goetz, 2006). The SAM focuses on readability, cultural appropriateness, and self-efficacy of the reader. The CSAT provides a quick checklist of items to consider when determining the cultural sensitivity of health information materials; it has been used with English-language Canadian ethnic newspaper articles on cancer and with online decision aids for cancer treatment.

> **REVIEW AND REFLECT**
>
> Describe one way in which cultural competence and cultural safety differ.

MULTICULTURALISM AND THE CANADIAN CULTURAL MOSAIC

Canada is often referred to as a *multicultural* society and as a *cultural mosaic*. What do these terms mean? How do they differ? How can they be applied to health literacy? Although it is beyond the scope of this chapter to review the broad range of social, political, legal, and economic meanings of "multicultural society," "multiculturalism," and "cultural mosaic," a general overview is provided to better understand the opportunities and challenges for health literacy initiatives in Canada.

Multiculturalism has many meanings. Dewing (2009) described four interpretations of Canada as a multicultural society: sociological, ideological, public policy, and process. The perspective of the authors of this text is based largely on Dewing's insights and framework, and informed by the work of Kunz and Sykes (2007). The sociological perspective defines multiculturalism as the presence and persistence of diverse racial and ethnic (as well as religious) minorities who self-define as a group and who wish to remain so. The basic cultural drivers of "demographic" multiculturalism are the First Nations peoples, the English and French "Charter" groups, and immigrants from around the world, who account for the increasingly diverse ethnic, cultural, religious, and language mix of Canada (Kunz & Sykes, 2007). For example, in 2010, of the 280,681 new permanent residents, more than one-third came from Asia, including the Philippines (36,578), India (30,252), and the People's Republic of China (30,197). Fewer individuals emigrated from countries representing the original Charter countries of the United Kingdom (9,499) and France (6,934), according to 2010 statistics (Citizenship and Immigration Canada, 2010).

A second perspective on the concept of multiculturalism is as an ideology (again, drawing on the seminal works of Dewing and of Kunz and Sykes). Multiculturalism is viewed as a set of goals, beliefs, and ideals celebrating Canada's diversity and informing the political, economic, and social systems of Canada. Prime Minister Harper's comments reflect this perspective: "Because what defines Canada ... is a land of opportunity where everyone—regardless of their ethnicity or religion—works and lives and succeeds together. A place in which where you are going matters more than where you came from ... preserving and strengthening the cultural diversity that makes us strong" (Prime Minister of Canada Stephen Harper, 2006).

Another orientation of multiculturalism is that of public policy. Here, multiculturalism refers to a set of formal initiatives structured to manage diversity in federal, provincial, and municipal society. This perspective is illustrated by bills, laws, and policy statements from all levels of government. For example, two hallmark documents identify multiculturalism as a framework for governance—the Canadian Charter of Rights and Freedoms (Government of Canada, 1982) and the Canadian Multiculturalism Act (Government of Canada, 1985).

As a process-level concept, multiculturalism reflects the actions of diverse groups to achieve certain goals and aspirations identified by those groups. Regardless of the level of analysis of multiculturalism, the focus has changed substantially over time: from celebrating differences in the 1970s ("culture"), to managing diversity in the 1980s ("structure"), to constructive engagement in the 1990s ("society building"), and, most recently, to integrative and inclusive citizenship ("Canadian identity") in the 2000s (Kunz & Sykes, 2007).

Canadian population diversity is also captured by the term *cultural mosaic,* which was adopted following the publication of the 1965 book by sociologist John Porter, *Vertical Mosaic: An Analysis of Social Class and Power in Canada.* The vertical mosaic showed that some groups in society had access to power and influenced decision making, reflecting ethnic, language, regional, and religious advantages, whereas other groups were disadvantaged, disempowered, and disenfranchised. (The concept of empowerment is defined and discussed in Chapter 4.) Another important contribution to the idea of a cultural mosaic comes from John Murray Gibbon's classic book entitled *Canadian Mosaic: The Making of a Northern Nation,* which was published in 1938. According to Gibbon, the Canadian mosaic reflected a society where each cultural group retained its distinctive identity while contributing to the nation as a whole. This perspective differs from the "melting pot" society of the United States, where assimilation is the goal.

REVIEW AND REFLECT
Explain the four interpretations of the term *multiculturalism.*

Is there a difference between "multiculturalism" and "cultural mosaic"? Although the terms have been used interchangeably, there are subtle distinctions that can influence health literacy initiatives (described in the next section). Multiculturalism identifies diversity within the demographics of a particular societal space and time. The concept of a multicultural society is built on policies aimed at maintaining discrete identities. A cultural mosaic has a different emphasis. According to the Oxford English Dictionary (2012), a mosaic is "a picture or pattern produced by arranging together small colored pieces of hard material, such as stone, tile, or glass." Mosaics allow us to see an overall picture while viewing each individual and unique piece. Chao and Moon (2005) developed a taxonomy that is useful in illustrating a cultural mosaic approach. The taxonomy consists of three primary factors (see Table 5.4). The first two factors (demographic and geographic) have some overlap with multiculturalism, whereas the third factor (associative) has less. Cultural mosaics change over time and place and with respect to social contexts and relationships to other groups in the mosaic. Moreover, the individual components of a cultural mosaic fit together in unique ways. Nevertheless, multiculturalism may be more defined in scope and allow for easier segmentation of the population to address health literacy gaps.

TABLE 5.4: CULTURAL MOSAIC PERSPECTIVE

Primary factor	Definition	Component	Specific example
Demographic	Physical characteristics and social identities from parents	Age, ethnicity, gender, language	Canadians over 65 years
Geographic	Physical features of an area that shape group identities	Climate, temperature, urban/rural	Canadians living in Nunavut
Associative	Groups that people associate or identify with	Family, religion, politics, activities	Canadians who play hockey

Source: Adapted from Chao, G.T., & Moon, H. (2005). The cultural mosaic: A metatheory for understanding the complexity of culture. Table 1. *Journal of Applied Psychology, 90*(6), 1130.

Canada has a rich representation of people from more than 200 different ethnic origins. The 2006 Census reported that 41.1 percent of Canadians had multiple ethnic ancestries, 16.2 percent self-identified as belonging to a visible minority, and 75 percent of recent immigrants were visible minorities (Statistics Canada, 2008). Of importance is that, even within any defined group, there is tremendous diversity. For example, people may identify themselves as "South Asian visible minority." Or, they may identify as a specific ethnic group within the South Asian visible minority, such as East India, Pakistan, Sri Lanka, the Punjab, or Bangladesh. And, within ethnic identities, diversity occurs. For example, of Canadians who identify themselves as South Asian visible minority and Pakistani, this could also mean Punjabi, Pashtun, Sindhi, Sariaki, Muhajirs, Balochi, or another group—with different first languages, political–historical experiences, values, and belief systems (Central Intelligence Agency, 2012). As described earlier, ethnicity and culture are fluid concepts. People's knowledge, understandings, attitudes, and values about their ethnicity and culture (and that of others) and the current, and historical, social context of Canada adds both complexity and diversity. This complexity and diversity pose challenges for the design of health literacy programs that include a multicultural or cultural mosaic approach.

Canadians are also quite linguistically diverse, as evidenced by the number of first or primary languages spoken. Traditionally, language has been described as a system of codes and signals (verbal, gesture, written) with specific rules that connect the signals and symbols to each other. Language is fundamental to the cultural framework whereby people make meaning and interpret the world (Kramsch, 1998). The relationship between language and culture can be illustrated by using food as a cultural medium. Indeed, conversations about food have been seen as a cultural vehicle to enhance the health literacy skill of immigrants to Canada for whom English is not their first language (Thomson & Hoffman-Goetz, 2011). Jiang (2000) asked 28 native Chinese speakers (NCS) and 28 native English speakers (NES) to describe what they thought about (associations) when they read a word. The NES described the process of cooking in response to the word *food*. The NCS did not associate the word *shiwu* (food) with cooking. *Pengren* (translated as *cuisine* in English) was better associated with the process of cooking and suggested a more delicate, subtle, and nuanced meaning. The NCS also associated the word *food* with more specific food items (e.g., steamed bread) compared to the NES (e.g., dessert).

Language contributes to multiculturalism and the cultural mosaic in Canada. With more than one-quarter of a million new immigrants to Canada every year, the linguistic landscape is indeed very diverse. In 2012, for example, between 240,000 and 265,000 immigrants were admitted to Canada (Citizenship and Immigration Canada, 2012). Figure 5.2 shows the change over time in the number of Canadians whose mother tongue (first language) was other than English, French, or an Aboriginal language. The 2006 Census indicated that more than seven out of ten immigrants had a first language other than English or French. While the vast majority of immigrants are able to communicate in one of the official languages, about 6 percent could not speak English or French well enough to conduct a conversation (Lachapelle & Lepage, n.d.). In the context of health literacy, these findings indicate that clear, language-appropriate information is needed for everyone but that the approaches may differ even within a "language group." Cultural meanings and nuances may not be the same for people without any English or French language skill compared with those who have some English or French language proficiency. Language and culture interact dynamically, with words taking on new meaning as one's lived experiences in Canada shift over time and place.

FIGURE 5.2: CANADIAN POPULATION WITH "OTHER" MOTHER TONGUE, 1971–2006

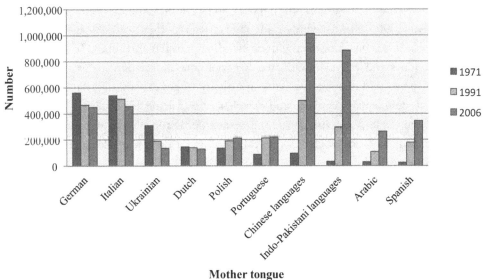

Mother tongue

Source: Modified from Canadian Heritage. (n.d.). *Evolution of population of some "other" mother tongues, Canada, 1971 to 2006.* Chart 1.2. Retrieved from http://www.pch.gc.ca/eng/1359983458549/1359983649745 [accessed: 13 June 2013].

To summarize, Canada is a multicultural society *and* a cultural mosaic. These two terms have subtle but important distinctions. Multiculturalism reflects a sociological (demographic) perspective, and includes the legal framework and policies necessary to ensure protection of the rights and freedoms of diverse ethnic, cultural, language, and religious groups. Multiculturalism emphasizes a rights-based approach to diversity and is linked to the Canadian Charter of Rights and Freedoms. A cultural mosaic is a more fluid concept and captures the idea that the whole (Canada) and the parts (the individual ethnic, cultural, religious, language, and other self-defining groups within Canada) have weight and visibility. How the individual mosaic pieces fit together can change over time and in relation to each other. The cultural mosaic perspective emphasizes a values-based approach to diversity.

CULTURE AND HEALTH LITERACY OF CANADIANS

Most research, practice, and policy initiatives on culture and health literacy of Canadians have adopted a multicultural perspective. This orientation allows researchers, practitioners, and policy-makers to identify issues and barriers that specific ethnocultural and language groups face in an effort to become health literate. To be health literate in Canada, one needs to be able to effectively apply a variety of skills to accomplish health-related tasks that are (or can be) challenging. These skills include reading and writing in English or French, speaking and listening in English or French, numerical computing, critical thinking, and decision making (Singleton & Krause, 2009). Culture affects how people acquire and use these skills and the degree of comfort they have in integrating and aligning their own values and beliefs to those of the larger dominant health and health care system.

The relationship between culture and health literacy in Canada has been explored primarily with two population subgroups: immigrants and people of Aboriginal heritage. Zanchetta and Poureslami (2006) make the important observation that these relationships are complex, have multiple dimensions, and require understanding of different realities. To illustrate this complexity, Jones and colleagues adapted hypertension information materials written in English for Indo-Asian populations living in Calgary (Jones et al., 2011). Among the findings was that, despite using certified and experienced translators for materials from English into one of four Indo-Asian languages, "numerous words and phrases were inappropriate, not understandable or did not convey the real meaning for the less acculturated community members" (p. 6).

Language is often used as a proxy or substitute for culture in clinical and community settings since it is easier to define and measure. Identifying language barriers for health literacy is an important first step. Consider the following example. In Cambridge Bay, a village of 1,500 people about 60 kilometres north of the Arctic Circle, the Nunavut Literacy Council produces *Read to Me* kits for new parents, available in English or French and in Inuktitut/Inuinnaqtun, and distributed through community health centres (Crockatt & Symthe, n.d.). This is an important step but potential health literacy challenges remain. Some Inuinnaqtun speakers may not be able to read translated syllabics (as Inuinnaqtun was originally an oral language). Nonetheless, there are a number of practices that help to address language barriers among communication-vulnerable individuals and groups (see Table 5.5). Several of these practices are relevant to health literate individuals for whom language barriers are not an issue. Can you identify which ones would apply to all Canadians?

TABLE 5.5: LANGUAGE PRACTICES TO ENHANCE HEALTH LITERACY

Clear, plain, accessible writing for printed materials
Printed health information at grade 6 or lower
Use of oral communication strategies (storytelling, role-playing, singing)
Use of visual communication strategies (cartoons, images, illustrations, photography, dance)
Principles of good design for word and sentence placement (white space, font, colour)
Community members as language and social network facilitators
Multiple translation/back-translation of printed materials into language of interest
Use of formal and informal aspects of language

Note: The information on principles of good writing to enhance health literacy can be explored in further detail in Wizowski, L., Harper, T., & Hutchings, T. (2008). *Writing health information for patients and families* (3rd ed.) Hamilton, ON: Hamilton Health Sciences.

Language effects may also differ from culture effects on health literacy skill. The findings of three studies—two from Canada and one from the United Kingdom—illustrate this point. Language and culture were explored as predictors of health literacy with 106 Chinese immigrants living in the Greater Toronto Area. Participants (older women) were randomized to receive colon cancer information in their first language (Mandarin or Cantonese) or their second language (English). More than 60 percent of the women had low scores on the Short Test of Functional Health Literacy in Adults (S-TOFHLA), which was used to measure their general health literacy. Of importance was that their specific health literacy skill was affected by language: the immigrant women who received the cancer information in English had lower health literacy (understanding of the information) compared to those who received it in Chinese. However, for both language groups, the specific health literacy of the women was not adequate. Thus, overcoming language barriers improved, but did not eliminate, low health literacy among immigrants to Canada, suggesting that unaccounted cultural factors were involved (Todd & Hoffman-Goetz, 2011).

In a sample of Pakistani immigrants to the United Kingdom, the use of pictorial flash cards (which removed language barriers) improved diabetes knowledge and glycemic control among women with higher literacy; however, the knowledge and understanding about diabetes was still low for immigrant women with low literacy, even after removing language/prose literacy barriers with the flash cards (Hawthorne, 2001).

Language, culture, and health literacy were explored among asthma patients from new immigrant groups in Vancouver (Poureslami, Rootman, Doyle-Waters, Nimmon, & Fitzgerald, 2011). Immigrants spoke to whether the health care system was culturally competent: "I think that culturally I am lost here" (p. 317); they also spoke separately about language barriers: "The information I try to access here is very difficult to understand because they were written in English. I normally ask my daughter to translate the information for me" (p. 318). The authors concluded that health literacy includes (presumably separate) components of different factors related to people's identity and cultural beliefs and practices.

What these studies suggest is that even if health materials are translated into their first language, and presented in easy-to-read words and in pictures and cartoons, immigrants from diverse cultures may still not understand the materials if "Western" constructs of health, illness, and health care are assumed or if their encounters with the health care system do not resonate culturally. Simich (2009) eloquently sums up this critical perspective:

> A narrow understanding of health literacy as functional verbal skills unfortu-
> nately still prevails among service providers. When this approach is applied
> to immigrants in Canada who are not proficient in official languages, the
> social and cultural context of communication practices are neglected and the
> meanings of important messages are lost. Consideration of cultural diversity
> must extend beyond language to a broader appreciation of cultural values,
> help-seeking beliefs and community engagement. (p. 8)

Although researchers, practitioners, and policy-makers agree that language and culture are fundamental determinants of health and health literacy, we simply do not know their separate influences. By considering each as a unique input, as well as recognizing that they intersect in theory and practice, we may be better able to address ongoing gaps and challenges for immigrants with low health literacy.

REVIEW AND REFLECT

Reflect on why language diversity is used as a proxy for cultural diversity in health literacy research.

MAKING MEANING: A CLINICAL VIGNETTE ILLUSTRATING THE INTERFACE BETWEEN CULTURE, LANGUAGE, AND HEALTH LITERACY

Physician–patient communication can be difficult. If the physician and patient are from cultures that emphasize different ways of understanding health and illness, the potential for misunderstanding and miscommunication increases (Kleinman, 1980). In Canada, the bio-medical model taught in medical schools is associated with a suite of culture-based values, such as ethical principles (e.g., the importance of individual autonomy), rules (e.g., when to use the emergency room versus the family doctor), and expectations of behaviour (e.g., role of the patient versus physician). When patients and physicians do not share similar cultural models, misunderstanding and miscommunication can pose grave risks to health outcomes. Fadiman (1997) chronicles such misunderstandings regarding the care of a young Hmong child with epilepsy in the United States. In her account, health care providers and hospital staff repeatedly failed to contextualize the actions of the child's parents in terms of the choices available to them given their personal situation (the social, political, and economic realities of daily life) and Hmong values, medical beliefs, literacy, and English language skill. These misunderstandings contributed to the parents being labelled as non-compliant, further complicating the medical care of the child and placing additional burden on an already struggling family. When communication between health care providers and patients includes a discussion about the assumptions and beliefs about the medical problem and a negotiation about what should be done, positive and mutually acceptable health outcomes are more likely to be achieved (Dutta, 2007). A guide to writing clear and easy-to-understand health information materials for patients and their families has been developed by Wizowski, Harper, and Hutchings (2008) from McMaster University; the "how to" section on translating materials into multiple languages with attention to cultural relevance is particularly useful for students involved in health literacy.

The vignettes described in Box 5.1 illustrate three approaches to a clinical encounter where health literacy is critical. Each successive encounter represents a greater attempt to recognize the role of culture, language, and literacy in the interaction.

BOX 5.1: IMPORTANCE OF HEALTH LITERACY IN CLINICAL ENCOUNTERS

THE SETTING

Maly, a 25-year-old Cambodian woman who recently immigrated to Canada, is expecting her second child. This will be her first child born in Canada. While Maly speaks fluent Khmer and conversational English, she cannot read in either language, and her prose literacy is low. Her female family physician, Dr. Jane Cooper, has been seeing Maly for about two months. Maly is the only Cambodian patient on Dr. Cooper's roster.

VIGNETTE 1

During her recent visit to her family physician, Maly was given prenatal vitamins and a leaflet in English listing foods to avoid while pregnant. Throughout the visit, Dr. Cooper did most of the talking and she interpreted Maly's lack of questions as a sign that Maly understood all of her instructions. After the visit, Maly was uncertain whether the vitamins were medication and she decided against using them. She tucked the leaflet into her purse to throw away at home. She was surprised that there had been very little conversation about proper foods, especially near the end of the pregnancy, as diet had been important during her previous pregnancy in Cambodia.

This vignette illustrates a

- lack of cultural awareness by the health care provider,
- significant miscommunication in the clinical encounter, and
- low health literacy for the patient, who could not read in English.

VIGNETTE 2

Realizing that English was not Maly's first language, Dr. Cooper contacted a local multicultural centre to obtain prenatal nutrition information in Khmer.

Dr. Cooper felt confident that Maly would have no difficulty understanding the translated text, since she had observed Maly speaking Khmer with her first child. At the visit, Dr. Cooper gave Maly some prenatal vitamins, advising her to take one every day. At the end of the visit, Dr. Cooper stood up, gave Maly the Khmer-language information leaflet, and asked if she had any questions. Sensing that Dr. Cooper was in a hurry, Maly decided not to ask about the vitamins or whether there were any diet recommendations. As Maly could not read Khmer, she tucked the leaflet into her purse to discard later and left somewhat frustrated. She wasn't sure if she would take the vitamins but felt that she at least knew about dietary expectations from her prior pregnancy in Cambodia.

This vignette illustrates

- some cultural competence by the health care provider,
- continuing miscommunication in the clinical encounter, and
- low health literacy for the patient, who could not read in English or Khmer.

VIGNETTE 3

Aware that Maly had recently emigrated to Canada and that English was not her first language, Dr. Cooper booked extra time for her visit. Upon giving Maly prenatal vitamins, she explained what they were, how to take them, and why they were important. When Dr. Cooper asked Maly about her prenatal nutrition knowledge, she was surprised to learn about the importance of hot and cold food and, specifically, about consuming coconut juice in late pregnancy. Together, Maly and Dr. Cooper came to an understanding of the types of foods to avoid and the foods that would be good to eat.

Dr. Cooper: Tell me about the foods you feel are important to eat for the baby.

Maly: Well, coconut juice is important at the end of pregnancy, so I will make sure I eat that. I will also eat vegetables and beans to get enough fibre, like we talked about.

At the end of the visit, both women felt confident that they had been understood and that Maly had a healthy and mutually acceptable plan for her dietary needs throughout her pregnancy.

This vignette illustrates

- collaborative discussion during the clinical encounter,
- cultural competence on the part on the clinician,
- cultural safety for the patient, and
- better health literacy for the patient.

KEY LEARNING POINTS

In this chapter, the concepts of culture and ethnicity were introduced. Despite many discipline-based approaches, there is no single and accepted definition for either concept. Crafting definitions has been contentious, since culture and ethnicity have been used to support differences in power relationships. According to the 2006 Census, Canada is extremely heterogeneous culturally, with about 20 percent of the population born outside of the country. Language diversity is also characteristic, with more than 80 languages spoken. Canada is both a multicultural country and a cultural mosaic; the former term relates to demographic and policy perspectives and the latter focuses on ideological perspectives and process. Approaches to health literacy have included cultural awareness, cultural competence, and cultural safety. Cultural awareness and competence are oriented to the health care provider or health organization. Cultural safety is vested in the individual who is seeking health information, care, and support. While often used as a proxy for culture, language appears to have separate (but related) effects on health literacy. Most would agree that culture- and language-based approaches are needed to address inequities in health literacy for communication-vulnerable groups in Canada. Health literacy has been operationalized as a set of skills, primarily addressing language barriers. The ways in which language diversity has been addressed in health literacy include translation, use of simple and plain words, and inclusion of pictures and images. Cultural values and realities have been more difficult to address within the context of health literacy. As Smylie, Williams, and Cooper (2007) ask, "What exactly are culture-based approaches to literacy and health; and how can they be effectively and practically applied?" (p. S24). The challenges are significant and will require thinking about health literacy at the intersection of different cultural realities and spheres of meaning.

A CANADIAN MILESTONE

In March 2009 the Indigenous Physicians Association of Canada and the Royal College of Physicians and Surgeons of Canada released a curriculum framework for continuing medical education. The rationale for the framework follows from the principles of social justice and the continuing health disparities that exist between the First Peoples of Canada and the general Canadian population. The report highlighted that the First Peoples of Canada are diverse in their languages, beliefs, histories, and health practices. And, while many immigrant groups to Canada also face health disparities arising from varied languages, cultural beliefs, and histories, the First Peoples of Canada are not a "cultural group." They are distinct, constitutionally recognized peoples with Aboriginal and treaty rights. The framework identified 29 core competencies for physicians to enable cultural safety. Many of these cultural competencies directly intersect with enhancing health literacy. For example, physicians should be able to have "effective and culturally safe communication [that] encourages reciprocity, equality, trust, respect, honesty and empathy" (competency 2.2). As well, physicians should be able to "deliver information to [the First Peoples of Canada] that is understandable, respectful and encourages participation in decision-making" (competency 2.3).

Source: Indigenous Physicians Association of Canada and the Royal College of Physicians and Surgeons of Canada. (2009). *First Nations, Inuit and Métis health core competencies.* Winnipeg & Ottawa. Retrieved from www.afmc.ca/pdf/CoreCompetenciesEng.pdf [accessed: 18 June 2013].

ADDITIONAL RESOURCES OF INTEREST

Nunavut Department of Culture and Heritage

http://www.cley.gov.nu.ca/en/home.aspx

This website provides information and resources to support the development and implementation of policies, programs, and services aimed at strengthening the culture, language, heritage, and physical activity of Nunavummiut. The mission of this department is, in part, to promote the use of Inuit language in the workplace and throughout the territory; promote access to information and resource materials in Nunavut's official languages in all communities; and to enhance public library services across Nunavut.

First Nation Literacy: Ningwakwe Learning Press

http://www.firstnationliteracy.com/about-us/mission-statement/

This is a resource for literacy and learning materials that emphasize holistic and culturally centred learning.

Northwest Territories (NWT) Literacy Council

http://www.nwt.literacy.ca

The NWT Literacy Council works with individuals and groups to promote and support literacy and essential skills in all the official languages of the NWT. The website provides literacy resources and research specific to citizens of the NWT.

CHAPTER 6

INFORMATION TECHNOLOGY
AND HEALTH LITERACY

The potential of the internet to assist and empower individuals by providing high quality information in multiple forms of media, and to provide access to personal social support in real and cybertime, when it is needed, is an extremely positive aspect of the internet. Similarly, the internet's capacity to collectively link people with common interests and concerns across time and space, as well as to provide timely access to a wide range of people, organizations and information gives it the potential to help the development and maintenance of collective action to promote healthy policies, programs and living conditions.

—HEALTH CANADA, *HEALTH PROMOTION AND NEW INFORMATION TECHNOLOGIES*, 1997

CHAPTER LEARNING OBJECTIVES
- Define eHealth and eHealth literacy
- Describe the online culture of health and health care
- Clarify the relationship between information literacy skill and health literacy skill
- Consider the roles of access, understanding, and trust in eHealth
- Consider the role of social media in health literacy for Canadians
- Describe concepts of "digital divide" and "literacy divide" in relation to health literacy skill

INTRODUCTION

Information technologies are found virtually everywhere in Canadian society. Many aspects of our lives are mediated by the use of some "high-tech" tool or another, whether it be banking, shopping, or our health. We interact with a technological device whenever we withdraw money from an automatic teller, pay with a credit or a debit card when we buy our groceries, register for courses at university from our home using an electronic connection, or even buy computers through vending machines at airports. We are surrounded by electronic devices in all facets of our lives.

As information technology becomes more commonplace, its application and use as a vehicle for health literacy becomes increasingly important. Health care in all its forms, but especially when it comes to prevention, communication, and education, is not exempt from diverse technology tools. Smart homes, smart cars, smartphones, smart information systems, and smart health care will become the new "normal" for society.

As students, researchers, and practitioners, it is important for us to consider the use of information technologies if effective use of health resources is to be achieved by the Canadian population and disparities in health are to be minimized. Information technologies, such as the Internet, are already seen as a major reservoir of virtual health care and health-relevant information on diseases, treatments, medications, nutrition, exercise, and services.

This chapter presents an overview of the relation between information technology and health literacy. Our aim is to outline the links between health literacy and information and communication technologies, and how technologies affect Canadians, mainstream or marginalized, in their interaction with health information and the health system. We describe the digital divide and the "online culture" of health communities.

INTERNET ACCESS AND LITERACY DEMANDS IN CANADA

There has been a marked increase in Internet access across social groups in North America. In the year 2010, almost 80 percent of adult Americans reported having online access, with over 60 percent having searched for health information using mobile cellular phones rather than the traditional computer (Zach, Dalrymple, Rogers, & Williver-Farr, 2011). The situation is similar in Canada, with 79 percent of Canadian households reporting Internet access in 2010 (see Table 6.1). The percentage of Canadians seeking online information is likely to increase in the coming years as more access opportunities become available (Statistics Canada, 2011a). Canadians have access to pamphlets, leaflets, and personal communication with health care providers, but they also have access to information on thousands of websites devoted to health and health care. For example, according to the 2010 Canadian Internet Use Survey, approximately 80 percent of Canadian adults ages 16 and older accessed the Internet for personal reasons, and 64 percent of these individuals used the Internet to search for health information (Statistics Canada, 2010b).

Our highly technological society places increasingly greater literacy demands on Canadians. We will be required not only to understand and use health information but also to communicate with the health care system through technological means, such as smartphones; to make effective use of applications or "apps" that monitor health states, such as blood glucose meters; or to take part in technology-aided personal health activities, such as walking with pedometers and using tools to monitor sleep patterns. And, as information technology becomes more affordable, these sources of information are also likely to increase. All Canadians need, at minimum, adequate levels of prose and numeric literacy for understanding health information (recall that this minimum level is Level 3 according to the IALS). They will also require knowledge about how to access reliable health information and the skills necessary to interact effectively with information technology tools.

TABLE 6.1: PERCENTAGE OF CANADIAN HOUSEHOLDS WITH INTERNET
ACCESS AT HOME, 2010

Province	Percentage (%) of households with Internet access
Alberta	83
British Columbia	84
Manitoba	73
New Brunswick	70
Newfoundland and Labrador	74
Nova Scotia	77
Ontario	81
Prince Edward Island	73
Quebec	73
Saskatchewan	76

Source: Modified from Statistics Canada. (2011, May 25). Canadian Internet use survey 2010. Table 1. *The Daily.* Retrieved from www.statcan.gc.ca/daily-quotidien/110525/t110525b1-eng.htm [accessed: 17 June 2013].

The number of Canadians relying on the Internet to search for health information, to make use of information technology tools for health purposes, or to access health care systems through online media, such as patient portals, is likely to increase in the coming years. The growing availability of digital access points into health care services and activities poses some problems, especially for vulnerable populations such as non-English- or non-French-speaking immigrants, people living in isolated rural communities, First Nations people, or the elderly. Since computer and media literacy depends in part on access (Howard, Busch, & Sheets, 2010), these groups are less likely to benefit from the deployment of innovative information technologies for health care. Without intervention, non-familiarity with these technologies may present an obstacle for individuals in these groups in becoming full participants of the health care system of the future.

The emergence of Health 2.0, with its reliance on advances in Internet technology supporting people's ability to interact with others online—especially in relation to peer-to-peer and social networking—is indicative of the need for all Canadians to become eHealth literate. Health 2.0 functions allow Internet users the ability to create and generate content, share ideas, and connect with others. Collaborative Web platforms such as blogs, wikis, video sharing, and other social networking sites are where users can access information from Internet sources but also share (health) information with others. Health 2.0 represents a major shift in the way that health information is created and disseminated, and in the manner in which health care is provided. However, meaningful use of Health 2.0 technologies requires informed consumers who are ready to use collaborative tools, such as online social networking and other Internet-based health resources, to engage with health professionals to manage their personal health issues (Eysenbach, 2008).

In a 2008 editorial in the *Journal of Medical Internet Research*, Gunther Eysenbach proposed a new model of health communication processes that accounts for Web 2.0 applications (e.g., online social networking). Despite differences in educational experience, knowledge, and skills related to issues of health and illness, Eysenbach recognizes all patients, health care providers, and researchers/scientists as experts in their own right, and "according to the Web 2.0 philosophy—their collective wisdom can and should be harnessed: the health professional is an expert in identifying disease, while the patient is an expert in experiencing it" (Eysenbach, 2008, p. 3). The Internet and especially online social networking sites such as Facebook and PatientsLikeMe have significantly transformed where, how, and from whom we access health information (Eysenbach, 2008). It is because of Web 2.0 interactive capabilities that individuals are no longer reliant only on their physician for health information but are able to access it from a broader global community of individuals, health care providers, and researchers. Eysenbach (2008) talks about this broader source of information access as a process of *apomediation*—people or applications that guide health information access. He describes apomediaries as

> users and friends ... [who] can help users navigate through the onslaught of information afforded by networked digital media, providing additional credibility cues and supplying further metainformation. Other examples of apomediaries and apomediation tools include consumer ratings on amazon.com or epinions.com; technologies like PICS or MedPICS ... collaborative filtering and recommender systems as exemplified by StumbleUpon.com; and other second generation Internet-based services and tools that let people collaborate on a massive scale and share information online in new ways, including social networking sites, social bookmarking, blogs, wikis, communication tools, and folksonomies. (p. 5)

We have already started to see examples of personal health information and data sharing among online health care consumers—a process that Eysenbach refers to as "crowdsourcing," or the collective wisdom of patients and/or professionals. The website PatientsLikeMe (www.patientslikeme.com/) exemplifies "crowdsourcing" whereby individuals can share their personal health experiences within an online site to help themselves, other individuals dealing with the same health concerns and illnesses, health care organizations caring for others with similar conditions, and researchers investigating health and illness. The developers of PatientsLikeMe have built an online "health data-sharing platform" that captures thousands of patients' health knowledge and experience, thereby transforming the way patients manage their own conditions. While the literacy demands needed to access much of the online health information is high (grade 12 or greater) (Friedman, Hoffman-Goetz, & Arocha, 2004), collaborative online resources such as PatientsLikeMe and many of the health- and disease-based groups on Facebook accommodate a range of health literacy skill (Donelle & Hoffman-Goetz, 2008).

This manner of accessing health information represents a core shift from the traditional Internet, or Web 1.0, which is based on static Web pages. Such a landscape may be conceptualized as the "Internet age" of health care, one that highlights the need for adequate health literacy skill that incorporates eHealth literacy competency. eHealth literacy skills are increasingly important in ensuring equitable access to health care information and services.

REVIEW AND REFLECT

In earlier chapters, provincial differences in literacy were described. Consider the statistics in Table 6.1. Does Internet access by province reflect differences in literacy from the Maritime provinces to British Columbia? Why or why not?

DEFINING EHEALTH LITERACY

Reducing health literacy disparities in Canada is an enormously difficult problem and one that we considered in Chapter 4. The reasons for doing so should be obvious: low levels of literacy are associated with poorer health outcomes (Berkman, Sheridan, Donahue, Halpern, & Crotty, 2011; Canadian Council on Learning, 2008a). Attending to such disparities should become a major focus of health policy and practice, and information technology can play an important role in solving this problem. Yet, the implementation and effective utilization of information technology for the task of increasing the health literacy levels of the population and bridging the literacy gaps between groups introduce difficulties of their own.

Although the concept of eHealth has been defined in various ways (Oh et al., 2005), the basic idea includes the concepts of "health" and "technology." One of the Canadian leaders in eHealth is Gunther Eysenbach (2001), who defined eHealth as

> an emerging field in the intersection of medical informatics, public health and business, referring to health services and information delivered or enhanced through the Internet and related technologies. In a broader sense, the term characterizes not only a technical development, but also a state-of-mind, a way of thinking, an attitude, and a commitment for networked, global thinking, to improve health care locally, regionally, and worldwide by using information and communication technology.

eHealth represents a major change in health care and offers the promise of a unification of the now separate areas of health and health care. Through eHealth, preventive health practices—nutrition and exercise, patient education resources provided by health libraries, patient-to-patient and doctor–patient communication, on-demand access to personal health data—are likely to change as information technologies are adopted by the general population and health professionals.

A chief component of such unification involves the role that information technology plays in the provision of health care, in the way health information is communicated, in how patients and the general public are educated in matters of health, and in enhancing health and preventing disease, all while more effectively reaching the larger population (Alvarez, 2002; Atkinson & Gold, 2002). eHealth should also be characterized by increasing efficiency, enhancing the quality of health care, educating and empowering patients and consumers, encouraging a new relationship between users and providers by enabling new forms of information exchange between the parties involved, and extending the scope of communication to facilitate interactions with global online health services (Eysenbach, 2001). However, these promises bring new challenges posed by the implementation of sophisticated information technologies. This implementation potentially affects equitable access, increasing the digital divide between rural and urban communities (Sawada, Cossette, Wellar, & Kurt, 2006) or between rich and poor (Looker & Thiessen, 2003).

Central to eHealth is the concept of eHealth literacy, which is defined as "the ability to seek, find, understand, and appraise health information from electronic sources and apply the knowledge gained to addressing or solving a health problem" (Norman & Skinner, 2006). This definition highlights an important characteristic of eHealth literacy: it is a process that depends in part on access to health information technology (e.g., computers, hand-held devices, online applications, etc.). It also requires that users be able to use these technological devices and processes. However, eHealth emphasizes shifting knowledge and abilities, since eHealth skills may change along with the technology. Furthermore, because use of a computer or other digital device is essential to eHealth literacy, the skill set does not depend exclusively on access but on the knowledge needed to use the device effectively.

REVIEW AND REFLECT

Are there any characteristics or features of eHealth that you would add to the definition by Norman and Skinner (2006) found above?

THE MULTIPLE COMPETENCIES FOR EHEALTH LITERACY

The notion of eHealth literacy can be seen as a component of the more general concept of health literacy. The concept of eHealth literacy emphasizes the knowledge and skills that people need to interact with electronic media, such as the Internet, and use such media to effectively improve their health. However, the concept of eHealth literacy also involves additional skills not usually associated with the traditional concept of literacy. A number of models and approaches incorporate key components of eHealth literacy, including computer literacy, science literacy, functional health literacy, media literacy, and information literacy (e.g., see Zarcadoolas, Pleasant, & Greer, 2005). One of the best known Canadian models of eHealth literacy is that proposed by Norman and Skinner (2006), who distinguish six different competencies for eHealth literacy, represented in their lily model. These six competencies are illustrated in Figure 6.1.

FIGURE 6.1: EHEALTH LITERACY LILY MODEL

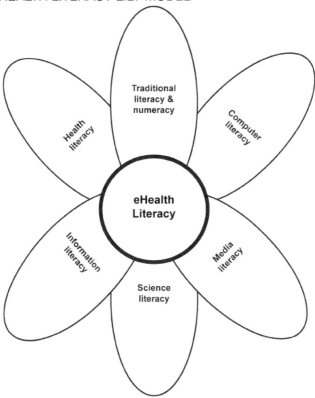

Source: Norman, C.D., & Skinner, H.A. (2006). eHealth literacy: Essential skills for consumer health in a networked world. Figure 1. *Journal of Medical Internet Research, 8*(2), e9. Retrieved from http://www.jmir.org/2006/2/e9/ [accessed: 14 June 2013].

One essential component of eHealth literacy is traditional literacy and numeracy, which involves the ability to read and understand general verbal and numeric information. A person who has difficulty in reading and understanding general information will also have difficulty interacting with information technologies and with the health care system.

A second component is computer literacy (Epperson, 2010), which refers to the ability to use a computer to solve problems, or the ability to interact with information systems such as computers to perform basic tasks. Using a word processing or an email program to write a letter or a message, adding numbers on a spreadsheet to finish a budget, or installing a virus-protection program are all considered tasks of basic computer literacy. The concept of computer literacy was originally used to refer to the skills and knowledge needed to use computers and computer programs (Thompson, Dorsey, Miller, & Parrott, 2003). More specifically, the term refers to "an individual's ability to operate a computer system, have basic understanding of the operating system to save, copy, delete, open, print documents, format a disk, use computer applications software to perform personal or job-related tasks, use Web browsers and search engines on the Internet to retrieve needed information and communicate with others by sending and receiving email" (Gupta, 2006, p. 115). Historically, the concept of computer literacy included basic knowledge of computer hardware and software, and knowing how to operate a computer, or how to use word processing or spreadsheet programs, within the changing landscape of information and communication technologies. Different authors (Epperson, 2010; Hoffman & Blake, 2003) have expanded the concept to include skills needed for solving problems with the use of a computer, knowledge of data privacy and security, and the ability to negotiate online networking sites (e.g., Twitter, Facebook) that require critical knowledge and skills about the psychological and social consequences of computing devices. An expanded concept of computer literacy entails a higher degree of knowledge and skill than currently exists among the Canadian population.

A third component is media literacy (Adair, 2006; Thoman, 2004), which involves the application of critical thinking to assess information gained from mass media: television, radio, newspapers and magazines, and (increasingly) the Internet. Thinking critically about media and their effective use to understand or convey a verbal, aural, or visual message involves "learning how to identify key concepts, make connections between multiple ideas, ask pertinent questions, identify fallacies, and formulate a response" (Thoman, 2004, p. 23). Similar to information literacy, media literacy involves the development of a critical approach to *accessing* (e.g., exploring content beyond the first six "hits" on a search, managing the "multimedia flow," and ability to contact others online [online networks] to get information and help); *assessing* (e.g., questioning the information source, determining the usefulness, timeliness, accuracy, and integrity of information, and judging the validity and completeness of material referenced by hyper-text links); and *using* information (Bawden, 2001; Eysenbach, 2008). Media literacy is considered in greater detail in Chapter 7.

A fourth component of eHealth literacy is science literacy (Laugksch, 2000), which comprises the skills and abilities necessary for basic scientific understanding. Science has become an integral part of modern societies, and, thus, the ability to understand how science is conducted, and its purposes, methods, and limitations, is necessary for interpreting much of health information, such as assessing one's own risk for disease. This could include knowing the place of evidence in health and how to differentiate between scientifically supported information and opinion (or even worse, scientific quackery), how to draw inferences from evidence and use the information to inform health decisions, and understanding the difference between science and technology. Basic knowledge of the scientific method is essential to critically evaluate the quality of health information. We will consider scientific literacy in further detail in Chapter 8 in our discussion of the relationship between public understanding of science, risk communication, and health literacy.

A fifth component of the eHealth literacy model is information literacy (Barnard, Nash, & O'Brien, 2005; Saranto & Hovenga, 2004). This includes the knowledge and skills necessary for searching and using information effectively; that is, knowing where to find information one is interested in and the basic strategies necessary for extracting the desired information from the search.

Finally, the sixth component or aspect of eHealth literacy is that of health literacy. In the context of eHealth literacy, traditional health literacy refers to the ability to understand health information, such as knowing what medical terms mean and how to interact with the health system.

As is often the case in emerging fields, the concepts of information, computer, or media literacy are complex, sometimes confusing, and often overlap. To appreciate the complexity of the concept of information literacy in the context of health information, let us consider three broad categories of related concepts put forward by Saranto and Hovenga (2004). In a review of the literature, Saranto and Hovenga looked for the concepts of computer and information literacy and related notions. They found that most concepts were not defined but similarities were found among some terms used in the literature, such as *computer experience*, *computer awareness*, and *information awareness*. Such concepts appear to match those listed in Norman and Skinner's (2006) lily model of eHealth literacy. In particular, Saranto and Hovenga showed the presence of three related concepts: one concept, associated in meaning to computer literacy, covered basic knowledge and skills needed for operating computer equipment, and how to use different software tools, such as spreadsheets and word processors. The second concept referred to an awareness of computer tools in the context of professional practice, such as using search engines and databases to locate desired information. The third concept focused on "awareness of literature, the skills to locate, retrieve and evaluate, and apply information in critical thinking and problem solving" (Saranto & Hovenga, 2004, p. 507), and, in general, is the ability to manage knowledge in practical situations.

The lack of explicit definitions in the literature underscores the need for a conceptual overview that clarifies the scope of the different skills and abilities involved in eHealth literacy. Despite the complexity of the concept, it is clear that for people to be at high levels of eHealth literacy, they need to possess the knowledge and skills necessary to fully and effectively participate in society and its institutions, including the health care system.

To determine the levels of eHealth literacy of Canadians, a first step is to devise tools that allow us to assess the current eHealth status of our population. Although instruments to assess health literacy have existed for some time, tests that can be used to determine eHealth literacy are only now beginning to appear.

REVIEW AND REFLECT

Consider what you have learned about literacy, health literacy, numeracy, media literacy, and science literacy in earlier chapters. Which components (if any) of eHealth literacy are unique to the lily model?

ASSESSING EHEALTH LITERACY

As described in Chapter 2, there are tests to assess health literacy that allow practitioners and researchers to evaluate a person's level of skill in understanding health information.

In general, health literacy is difficult to evaluate without the use of specifically developed tools for assessing the skills involved. Research suggests, for instance, that medical doctors often fail to estimate the literacy skills of patients, frequently overestimating their abilities (Bass, 2005).

In addition to the measurement instruments discussed in Chapter 2, Norman and Skinner (2006) have developed an instrument to assess eHealth literacy, the eHealth Literacy Scale, eHEALS (Norman & Skinner, 2006). The instrument consists of eight statements that are ranked on a 5-point Likert scale designed to assess a person's declared knowledge of eHealth skills, such as knowledge of where to find health information, confidence in how to evaluate the searched health information, and the ability to understand and make use of health information found on the Internet. The eHEALS instrument is shown in Table 6.2.

Even though young people tend to be "super-users" of computers and tend to be the most familiar with information technologies, research has shown that they lack the skills needed to use their knowledge to access reputable sources of health information. Skinner and colleagues (2003) showed that searching for health information was often found to be "overwhelming" for young people. Furthermore, they had difficulties discerning sources of reputable health information from disreputable sources. If young Canadians, who are knowledgeable and skilful users of information technology, present difficulties in accessing valid online health information, we can anticipate that older Canadians are not likely to fare better.

The gap in information technologies skills needed for eHealth literacy is likely to be even more troubling for older adults. Surveys conducted by Statistics Canada (Sciadas, 2002) have shown the gap that exists in Canadians' use of the Internet is a function of age. Whereas over 90 percent of Canadian teenagers and 60 percent of middle-age Canadians used the Internet in the year 2000, only 5 percent to 10 percent of Canadians 75 years and older reported using the Internet that year (Sciadas, 2002). Although there has been an increase in Internet use in recent years across all age groups, by the year 2009 only 27 percent of adult Canadians age 75 years and older reported daily use of the Internet in comparison to 83 percent for those under 35 years of age (Statistics Canada, 2011b).

THE CHANGING LANDSCAPE OF EHEALTH LITERACY

In the realm of health, using the Internet to access reliable information can lead to informed patients (Murray et al., 2003a; 2003b) and potentially better health outcomes (Liira, 2011). As eHealth is conceived of as a process dependent on the state of available technology, it is critical that users of health information adapt to new ways of communication. In the short history of the Internet and the World Wide Web, we can see a shift from a system in which users simply access static health information to one in which they actively generate information. Although the most common use of health content on the Internet consists of accessing and reading consumer-focused health information provided by both public and private health organizations, there is increasing use of social media technologies that enable connection and interaction among online health consumers and provide patient education and care (Hawn, 2009; Rich, 2011a)

TABLE 6.2: THE EHEALTH LITERACY SCALE

Questions used in the eHealth Literacy Scale					
1. How useful do you feel the Internet is in helping you in making decisions about your health?	Not Useful At All	Not Useful	Unsure	Useful	Very Useful
2. How important is it for you to be able to access health resources on the Internet?	Not Important At All	Not Important	Unsure	Important	Very Important
3. I know what health resources are available on the Internet.	Strongly Disagree	Disagree	Undecided	Agree	Strongly Agree
4. I know where to find helpful health resources on the Internet.	Strongly Disagree	Disagree	Undecided	Agree	Strongly Agree
5. I know how to find helpful health resources on the Internet.	Strongly Disagree	Disagree	Undecided	Agree	Strongly Agree
6. I know how to use the Internet to answer my questions about health.	Strongly Disagree	Disagree	Undecided	Agree	Strongly Agree
7. I know how to use the health information I find on the Internet to help me.	Strongly Disagree	Disagree	Undecided	Agree	Strongly Agree
8. I have the skills I need to evaluate the health resources I find on the Internet.	Strongly Disagree	Disagree	Undecided	Agree	Strongly Agree
9. I can tell high quality health resources from low quality health resources on the Internet.	Strongly Disagree	Disagree	Undecided	Agree	Strongly Agree
10. I feel confident in using information from the Internet to make health decisions.	Strongly Disagree	Disagree	Undecided	Agree	Strongly Agree

Note: Questions 1 and 2 are used to gather information about the respondents' interests about eHealth and are not part of the eHealth Literacy Scale.
Source: Modified from Norman, C.D., & Skinner, H.A. (2006). eHEALS: The eHealth Literacy Scale. *Journal of Medical Internet Research, 8*(4), e27. Multimedia Appendix 1. eHealth Literacy Scale [DOC (MS Word) file, 51 KB]. Retrieved from http://www.jmir.org/2006/4/e27/ [accessed: 17 June 2013].

Since the early beginnings of the computer revolution that brought us home-based personal computers, there has been a dramatic increase in the power and variety of computer technologies. High-end computers of just a few years ago are not capable of processing all the data that is required in many tasks today. While earlier computer technology was limited to the desktop computer, more suitable for office work, now we have access to a large array of electronic devices of various types that have blurred the distinction between traditional computers and other electronic media sources, such as television and radio. The way we communicate with these devices has also changed: early computer systems only allowed for the use of a keyboard, whereas now there are various forms of interaction, such as with a mouse, touch screens, and voice. These forms of communication make it potentially easier for individuals with less computer confidence (less self-efficacy) to use the devices in a more natural way.

In the following short section, we briefly review the history of the Internet and the World Wide Web in order to set the stage for understanding the eHealth literacy landscape. The Internet and associated technologies have their roots in ideas of interconnected computers that first arose during the early 1960s. These early developments and ideas led to the first communicating computers, with the creation of a network connecting two computers located some distance apart, one in Massachusetts and the other in California (Leiner, Handal, & Williams, 2004; Leiner et al., 2009). The early research on these ideas was taken over by the Advanced Research Projects Agency (ARPA), a military organization of the United States government, and developed by researchers at the Massachusetts Institute of Technology, Stanford University, and Bolt, Beranek, and Newman, a private technology development firm. During the 1960s and 1970s, advances in computer technology led to the design and implementation of the Advanced Research Projects Agency Network (ARPANET), the first network connecting computers at four universities: the University of California, Berkeley; the University of Utah; the University of California at Santa Barbara; and the Stanford Research Institute, then part of Stanford University (Leiner, Handal, & Williams, 2004; Leiner et al., 2009). Later developments during the 1970s were peer-to-peer electronic mail, the file transfer protocol known as Telnet, and the Internet protocol known as the Transmission Control Protocol (TCP) (for further information on various Internet technologies, consult the online source Wikibooks at http://en.wikibooks.org/wiki/Internet_Technologies).

The World Wide Web also has a long history. A key term is *hypertext*, which conveys the notion of information connected through links, making non-sequential navigation possible. The term actually refers to a format where terms in a given document are linked to related documents in such a manner that they can be "navigated" in a non-linear way; for instance, clicking on a word brings the reader to a verbal, aural, or visual document relevant to that word. Although there were precursors to the idea of connecting information in networks (Bush, 1945), the term *hypertext* was coined by Ted Nelson to express his idea that computer systems could be designed to allow distributed information of all kinds—text, images, sounds, movies, and interacting multimedia—to present complex information for reading and learning. Practically, this meant that users could follow many different paths to knowledge, accessing information and learning in any desired or preferred format. The Internet truly became the common technology we know today after

Tim Berners-Lee developed the Hyper-Text Markup Language (HTML), the World Wide Web (WWW), and the first Web browser during the early 1990s. HTML is a computer markup language that allows the management and presentation of Web pages on computer screens while connecting Web pages in different locations. The WWW refers to the linked information that is on the Internet, so it is the information counterpart to the physical Internet. Unlike books and magazine articles, which have a very rigid and fixed presentation of concepts and ideas and are mostly designed to be read sequentially, the WWW with its underlying technologies allows for knowledge to be joined through "links" that lead to associated concepts. However, advances in Internet technology are not limited to the browsing of linked Web pages.

REVIEW AND REFLECT

What is hypertext? How does it change the way we look at and access information?

WEB 2.0: SOCIAL MEDIA AND HEALTH LITERACY

Although limited in many respects, the traditional Web or Web 1.0 was the first step in connecting people worldwide. Web 2.0 changed the Web landscape by the use of more interactive technologies (see Table 6.3). Much of what we call "social media" is part of Web 2.0, and this has large implications for eHealth. We have all heard the term *social media* and many, especially young people, are familiar with these widely used Web technologies. In general terms, social media can be defined as "web-based services that allow individuals to (1) construct a public or semi-public profile within a bounded system, (2) articulate a list of other users with whom they share a connection, and (3) view and traverse their list of connections and those made by others within the system" (Boyd & Ellison, 2007, p. 211).

Social media networks allow people with similar interests to share knowledge and experiences, and to help one another. Because of its unique features in information sharing among multiple parties, social media can often help patients and consumers of health care services. First, patients can connect and exchange information and personal experiences with one another regardless of geographical location, as long as they have access to an Internet or a cellular phone connection. Second, personal aspects such as age or gender tend to be more diffuse in online communication, which could bridge the barriers between age groups. Third, because online social networks are often anonymous, people can express themselves more freely without fear of stigma. Given these characteristics and the potential for interactive communication, social media could be exploited as a tool for providing health care and help to consumers of health care services (Duffett-Leger & Lumsden, 2008; Hawn, 2009), as well as a tool for public health (Merchant, Elmer, & Lurie, 2011).

Newer technologies offer the promise of more personal connections between users by the sharing of personalized individual data (Crow & Ondrusek, 2012; Kreuter, Caburnay, Chen, & Donlin, 2004). The next wave of online technologies will allow for the interconnection of individualized data, rather than only the information provided by current Web pages. This is a consequence of the use of peer-to-peer technologies that serve to connect people and allow them to contribute to a common pool of data, which can then be used in health applications. This use of data has considerable implications for individual health and health care, as patients who have common interests or suffer similar illnesses are able to exploit the personal knowledge gathered by other individuals, forming some sort of "collective memory" or shared composite experience (Bush, 1945). For example, websites such as PatientsLikeMe (www.patientslikeme.com) allow patients with specific illnesses or symptoms to connect with other patients suffering from the same affliction and thereby learn from one another's experiences. The site also presents statistical information on its members, including treatments undertaken, drugs used, symptoms suffered, and treatment options.

A second example of the use of personalized health data is that of Google Flu Trends (www.google.org/flutrends), which provides information on the spread of the influenza and other respiratory illnesses across North America and other parts of the world. By tracking the references that Internet users make of terms such as *flu*, *virus*, *cold*, or *allergy*, the search engine Google follows the spread of the yearly influenza. In past years, it has been shown that Google Flu Trends has registered flu activity in the United States several days before the Centers for Disease Control reported an influenza outbreak (Ginsberg et al., 2009; Dugas et al., 2012); however, readers should be aware that such Internet tracking is not without a downside, as it raises issues of privacy.

The use of social media in health care, however, presents challenges in relation to health literacy, as the new technologies impose new ways of interacting and communicating to the user. As surveys have shown, not all Canadians are participating in the computer era. The 2010 Canadian Internet Survey showed that almost a quarter of Canadian households do not have access to a computer at home. The reasons for not having computer access vary, from not needing it, to the high cost of the service or the device, to a lack of confidence in the skills or knowledge needed to use computers (Statistics Canada, 2011a).

As individuals participate in generating the data that can be used to provide more personal information that is tied to the experiences of patients (as PatientsLikeMe shows), or data that can be used to monitor public health risks (as Google Flu Trends exemplifies), individuals may become more engaged in their own health care (Wicks et al., 2010) and become more eHealth literate (Pomerantz, Muhammad, Downey, & Kind, 2010). Such engagement may be critical to enhancing the health information literacy of the general public and patients, but it may also further perpetuate the knowledge gap hypothesis described in Chapter 4. Individuals with greater access to information (e.g., Internet access, adequate eHealth literacy skills, and greater education and income) are privileged in terms of access to health information and services.

REVIEW AND REFLECT

Although Web 2.0 technologies have the potential for improving health care, what dangers are posed by the implementation of such technologies in health care? How would these challenges both increase and decrease the knowledge or health information gap for Canadians?

FROM WEB 2.0 TO WEB 3.0

New information technologies can have an impact on health literacy as the technologies become more interactive and immersive, especially with Web 2.0 and the proposed Web 3.0 (see Table 6.3 for distinguishing features of Web 1.0, 2.0, and 3.0). For the general population, Web 2.0 is a reality that is changing the way people interact. Social networking tools, such as Facebook, Twitter, and YouTube, are used to convey information in a form that may be more attractive to many populations than the traditional Internet Web page. Because of its audiovisual nature, YouTube is one of the most popular sources of information and entertainment. For instance, in 2012, YouTube had an average of 800 million visitors each month who watched over 3 billion hours of video (Bullas, n.d.). The most visited social network site, Facebook, received one trillion visits in 2011 (Google, 2012). In Canada, according to WebFuel, it is estimated that over 17 million Canadians connect monthly to social media sites (Faber, 2011), with 15 million monthly users on Facebook alone (6S Marketing, 2012).

TABLE 6.3: CHARACTERISTICS OF WEB 1.0, WEB 2.0, AND THE PROPOSED WEB 3.0

Web 1.0	Web 2.0	Web 3.0
Static content	Dynamic content	Dynamic content
User as passive consumer	User as generator of information	User as generator of data
Information generated by organizations	Information actively generated by user	Information generated by user and organizations to summarize and analyze trends
Personal Web pages	Web blogs	Data from multiple sources
General disease information	Personal experiences with illness	Personal experiences and data shared among users
Focus on the single individual	Focus on the social	Focus on intelligent agents
Isolation	Fragmentation	Integration
Keyword search	User-aided search (e.g., Google)	Semantic findings
Monologue	Dialogue	Data sharing
Simple	Anarchic	Structure, standards, and protocols
Encyclopaedia Britannica	Wikipedia	Wolfram Alpha

Source: Modified from Boulos, M.N.K., & Wheeler, S. (2007). The emerging Web 2.0 social software: An enabling suite of sociable technologies in health and health care education. *Health Information & Libraries Journal, 24*(1), 2–23; and from Giustini, D. (2007). Web 3.0 and medicine: Make way for the semantic web. *British Medical Journal, 335*(7633), 1273–1274.

These numbers highlight the power of Web 2.0 information technologies, which have not yet been fully exploited by the health care system to provide information and educate Canadians. Although Web 2.0 technologies are promoted and used by millions of people around the world to communicate with one another, because of its interactive nature, it can also become a vehicle for informing and educating the user about health matters. Such potential has not been completely ignored by health professionals: a small survey conducted by the Canadian Medical Association (CMA) showed that 26 percent of physician members belonged to a social network for the purpose of communicating with other physicians (Hines, 2011; Rich, 2011a). Similarly, in the United States, an email survey of primary care physicians and oncologists revealed that 17 percent of the respondents made use of email, 52 percent used restricted online communities, and 33 percent used Twitter in some form to support their practice, especially to communicate with other professionals (Rich, 2011b). Some Canadian organizations, such as the Canadian Federation of Medical Students, have been using Web 2.0 technologies to increase medical students' participation in online discussions of medical school course content and practical skill development. The Canadian Medical Association has recognized Web 2.0 technologies, particularly social media applications such as Facebook, Twitter, and YouTube, and is embracing them while providing guidance for their use. (This is described further at www.cma.ca/advocacy/social-media-canadian-physicians; see "Additional Resources of Interest" at the end of this chapter).

While Web 2.0 applications provide access to inordinate amounts of data generated from the collaboration of thousands or millions of users, Web 3.0 promises to organize such data into effective knowledge (Eysenbach, 2008). Web 3.0 is basically characterized by two related developments. The first is the organization of the massive amounts of data provided by Web 2.0 into meaningful information; the second is the development of the semantic web. Organization of vast amounts of data into usable knowledge is to be accomplished by categorizing all information into semantic or meaningful chunks of information. The underlying idea is that digital devices will be able to search and find information in the same way that humans do: by attaching meaning to data. Some health projects feed into Web 3.0 technologies, particularly those that rely on the development of medical ontologies for organizing areas of health, such as cardiovascular diseases or diabetes (Hoehndorf, Loebe, Kelso, & Herre, 2007). Medical ontologies are clusters of concepts about a medical topic that are hierarchically organized by means of "tags" attached to such concepts (Robu, Robu, & Thirion, 2006). Ontologies act by imposing a structure on data. For instance, in conducting a search, the concept of "heart attack" and its associated concepts can be retrieved together by virtue of the fact that the concept has been tagged as a type of cardiovascular disease, rather than by matching the keywords "heart" and "attack." Although organizing information into categories may prove to be beneficial in providing a more intuitive approach to information retrieval, the use of Web 3.0 technologies is, at this point in time, only a promise (Rowell, 2008). Time and technological advances will tell if such promises are realized. In a broader sense, Web 3.0 characterizes not only a technical development, but also a state of mind, a way of thinking, an attitude, and a commitment to networked global thinking to improve health care locally, regionally, and worldwide by using information and communication technology.

> **REVIEW AND REFLECT**
>
> Search for information using Wikipedia and Wolfram Alpha. Do you notice any difference in the way these two databases answer your questions?

THE CULTURE OF ONLINE HEALTH INFORMATION

The World Wide Web is filled with sites that provide health information. The exact number is unknown, but they probably number in the millions given that the total number of all websites was estimated to be 666 million in 2012 (Netcraft, 2012). And, as we stated earlier, health is one of the most popular online topics. The most typical sites offer health information provided by government agencies, health care providers, and pharmaceutical companies. Blogs, started by private individuals to share their experiences, are sometimes taken over by companies (e.g., http://healthblog.ctv.ca) or health care organizations (e.g., http://sunnybrook.ca/). Online communities are another type of Internet site used for health purposes. Despite the dramatic advances in Web technologies, for eHealth to become universally used, we require high-speed network connections. To be usable by all Canadians in an increasingly interconnected world, many Web services, such as online health communities and timely access to health information, require universal access, regardless of socio-economic level, age, or geographical location. Although Internet use has been increasing steadily across all levels of Canadian society, many barriers remain. Some Canadians, particularly marginalized populations and those in isolated communities, are at a disadvantage in terms of access to the Web (Sawada, Cossette, Wellar, & Kurt, 2006). Whereas all households in such provinces as Ontario and Alberta had access to broadband Internet, only 27 percent of households in Nunavut share such access. When speed is used as a criterion, only 20 percent of households in rural communities have access to Internet speeds of 25 megabits per second or higher. This compares with 90 percent of households in urban areas (Canadian Radio-television and Telecommunications Commission, 2011).

The small population of rural communities makes it more expensive to deploy regular Ethernet connection, such as fibre optic, cable, or fast DSL (i.e., broadband communication through telephone lines). Often the only medium available is satellite access, which is more expensive and less reliable than alternative technologies (Marlow & McNish, 2010). Recognizing such disparities, however, a government-led program, Broadband Canada: Connecting Rural Canadians, designed to bring Internet access to remote rural communities across the country, was implemented from 2009 to 2012 and resulted in over 200,000 new households having online access (Industry Canada, 2012). In the next section, we will relate the issues of computer access and computer and information literacy to eHealth literacy, and explore what this means for Canadians.

HEALTH LITERACY AND MINORITY POPULATIONS: THE DIGITAL DIVIDE

The concept of the "digital divide" is often used to indicate the difference in access and use of information technologies by different populations as determined by economic, social, cultural, educational, and linguistic factors. More specifically, the digital divide refers to the disparity that exists between societal groups in the access to, and knowledge and use of, information and communication technologies, such as computers and smartphones (Warschauer, 2003; Wyatt, Henwood, Hart, & Smith, 2005).

There are different aspects to the digital divide and no single definition can be given without a consideration of context. In highly technological societies, a person who accesses the Internet at a public library may be considered at the lower end of the digital divide and a "digital have-not." However, a person in the same situation in a developing country may be considered to be at the higher end of the scale, and therefore be among the privileged for that society (Warschauer, 2003) Thus, the concept of digital divide must always be examined within the broader social and cultural context.

How can we therefore understand the "digital divide" if there is no clear-cut definition or universally agreed-upon benchmark of the concept? One useful approach is to consider the digital divide as having different dimensions or layers along which social groups can be placed. Probably the most basic level is access to electronic media. For example, this could be cell phones in Grise Fiord (Nunavut) or computer labs in adult education centres in Kitchener (Ontario). However, we know that not all populations have equal access to computers and other Internet-capable devices. Indeed, access to information technology is associated with many factors, such as income, geographical location, age, and education. A large number of these factors are socially determined (i.e., social determinants).

Economics plays an important role. Typically, wealthier individuals have more opportunities for owning or accessing computer technologies. For instance, a survey conducted in the United States in 2001 showed that, among families earning more than $75,000, 80 percent had computer access, whereas among the poorest Americans, only 25 percent had access (Chang et al., 2004). Among adults, computer use was lower among economically disadvantaged individuals (66 percent for people with incomes below $50,000 versus 86 percent for people with incomes above $50,000) (Brodie et al., 2000). In Canada, by the year 2000, only 24 percent of Canadians at the lowest economic quintile used the Internet, whereas 81 percent of those at the highest quintile did so. More recently, the 2010 Internet Use Survey (Statistics Canada, 2011a) revealed that, whereas 97 percent of the households with incomes above $87,000 had Internet access at home, only 54 percent of households with incomes of $30,000 or lower had access.

Geographical location also plays an important role. Partly due to isolation and distance from urban centres, people living in rural communities have less access to electronic media. Studies show that in the United States, a higher percentage of urban dwellers use computers in comparison with rural dwellers (65 percent versus 48 percent, respectively). The situation is similar in Canada, where 82 percent of individuals living in large metropolitan areas have access to the Internet at home compared to 72 percent of those living outside these areas (Statistics Canada, 2011b).

Other surveys have shown age to be another dimension relevant to the digital divide. A study designed to investigate computer and Internet use among American youth and adults of various ethnicities (Brodie et al., 2000) showed that those Americans below 60 years of age utilized computers and surfed the Internet more than older adults. Similarly, in Canada, surveys have shown that Internet use substantially decreases with age: while over 90 percent of Canadian teenagers used the Internet in 2002, only 5 percent of older individuals made use of the technology (Sciadas, 2002; Statistics Canada, 2010b). Although there has been an increase in Internet use across all age groups, older individuals still trail younger Canadian adults in Internet use, accounting for half of all non-users. Whereas 97 percent of adults under 34 years of age reported Internet use from any location (e.g., home, libraries, work, etc.), only 41 percent of older adults aged 65 and older went online in 2009 (Statistics Canada, 2010b).

Even if age is factored out, results consistently show socio-economic factors as a key determinant of computer use (Howard & Busch, 2011; Looker & Thiessen, 2003). Young people of different socio-economic levels show results similar to their adult counterparts, with those children in low-income homes reporting 31 percent using computers, in contrast to 61 percent for those in high-income homes. If the difference in computer use reveals the digital divide between income levels of households, one can only expect that the distinction will be maintained when it comes to health information. This differential use of computers, it is assumed, puts some social groups at a disadvantage when it comes to access to information and makes it difficult to acquire needed skills in a modern society that is increasingly reliant on information and communication technologies.

It appears, then, that access is a very important aspect of health and eHealth literacy. Once people have access to computers and the Internet, the digital divide diminishes, as a survey by Brodie and colleagues (2000) shows. However, regardless of access, younger users appear less prepared to search for health information than do older adults. Yet regardless of ethnicity or level of income, about half of the adults between the ages of 18 and 59 who participated in a survey about Internet use reported using it to search for health information. In contrast, only 19 percent of persons surveyed age 17 years or younger used it for that purpose (although this could also reflect the relative lack of ill health among younger people). The digital divide, therefore, is not only dependent on social groups having access to computer technology or usage of the Internet, but also on making effective use of the technology. To be effective, several different skills are needed. One can argue that bridging the gap between economic, social, or ethnic user groups (Lorence, Park, & Fox, 2006) necessitates possessing the six competencies identified in eHealth literacy.

Thus, to be fully engaged in eHealth, Canadians need to be able to read and understand general information (traditional literacy), possess the knowledge and skills to use computers and digital devices (computer literacy), critically understand and assess media messages in all its forms, verbal, aural, and visual (media literacy), be able to discern reliable and valid information from mere opinion or quackery (scientific literacy), search and use information skilfully (information literacy), have the knowledge necessary to promote their own health and be able to navigate the health care system (health literacy), and apply meaning and values to the health information and health care decisions that are made (cultural literacy). Although no person is likely to possess all these literacies at their optimal levels, it is important to work toward achieving them. Using and becoming familiar with new information technologies as they become available can aid in this goal.

REVIEW AND REFLECT

What are the component literacies that contribute to Canadians having adequate eHealth literacy? On reflection, and from your perspective, would some of these component literacies be "easier" to address than others?

KEY LEARNING POINTS

In this chapter we presented the concepts of eHealth, eHealth literacy, the Internet and its changing landscape, and the digital divide. eHealth literacy is a dynamic concept, requiring different skills as the technology advances and the social context of health changes. In a brief period we have witnessed the dramatic change in the Internet from a tool for static health information retrieval to one of active health information provision. Despite the rapid advances in online technologies, the optimal implementation of eHealth for all Canadians is still a work in progress and will probably remain so as long as the technology continues to change. Furthermore, difficult challenges remain for inclusion in this eHealth evolution for many segments of the Canadian population and especially for those living outside most metropolitan areas. Still, there are multiple opportunities for engaging all Canadians in an improved health care that serves to satisfy patients and health providers alike. We have seen that eHealth literacy cannot be isolated from other literacies (e.g., computer literacy and traditional literacy) or from the broad social determinants that affect health and health literacy.

A CANADIAN MILESTONE

In 1999, the Government of Canada, under the Minister of Health, the Honourable Allan Rock, delivered a bold and strategic vision for health information and health care in the digital age. This vision was articulated in the Canada Health Infoway report:

Developing a Canadian health infostructure can be compared to building a transcontinental railroad or highway, but this time it is our health care system in the knowledge society and digital world of the 21st century.... We believe investments in the Canada Health Infoway will be of similar benefit for the health care system and the health of Canadians....

Health Canada, in partnership with provincial and territorial ministries of health, takes a leadership role in ensuring that health information and health care applications for the general public are developed in such a way to be accessible to all citizens, irrespective of their geographic location, income, language, disability, gender, age, cultural background or level of traditional or digital literacy.

Source: Advisory Council on Health Infostructure. (2000, pp. 2–9). *Canada Health Infoway: Paths to better health, final report*. Retrieved from http://publications.gc.ca/collections/Collection/H21-145-1999E.pdf [accessed: 18 June 2013].

ADDITIONAL RESOURCES OF INTEREST

The Canadian Medical Association's (CMA) position on the use of social media by health care professionals

http://www.cma.ca/advocacy/social-media-canadian-physicians

Recognizing the importance of Web 2.0 technologies for health care, the CMA has provided some guidelines for their safe use.

Medicine 2.0

http://www.medicine20congress.com/ocs/index.php/med/med2013

This is a yearly academic conference devoted to research about the use of Web 2.0 technologies in health care. The conference is organized by Dr. Gunther Eysenbach, a Canadian leader in information technology in health care.

Canada Health Infoway

http://www.infoway-inforoute.ca/index.php

This is an independent, not-for-profit corporation funded by the Government of Canada to provide leadership in transforming the Canadian health care system using information technologies.

Broadband Canada: Connecting Rural Canadians

http://www.ic.gc.ca/eic/site/719.nsf/eng/home

This is an initiative of the Government of Canada to extend the use of broadband coverage to underserved rural and isolated populations across the country. The program, in place between 2009 and 2012, funded 86 projects in seven provinces.

CHAPTER 7

MASS MEDIA AND HEALTH LITERACY

This is a new area of research and relatively few studies have, thus far, moved beyond assessments of written materials. More work needs to be done to link outcomes to materials and processes and measure health behaviours and outcomes. Furthermore we need to expand beyond the written word and look more closely at oral and aural skills, the value of visuals as pictograms, and the benefits of new technology such as the internet.

—RIMA RUDD, *LITERACY AND HEALTH RESEARCH WORKSHOP*, 2000

CHAPTER LEARNING OBJECTIVES
- Describe the relationship between mass media and health literacy
- Describe media literacy and consider media literacy initiatives in Canada
- Review how learning to analyze, evaluate, and create health-related media messages can help health literacy efforts
- Consider ethnic media as an opportunity to close the health literacy gap among culturally and linguistically diverse groups in Canada

INTRODUCTION

In today's media-rich environment, we can be overwhelmed by the many different sources and forms of health information. On a daily basis, we encounter print and billboard advertisements, radio and television programs, and newspaper articles and books that promote different products, ideas, and services related to or with implications for our health. For example, consider the Special K° advertising campaigns by Kellogg: "If you can pinch more than an inch, you may need to watch your weight"; "What will you gain when you lose?"; and the "Drop a jean size" challenge.

Do these Special K° advertisements equate slimness with health for women? Would the viewer likely infer that being skinny is ideal and healthy? Ironically, the biggest brands and advertisers often market and endorse products that undermine the importance of a healthy lifestyle. Never before in our technology-intense information society have we been so exposed to, and become such avid consumers of, media. Accordingly, with so many media choices, obtaining health information has never been an easier task; on the other hand, never before has media literacy—"the ability to access, analyze, evaluate, and create media in a variety of forms" (Thoman & Jolls, 2003, p. 21)—been so crucial in aiding health literacy.

In this chapter, we will look at the relationship between mass media and health literacy, and discuss the concept of media literacy (introduced in Chapter 6). We will explore media literacy initiatives in Canada and examine how learning to analyze, evaluate, and create health-related media messages help health literacy efforts. Finally, we will consider ethnic media as an opportunity to close the health literacy gap among culturally and linguistically diverse groups in Canada.

MASS MEDIA AND HEALTH LITERACY

In a seminal work highlighting the role of mass media in public health, Griffiths and Knutson (1960) noted how "vast sums are spent annually for materials and salaries that have gone into [the] production and distribution of booklets, pamphlets, exhibits, newspaper articles, and radio and television programs" (p. 515). They postulated three effects of mass media in achieving desired public health goals: (1) "the learning of correct health information," (2) "the changing of health attitudes and values," as well as (3) "the establishment of new health behavior" (p. 515). Even half a century ago, there was abundant research evidence suggesting that, while mass media might reach enormous numbers of people, they tend to reach selected groups of audiences, and even when the desired groups of audiences are reached, the effects of mediated intended messages might be limited.

Although the popularity of new media, especially social media—YouTube, Wikipedia, Facebook, Twitter, and blogs—has swept the world, "the traditional media are here to stay to a surprising extent … books, magazines, film, television, and radio will never go away" (Moggridge, 2008, p. 5). While we examined the role of technology in health literacy in Canada in Chapter 6, this chapter focuses on the role of traditional mass media in health literacy in Canada.

Mass media are important sources of health information, and the term used to describe these sources is *mediated health information*. Mediated health information is available in the form of news stories; specialized journals and magazines for health, wellness, and fitness; health books; health shows on television and radio; and commercials and advertising about products with an added health value. As a member of this media-rich society, are you able to access, understand, evaluate, and communicate this mediated health information in a way that promotes good health? Schaefer (2008) argued that "media can help in the fight against health illiteracy through their ability to entertain and promote health awareness at the same time" (p. 27). However, mass media can be a double-edged sword, influencing health behaviour in both positive (health-enhancing) and negative (health-compromising) ways. The general public considers news media to be a major source of medical and health information (Karpf, 1988; Maibach & Parrott, 1995, Parrott, 1996), and studies have documented the role of health news media coverage in shaping health behaviours (Niederdeppe & Frosch, 2009) and influencing public health policy (Tong, Chapman, Sainsbury, & Craig, 2008). Research has also found, however, that media coverage of health issues, especially media reporting of medical and health news, is of poor quality (Gasher, Hayes, Hackett, Gutstein, & Dunn, 2007; Hayes et al., 2007; Johnson, 1998; Radford, 1996; Shuchman & Wilkes, 1997) and often poorly related to the actual empirical scientific evidence (MacDonald & Hoffman-Goetz, 2002).

Yet the important role of mass media in enhancing public health cannot be undermined. A case in point is the media coverage (e.g., newspaper and television reporting) about Reye's Syndrome and the use of aspirin in children (Soumerai, Ross-Degnan, & Kahn, 1992; Moynihan et al., 2000). Soumerai, Ross-Degnan, and Kahn (1992) argued that "the professional and lay media were important communication channels in alerting health professionals and parents about the relation between aspirin and Reye's Syndrome, particularly during the early years of the controversy (1981–1983)" (p. 283). Box 7.1 shows an example of a news report from the *New York Times* describing how aspirin can be linked to Reye's Syndrome, a fatal children's disease.

BOX 7.1: MEDIA REPORT: ASPIRIN LINKED TO CHILDREN'S DISEASE
Michael deCourcy Hinds, Special to the New York Times

WASHINGTON, April 27—There is growing concern in the medical profession about a link between aspirin and a rare but sometimes deadly children's disease called Reye's Syndrome.

In the last six years, Government agencies have released studies and issued guarded warnings, hoping to alert the public to the potential danger without causing undue alarm. But as each new case of Reye's Syndrome is recorded, the pressure builds on Government agencies to take stronger action.

The American Academy of Pediatricians has now decided to issue its own warning to its 23,000 members. Its June issue of *Pediatrics*, the academy's technical journal, will advise members not to prescribe aspirin or aspirin compounds to children suffering influenza symptoms or chicken pox. The recommendation, similar to those issued by the Centers for Disease Control in Atlanta, is based on evidence linking 137 cases of Reye's Syndrome to children who were administered aspirin in previous bouts with flu or chicken pox.

Ralph Nader's Health Research Group and the American Public Health Association have expressed concern with the way the Food and Drug Administration is exercising its regulatory authority. The two groups have individually petitioned the F.D.A. to require warning labels on children's aspirin, and both have threatened legal action if the agency does not respond by Friday.

Reye's Syndrome, which may annually affect 600 to 1,200 children, is characterized by the sudden onset of fever, vomiting and headaches, and progresses rapidly to convulsions and coma. About 25 percent of the victims, or up to 300 a year, die, and many others suffer permanent brain damage, according to the Centers for Disease Control, which is affiliated with the Department of Health and Human Services.

Dr. Sidney Wolfe, head of the Health Research Group, has said that without

Government delays some of the 14 deaths associated with the illness so far this year might have been prevented. Using the Freedom of Information Act, Dr. Wolfe obtained F.D.A internal memos indicating that the agency has almost as much evidence now as it had in November 1980. "Yet the endless reviews continue," Dr. Wolfe said.

Another F.D.A. memo also shows that aspirin manufacturers have been keenly interested in the agency's activities. Children's aspirin manufacturers, which have sales approaching $50 million annually, have maintained that the studies linking aspirin to Reye's Syndrome are flawed.

Wayne Pines, an F.D.A. spokesman, said the agency wanted to continue its review of the data before joining in the Centers for Disease Control's warning. In January, the F.D.A set up its own panel to review the data from the four studies and make recommendations to Dr. Arthur H. Hayes, the F.D.A. Commissioner.

The group's report is nearly complete, and Dr. Hayes may soon make a decision, according to Dr. Edward Mortimer, who worked on the Centers for Disease Control's panel and is an F.D.A. consultant.

Dr. Marion J. Finkel, associate director of the F.D.A.'s Bureau of Drugs, defended the agency's policy. Until recently, she said, the agency has not had a chance to review the raw scientific data—the actual questionnaires and statistics assembled in the various studies.

"The matter could not have been handled more expeditiously," she said. To have made a decision sooner, she added, would have "needlessly raised concerns on the part of the patients." A hasty judgment, if it proved wrong later on, might also damage the agency's credibility, she said.

Dr. Ralph Kauffman, a pediatrician who served on the Centers for Disease Control's advisory panel, said the public should be given stronger warnings about aspirin's link to Reye's Syndrome. But he said he did not think warning labels on aspirin would be effective.

"All that the label could say," he said, "is that preliminary studies have suggested an association of aspirin taken during the flu or chicken pox and the development of Reye's Syndrome. Would that help? I don't think that people read labels."

Dr. Kauffman suggested that the best way to get the message across was through medical channels and the press. Donald Berreth, spokesman for the Centers for Disease Control, said the mortality rate from Reye's Syndrome was only about 1 per 400,000 children under the age of 18; 25 children in the same sample die from cancer. Mr. Berreth said the Centers for Disease Control were continuing to do laboratory tests and to assemble case histories.

Source: deCourcy Hinds, M. (1982, April 28). Aspirin linked to children's disease. *The New York Times.* Retrieved from http://www.nytimes.com/1982/04/28/garden/aspirin-linked-to-children-s-disease.html [accessed: 18 June 2013].

REVIEW AND REFLECT

Do you think television drama series can help facilitate health education? View an episode of *Grey's Anatomy* or *House*. Do you think the episode delivered in clear and easily understood terms information on a health care topic that may have been unfamiliar to viewers?

TYPES OF MASS MEDIA

Mass media can be defined as technological tools for the transmission of messages to reach a large group of mixed audiences (Hanson, 2005; Hart, 1991). Hart (1991) identified three main types of media: presentational, representational, and mechanical/electronic. Presentational media are characterized by face-to-face communication; for example, speech and sign language. Representational media help store messages that can be reproduced with the help of technical devices, such as telegrams, books, newspapers, and magazines. Mechanical/electronic media are distinct because of their reliance on technical devices for sending as well as receiving messages. Telephone, music, film, radio, television, and the Internet are examples of mechanical/electronic media.

In today's health care system, health care providers are presented with unique challenges and opportunities in communicating health information to patients with different types of communication needs and preferences. To illustrate, since effective provider–patient communication is essential for health literacy (Koch-Weser, Rudd, & Dejong, 2010; Kripalani et al., 2010), computerized entertainment education (Jibaja-Weiss & Volk, 2007) and augmentative and alternative communication (AAC) tools and strategies—picture communication boards, alphabet boards, computers, and Speech Generating Devices (SGDs)—can be used to help address health literacy problems among communication-vulnerable patients—those with speech, language, hearing, vision, and cognitive impairments (Costello, Patak, & Pritchard, 2010). Hence, the type of media used might have different consequences on health literacy depending on whether presentational, representational, or electronic media is used to transmit messages.

MEDIA EFFECTS

As consumers of mass media, we ought to think about their power and ask ourselves in what ways—if, when, how, and why—we are influenced by newspapers, books, magazines, television, radio, film, music, and the Internet. Canadian communication scholar Marshall McLuhan (1973) called attention to the importance of the particular medium used for communicating messages. Scholars in communication, education, psychology, sociology, anthropology, and political science, among other fields, have been studying media effects. Decades of research on media influence show the complexity of measuring media effects because of its variance by medium (e.g., television, radio, print, Internet), consumption (e.g., time spent daily, weekly, or monthly watching television, listening to radio, reading newspapers, surfing the Internet), and other mediating factors, such as socio-demographics (e.g., age, gender, ethnicity, occupation, income, household size).

When considering media effects on health and the application of media use in public health promotion, Finnegan and Viswanath (2008) highlighted three important media effects: (1) the knowledge gap, (2) agenda setting, and (3) cultivation of shared public perceptions.

The *knowledge gap* (introduced in Chapter 4) refers to mass media's unequal distribution of information within a social system. For example, members of underserved populations may not be well informed about health issues because of limited access to relevant health information (Institute of Medicine, 2004; Welinrich et al., 2007). Hence, factors such as appeal, accessibility, and desirability of media content, and the amount of social conflict and diversity there is in a community, can influence the impact of mass media on audience knowledge gaps.

As an important media effects theory, *agenda setting* was advanced by McCombs and Shaw (see Shah, McLeod, Gotlieb, & Lee, 2009). In their investigation of the United States presidential campaigns in 1968, McCombs and Shaw (1972) found that the mass media wielded a powerful influence on what voters considered to be the major issues of the campaign. Focusing on the agenda-setting function of news media, McCombs (2004) argued: "Through their day-by-day selection and display of the news, editors and news directors focus our attention and influence our perceptions of what are the most important issues of the day. This ability to influence the salience of topics on the public agenda has come to be called the agenda-setting role of the news media" (p. 1). In other words, the agenda-setting theory suggests that "mass media decision makers decide what is news-worthy, what is entertaining, what is to be advertised and promoted. By doing so, they establish the topics that people think about" (Hiebert & Gibbons, 2000, p. 132). Accordingly, news media set the public agenda about what are considered to be important issues, including those related to health.

Cultivation refers to the extent to which media exposure shapes audience perceptions over a period of time. For example, heavy exposure to television may cultivate or lead to the belief in viewers that the real world is similar to the televised world (Gerbner, Gross, Signorielli, & Morgan, 1980). Think about the medical interactions that occur in popular television shows such as *Grey's Anatomy* or *House* or *ER* and compare these with the dynamics in actual community hospitals!

Scholars have also identified two other potential media effects: (1) priming, and (2) framing. *Priming* indicates that media messages may stimulate recall of stored ideas, knowledge, opinions, or experience associated in some way with the message content (Fiske & Taylor, 1991). *Framing* reveals how stories are told. According to Reese (2001), the framing approach began with sociologist Erving Goffman (1974) and anthropologist-psychologist Gregory Bateson (1972), and refers to "the way events and issues are organized and made sense of, especially by media, media professionals, and their audiences" (p. 7). Framing in the context of media effects research "denotes the idea that the media deal with certain issues in different ways and that, therefore, the issue is covered and reported to the public in different frames or perspectives" (Kohring & Matthes, 2002, p. 143). According to Entman (1993), "Framing essentially involves selection and salience. To frame is to select some aspects of a perceived reality and make them more salient in a communicating text, in such a way as to promote a particular problem definition, causal interpretation, moral evaluation, and/or treatment recommendation for the item described" (p. 52).

Thus, the framing of news in the media can influence the recipient's knowledge, perception, and opinion of that news (Price, Tewksbury, & Powers, 1997; Scheufele, 1999). Framing effects research has focused on the effect of news frames on the cognitive, attitudinal, and behavioural outcomes of those who receive them (Price et al., 1997; Shah et al., 2009). For example, studies have found that the framing of news stories influences readers' knowledge (Coleman & Thorson, 2002), decision making (Shah, Domke, & Wackman, 1996), and public opinion (de Vreese, Boomgaarden, & Semetko, 2011).

Scholars have examined how media framing of public health issues, such as avian flu (Dudo, Dahlstrom, & Brossard, 2007; Nerlich & Halliday, 2007) and the HPV vaccine (St. John, Pitts, & Tufts, 2010), shapes the public's understanding of health risks and health behaviour, and impacts health literacy. (See Chapter 8 for further discussion of the effects of media framing.)

In their study of news media attribution of blame associated with a controversial medical study linking the measles, mumps, and rubella (MMR) vaccination with autism, Holton, Weberling, Clarke, and Smith (2012) found that news media framing of public health issues plays a potentially vital role in shaping public behaviour, in this case, in rates of vaccination uptake. The study underscores the important role news media coverage plays in directing attention to and in framing important public health issues and the importance of effective communication about public health risks.

Hinnant, Oh, Caburnay, and Kreuter (2011) examined journalists' role in shaping health news story framing. Existing literature reveals that negatively framed news stories (e.g., disparities between racial groups) could have unintended consequences on African-Americans' general health-seeking behaviour (e.g., delays in seeking medical treatment). They found that informing journalists of audience reactions to race-specific health information could influence journalists' rating of the disparity-frame story more favourably, and thus potentially influence how health news stories are framed.

Hanson (2005) categorized media effects into four categories: (1) *cognitive*, in which the amount of learning from media content depends on consumer motivation; (2) *attitudinal*, where consumer thoughts about a product, person, or idea are shaped by media content; (3) *behavioural*, where consumers may adopt or emulate a certain behaviour that they see on television or in a movie; and (4) *psychological*, in which media content can arouse feelings of joy, fear, amusement, or revulsion in consumers.

MEDIA EFFECTS ON HEALTH

There is a growing body of research on media's influence on health, especially among young people, given their regular consumption of mass media (Manganello, 2008). The following brief selection of sample studies illustrates the influence of media on youth health.

ALCOHOL, TOBACCO, AND OTHER DRUGS

Snyder, Milici, Slater, Sun, and Strizhakova (2006) found that alcohol advertising contributed to increased alcohol consumption among youth. Those youth who were more exposed to alcohol advertisements drank more on average relative to those who did not view the advertisements. In fact, with each additional exposure to an advertisement there was a 1 percent increase in the number of drinks consumed by the youth. From a profitability perspective, youth exposed to greater alcohol advertising drank more, and each additional dollar spent per capita increased the number of drinks consumed by 3 percent.

BODY IMAGE, NUTRITION, AND FITNESS

Highly cited research comparing body shape and weight measurements of popular toy dolls (Barbie and Ken) to young adults reflects the unrealistic yet culturally acceptable standards for body shape and weight (Brownell & Napolitano, 1995). Using hip measurements as a constant, researchers calculated the change in body measurement and weight needed for a young, healthy adult woman and man to attain the same body proportions as the Barbie and Ken dolls respectively. The changes in body measurement required to conform to the Barbie and Ken ideal were significant (see Table 7.1).

TABLE 7.1: BODY MEASUREMENT CHANGES TO ATTAIN BODY IDEAL FOR MEN AND WOMEN

Gender	Height	Chest	Waist
Changes in female form to look like Barbie	24 inch increase	5 inch increase	6 inch decrease
Changes in male form to look like Ken	20 inch increase	11 inch increase	10 inch increase

Source: Modified from Brownell, K.D., & Napolitano, M.A. (1995, p. 297). Distorting reality for children: Body size proportions of Barbie and Ken dolls. *International Journal of Eating Disorders, 18*(3), 295–298.

Researchers have concluded that mass media (e.g., television, advertising) directed at children present unrealistic shape and weight ideals for boys and girls. Mass media persist as a powerful influence even today (Derenne & Beresin, 2006). Van den Berg, Neumark-Sztainer, Hannan, and Haines (2007) evaluated the association between reading frequency of magazine articles about dieting or weight loss and weight-control behaviours and psychological outcomes in a sample of adolescents. Their findings revealed that reading frequency of magazine articles about dieting or weight loss predicted unhealthy weight-control behaviours in adolescent girls, but not boys. The researchers urged for interventions for reducing exposure to media messages regarding dieting and weight loss.

AGGRESSIVE BEHAVIOUR AND VIOLENCE

Murray (2008) argued that television remains the most widely used screen media format, despite the emergence of new media technologies. Yet concerns have arisen about the effects of television on the health and well-being of children and adolescents. Existing research suggests that excessive television viewing is associated with negative effects on sleep, attention, and interpersonal relationships. For example, aggressive attitudes or behaviour in children and adolescents have been linked to viewing violent TV programs. The researcher called for more research and emphasized the importance of education on the appropriate use of media with youth.

SEXUAL BEHAVIOUR AND ATTITUDES

Highlighting the role of media as the leading sex educator for American children and adolescents (with more than 80 percent of the top teen shows containing sexual content, and the average teen exposed to nearly 14,000 sexual references on television alone), Strasburger (2005) called on parents and teachers to realize the educational power of the media and urged them to begin incorporating principles of media literacy into existing sex education programs.

OBESITY

The 2004 Canadian Community Health Survey reported a rapid increase in the percentage of children and adolescents who are overweight or obese (Shields, 2005; 2006). For example, while 12 percent of two- to seventeen-year-olds were overweight and 3 percent were obese in 1978/1979, the overweight and obesity rates for this age group had risen to 18 percent and to 8 percent, respectively, by 2004. "Screen time," meaning time spent on activities such as watching television, playing video games, and using the computer, is common among many Canadian youth and is a factor associated with overweight and obesity among young people. In 2004, the daily screen time for 36 percent of children age six to eleven was more than 2 hours (see Figure 7.1). These children were twice as likely to be overweight in comparison to children who logged a total of an hour or less screen time each day (35 percent versus 18 percent), and about twice as likely to be obese (11 percent versus 5 percent).

Shields (2005, 2006) reported that keeping track of screen time trends has become complicated with the rapid proliferation of video games and home computers. For example, according to the 1988 Campbell's Survey on Health and Well-being, average weekly television viewing for twelve- to seventeen-year-olds was 9 hours and increasing to 10 hours per week in 2004. However, the total average screen time for adolescents doubled to 20 hours per week with the inclusion of time spent on the computer and playing video games (as shown in Figure 7.2). The good news is that factors affecting overweight and obesity rates, such as spending less time watching television and playing video games, and increasing consumption of fruit and vegetables and engaging in physical activity, are considered modifiable. More importantly, media literacy can play an important role in helping advance health literacy efforts in this fight.

FIGURE 7.1: OVERWEIGHT AND OBESITY RATES AMONG CHILDREN AGE 6–11, BY DAILY HOURS OF SCREEN TIME, CANADA, EXCLUDING TERRITORIES, 2004

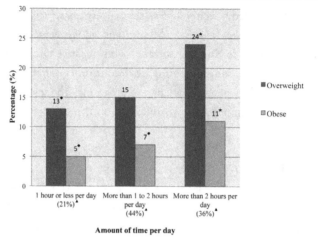

Source: Modified from Shields, M. (2005, p. 28). Measured obesity: Overweight Canadian children and adolescents. Chart 12. *Nutrition: Findings from the Canadian Community Health Survey.* Cat. No. 82-620-MWE. Ottawa, ON: Statistics Canada. Retrieved from http://s3.amazonaws.com/zanran_storage/www.calgaryhealthregion.ca/Content-Pages/18451313.pdf [accessed: 14 June 2013].

FIGURE 7.2: OVERWEIGHT AND OBESITY RATES AMONG ADOLESCENTS AGE 12–17, BY WEEKLY HOURS OF SCREEN TIME, CANADA, EXCLUDING TERRITORIES, 2004

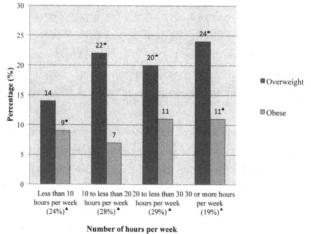

Source: Modified from Shields, M. (2005, p. 29). Measured obesity: Overweight Canadian children and adolescents. Chart 13. *Nutrition: Findings from the Canadian Community Health Survey.* Cat. No. 82-620-MWE. Ottawa, ON: Statistics Canada. Retrieved from http://s3.amazonaws.com/zanran_storage/www.calgaryhealthregion.ca/Content-Pages/18451313.pdf [accessed: 14 June 2013].

Studies have also investigated the health-promoting effects of media on young people's health behaviour. Rosenkoetter, Rosenkoetter, and Acock (2009) reported results from a year-long intervention undertaken with children in grade school in an effort to minimize the harmful effects of violent TV. The intervention resulted in a reduction in children's viewing of violent TV as well as in less identification with violent television characters. Developing TV literacy programs may help reduce some of the potentially harmful effects of violent TV on young viewers. The American Academy of Pediatrics (2010) recognizes the potential of media education to reduce the harmful effects of media (e.g., television, movies, video and computer games, the Internet, music lyrics and videos, newspapers, magazines, books, advertising) and support positive effects on children and adolescents' health.

Based on short-term early childhood educational achievement to long-term study results, the preschool television series *Sesame Street* is considered to be an effective health-promoting medium (Cole, 2009). Over the past four decades, *Sesame Street* has aired in over 130 countries. Literacy and health issues have been part of the special educational focus of selected *Sesame Street* international co-productions. Developed by local production teams, the international co-productions of *Sesame Street* feature indigenous puppet characters and sets that are based on educational frameworks designed to provide culturally relevant experiences and promote the unique learning needs of children around the world. Although few in number, studies offer insights into the impact of *Sesame Street*'s health intervention on children and their parents' knowledge and perceptions about health issues. Cole called for more research to gauge the educational potential of children's media, more specifically *Sesame Street*, to change children's health behaviour.

REVIEW AND REFLECT

Considering the potential impact of media proliferation on health literacy, do you see any possible danger associated with such issues as "accessibility," "misuse," or even "information overload"?

MASS MEDIA HEALTH CAMPAIGNS

When examining the impact of mass media on health literacy promotion, certain questions arise. Can media campaigns and the design of messages close the gap in health literacy? And what are the potential dangers associated with individuals' "access to" or "misuse of" information about their health? We live in a media-saturated world and are increasingly using the media as a key source of health information (Chen & Siu, 2001; Kickbusch, 2001; Manafo & Wong, 2012). Mass media are important channels for the delivery of health-related information. According to Noar (2006), "A compelling health communication intervention tool that potentially can address health attitude and behavioral change across numerous health problems and in numerous audiences is the mass media campaign" (p. 22). While mass media provide important communication tools in promoting health literacy goals, communicating mediated health information effectively is far more important than before. As consumers of an increasing amount of health information from multiple types of media, both traditional and new, we are called upon to critically evaluate the quality of this mediated health information. Ask yourself if you have the capacity to access, understand, evaluate, and communicate mediated information to promote health. Do you know which mediated information is important for you to take care of your health?

Mass media have an important role in presenting growing information regarding different aspects of prevention, health promotion, and treatment for patients, their families, and health care providers. In this regard, basic persuasion strategies such as advertising and information campaigns are pertinent to health literacy. Health communicators can employ a variety of mass media channels, such as newspapers, magazines, radio, and television, to design com-munication programs to inform and influence individual and community health. However, as argued by Payne and Schulte (2003), "mass media agendas and health communication objectives can be authoritative allies or forceful foes when it comes to supplying the public with accurate and timely health information" (p. 124). Rootman and Gordon-El-Bihbety (2008) argued for "developing and undertaking a coordinated multi-media campaign to increase awareness of the issue of health literacy in Canada among the public and specific audiences" (p. 6).

Silverblatt (2004) called attention to "the emergence of mass media as a social institution, which has assumed many of the functions formerly served by traditional social institution such the church, school, government, and family" (p. 35) and, hence, the case for media literacy.

REVIEW AND REFLECT

Think about recent health-related mass media campaigns in Canada. Select one campaign that you think has been successful, and explain its success.

MEDIA LITERACY

The importance of media literacy for a health-literate society cannot be overemphasized. Canada has been the pioneer in developing media literacy, a "term most commonly used in North America, especially in relationship to media education for youth" (Tyner, 2010, p. 3). A case in point is compulsory media education for students in grades 7 through 12 in Ontario since 1987 (Tyner, 2010).

What is media literacy? Why is media literacy especially important in this media-saturated world that we live in today? Buckingham (2003) defined *media education* as "the process of teaching and learning about media" and *media literacy* as "the outcome—the knowledge and skills learners acquires" (p. 4). On the most basic level, media literacy includes the skills to access, analyze, evaluate, and produce information in a variety of media formats (Pungente, 2002–2011; Silverblatt, 2001). According to Silverblatt's (2001) definition of media literacy, a media-literate person should have a number of characteristics (see Table 7.2).

TABLE 7.2: CHARACTERISTICS OF A MEDIA-LITERATE INDIVIDUAL

Characteristics
Possess critical-thinking skill for developing independent opinion about media content
Have an understanding of the mass communication process
Be aware of media's impact on the individual and society
Develop strategies for analyzing and discussing media messages
Be cognizant of media content that provides insight into our lives and culture
Greatly enjoy, understand, and appreciate media content
Acquire effective and responsible media message production skills

Source: Table modified from Silverblatt, A. (2001, pp. 23). *Media literacy: Keys to interpreting media messages* (2nd ed.). Westport, CT: Praeger Publishers.

The Ontario Media Literacy Resource Guide defined media literacy as being concerned with helping students develop an informed and critical understanding of the nature of mass media, the techniques used by them, and the impact of these techniques (Pungente, 1993). More specifically, it is education that aims to increase students' understanding and enjoyment of how the media work, how they produce meaning, how they are organized, and how they construct reality. Media literacy also aims to provide students with the ability to create media products.

From the above definitions it is important for us to recognize that media literacy does not protect us from superfluous messages. Rather, it teaches us the skills necessary to become critical consumers of media messages for our personal and social growth and development—an important aspect of health literacy. As argued by Buckingham (2003), media education "does not aim to shield young people from the influence of the media and thereby lead them to do 'better' things, but enable them to make informed decisions on their own behalf" (p. 13).

The Ontario Association for Media Literacy developed the following key concepts of media literacy that offer teachers a framework for helping students critically analyze media messages and which have important implications for health literacy. These are highlighted in Table 7.3.

TABLE 7.3: ONTARIO ASSOCIATION FOR MEDIA LITERACY KEY CONCEPTS

Key concepts
All media are constructions.
Each person interprets messages differently.
The media have commercial interests.
The media contain ideological and value messages.
Each medium has its own language, style, techniques, codes, conventions, and aesthetics.
The media have commercial implications.
The media have social and political implications.
Form and content are closely related in the media.

Source: Table modified from Pungente, J.J. (2002–2011; paras. 3–10). Canada's key concepts of media literacy. *Center for Media Literacy.* Retrieved from http://www.medialit.org/reading-room/canadas-key-concepts-media-literacy [accessed: 17 June 2013].

According to Potter (2004), media literacy involves cognitive processes and critical thinking skills that can be applied to media messages. He identified four dimensions of media literacy: (1) cognitive, (2) emotional, (3) aesthetic, and (4) moral. The cognitive dimension of media literacy involves the ability to intellectually process media information. The emotional dimension refers to the feelings evoked by media messages. The aesthetic dimension involves the skill to interpret media messages from an artistic or critical point of view. The moral dimension deals with the examination of the value of media messages. Given these four dimensions, media literacy has great potential to enhance health literacy efforts. As with media literacy, being health literate involves cognitive processes and critical thinking skills—developing communication skills, including listening; asking questions, finding, and evaluating quality health information; and using that information to lead a healthy life. Hence, in today's information-rich society, we can certainly exploit the potential of media literacy to facilitate our understanding of mediated health information, processes, and systems for advancing health literacy and improving public health.

MEDIA LITERACY INITIATIVES IN CANADA

Canada is recognized as an international leader in media literacy education. Table 7.4 illustrates the milestones in Canadian media literacy initiatives. The interested reader is encouraged to refer to the "Additional Resources of Interest" at the end of the chapter for details about each initiative.

TABLE 7.4: MILESTONES IN MEDIA LITERACY INITIATIVES IN CANADA

Year	Initiative
1978	The Association for Media Literacy (AML) was formed by Barry Duncan and colleagues and members of the National Film Board of Canada.
1979	Task Force on Sex Role Stereotyping was established.
1982	MediaWatch was founded to monitor issues on sex-role stereotyping in the media.
1984	Jesuit Communication Project was founded to promote media education across Canada.
1987	Ontario introduced media literacy into secondary school curricula.
1992	Canadian Association of Media Literacy Organizations (CAMEO) was created to promote media literacy across the country.
1996	Media Awareness Network was incorporated and launched on the World Wide Web.

Source: Modified from Ontario Health Promotion E-Bulletin. (n.d.). Media literacy. *OHPE Bulletin 37, 1998*(37). Retrieved from http://www.ohpe.ca/node/19 [accessed: 17 June 2013].

In 2004, the Canadian Media Research Consortium, a partnership of the University of British Columbia School of Journalism, the York Ryerson Graduate Program in Culture and Communications, and Centre d'études sur les médias at Université Laval, released the first independent national survey of Canadian attitudes and behaviour regarding news media and media credibility (Hayward, Pannozzo, & Colman, 2007). Just over 3,000 Canadian adults reported what they thought about the news and whether or not they trusted the media. The survey results regarding the use and source of news are presented in Table 7.5.

TABLE 7.5: SELF-REPORTED USE AND SOURCE OF NEWS BY CANADIANS

Use and source of news
Television news: While 67% of Canadians watch television news daily, and nearly 90% watch several times a week, only 6% of Canadians never watch the news.
Radio news: 57% of Canadians listen to radio news every day.
Newspaper: 42% of Canadians read a newspaper daily.
Internet for news: 33% of Canadians use the Internet for news, many of whom use mainstream media websites. Canadians under the age of 35 with a university education and incomes over $75,000 are most likely to use the Internet daily for news. 67% of Canadians reported rarely or never using the Internet for news.

Source: Modified from Hayward, K., Pannozzo, L., & Colman, R. (2007, p. 382). *Developing indicators for the educated populace domain of the Canadian Index of Wellbeing: Background information literature review.* Document 2, Parts IV–VI (of VI). Retrieved from http://uwaterloo.ca/canadian-index-wellbeing/sites/ca.canadian-index-wellbeing/files/uploads/files/Historical-Educated_Populace_Literature_Review_Doc2_August_2007.sflb_.pdf [accessed: 17 June 2013].

The survey results regarding perceived credibility, accuracy, and bias of news are presented in Table 7.6.

TABLE 7.6: PERCEPTIONS OF CREDIBILITY, ACCURACY, AND BIAS OF NEWS

Perceived credibility, accuracy, and bias of news
59% of Canadians thought the news was accurate.
While 37% of Canadians found the news was often fair, 62% found the news was often unbalanced, and 19% deemed the news to be rarely or not at all balanced.
Nearly 80% of Canadians consider reporters' bias to often or sometimes affect news.
While 54% of Canadians found the news media attempt to cover up their mistakes, 34% found the news media willing to admit their mistakes.

Source: Modified from Hayward, K., Pannozzo, L., & Colman, R. (2007, pp. 382–383). *Developing indicators for the educated populace domain of the Canadian Index of Wellbeing: Background information literature review.* Document 2, Parts IV–VI (of VI). Retrieved from http://uwaterloo.ca/canadian-index-wellbeing/sites/ca.canadian-index-wellbeing/files/uploads/files/Historical-Educated_Populace_Literature_Review_Doc2_August_2007.sflb_.pdf [accessed: 17 June 2013].

The survey results regarding perceived news independence are presented in Table 7.7.

TABLE 7.7: PERCEPTIONS OF NEWS INDEPENDENCE

Perceived news independence
While 19% of Canadians found news organizations to be generally independent, 76% of adult Canadians overall and 81% of Canadian youth ages 19 to 25 found powerful people and organizations as influencing news organizations.
Political interests (42%), which included local and federal governments, politicians, and bureaucrats, was the most frequently mentioned group as affecting the news. Economic interests (27%), including people with money and perceived influence, businesses, and large corporations, was the second-largest group mentioned as affecting the news.
While 12% of Canadians found media owners as having an influence on the news, and 56% of Canadians deemed consolidation of media ownership to negatively affect their trust in the media, 12% deemed lobby groups, 4% deemed advertisers, and 3% deemed protest groups to affect the news.

Source: Modified from Hayward, K., Pannozzo, L., & Colman, R. (2007, p. 383). *Developing indicators for the educated populace domain of the Canadian Index of Wellbeing: Background information literature review.* Document 2, Parts IV–VI (of VI). Retrieved from http://uwaterloo.ca/canadian-index-wellbeing/sites/ca.canadian-index-wellbeing/files/uploads/files/Historical-Educated_Populace_Literature_Review_Doc2_August_2007.sflb_.pdf [accessed: 17 June 2013].

Given that a large number of Canadians have a daily diet of mass media news, there is a great need for Canadians to be media literate. As Hayward, Pannozzo, and Colman (2007) argued:

> After all, if most Canadians think that the news is generally not fair and balanced, that the media try to cover up their mistakes, that reporters' bias influences reporting, that news sensationalism reduces their trust, and that news organizations are not independent but subject to influence by powerful people and organizations, then there is clearly a serious problem in public perceptions of the media and a correspondingly pressing need for Canadians to be able to evaluate the media critically and effectively. (pp. 383–384)

Simultaneously, the dearth of empirical data calls for more reliable and consistent data collection efforts (Hayward, Pannozzo, & Colman, 2007). Given that trust and credibility impact the processing of information (Covello, 1992), please see further discussion on their importance in Chapter 8.

MEDIA LITERACY FOR ADVANCING HEALTH LITERACY

Rootman et al. (2002) identified media literacy as one of the areas where more research is needed in Canada to improve health care providers' communicative abilities to improve health literacy among consumers. More specifically, they called for research on the impact of health communication and drug advertising on consumers. How can media literacy help advance health literacy? Payne and Schulte (2003) underscored the "mediated reality" and "misinformation that is often rampant in medical and health stories" and the need for steps "to minimize potentially harmful effects and provide consumers with the skills necessary to apply specific health information to their own lives" (p. 124).

As media applications have become a regular part of the public health environment, considering media literacy in light of health literacy is essential. In order to advance effective communication in health care to deliver effective health care and promote health, health care providers, consumers, and educators need to recognize and use the power of media. Media literacy education can address a variety of relevant health literacy concerns. As argued by Bergsma (2004), within a framework of media literacy and health promotion for youth, media literacy is an innovative health promotion and prevention strategy. Media literacy can be an effective approach for behaviour change among adolescents. In their study evaluating the effectiveness of a media literacy school-based health education intervention as a method of tobacco prevention for high school students, Gonzales, Glik, Davoudi, and Ang (2004) found that "a curriculum that integrates media literacy and health promotion gives high school students an opportunity to acquire the knowledge and skills needed to recognize social pressure that goes beyond peer pressure, one that is woven into the very fabric of everyday youth culture and social norms" (p. 198).

In their study of the promotion of health empowerment and health behaviour among adolescents, Levin-Zamir, Lemish, and Gofin (2011) developed the concept and measure of Media Health Literacy (MHL). According to Levin-Zamir, Lemish, and Gofin (2011), "The concept of MHL is based on the premise that the individual has the capability to control the determinants influencing his or her health through thought and action" (pp. 324–325). Rooted in the theoretical foundations of Nutbeam's (2000) model for both health literacy and media literacy (both based on models of empowerment), MHL provides "a new conceptual framework that integrates the fields of literacy, adolescent health, health behavior and media, providing a basis for a reliable, empirical measure to assess cognitive, attitudinal and behavioral characteristics that explain responses of adolescents to explicit and implicit health-related media content" (p. 324). Although a first-time effort, the findings of the study demonstrated MHL as measurable and scalable. Figure 7.3 illustrates the research model—the characteristics and measurements—of MHL.

However, Levin-Zamir, Lemish, and Gofin (2011) call for future research; further testing of the model by moving beyond Jewish urban adolescent public school settings in Israel to "consider the influence of MHL in achieving outcomes through promoting adolescents' critical thinking, reasoned choices and active participation in promoting their own health"; and to further apply MHL "to other media and among ethnically diverse populations" (p. 334).

FIGURE 7.3: RESEARCH MODEL OF MEDIA HEALTH LITERACY

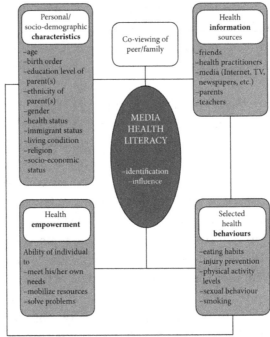

Source: Modified from Levin-Zamir, D., Lemish, D., & Gofin, R. (2011, p. 326). Media Health Literacy (MHL): Development and measurement of the concept among adolescents. *Health Education Research, 26*(2), 323–335.

Considering the social determinants of health perspective, being media health literate involves developing an understanding that mediated health information is shaped by social, economic, cultural, and political contexts. For instance, in looking into media representations of breastfeeding, studies have found that "the media are more often contributing to perceptions that breastfeeding is difficult for mothers and potentially dangerous for babies" (Brown & Peuchard, 2008, para. 1) and have attributed such media representations to market forces, with breastfeeding advocates lacking the money needed to spend on advertising compared to "the infant formula companies with large advertising budgets" (para. 6). Such media representations of breastfeeding reveal how media discourses are often driven by profit within commercial, ideological, or political contexts. Hence, the commercial implications of the media underscore the importance of developing media literacy skills to help promote health literacy.

The Consortium for Media Literacy (2012) considers media literacy education as a cognitive intervention strategy for health and accordingly delivers media education for youth, parents, educators, and community organizations for the advancement of media literacy in areas such as nutrition, body image, violence prevention, sexuality, and geriatrics, among others.

Media health literacy is as much a process as an outcome. It requires constant attention and upgrading, and is much like health literacy in being a practice-driven skill. It is not only about receiving health information and having the ability to understand and make sense of it; it is also about being able to identify or distinguish the source of that information. As described by Natharius (2004), "We have to treat all information with a certain degree of skepticism and caution, particularly regarding the source" (p. 245). Natharius (2004) emphasized the role of visual perception in media literacy, suggesting that "we are moving from a world of literacy to a world of visuality" (p. 242). Olson and Pollard (2004) bring our attention to the "digitalization of media [which] both requires and enables new ways of looking at media literacy education" (p. 248). Today's media-rich environment has greatly increased the availability of a wide array of communication channels and created new patterns of health information–seeking and usage. However, what good is this information if it is confusing and unreliable? How do we determine the accuracy of health news articles? How can we evaluate the credibility of television health news? How do we establish whether food advertisement messages are misleading? How can we find reliable health information on the Internet? Understanding the mediated context improves the potential for the health message to be understood and acted upon, increasing its effectiveness. Media literacy skills can aid us in critically processing health-related information from newspapers, television, advertising, and the Internet, and foster application of that understanding in our everyday lives; hence the link between media literacy and health literacy. In fact, Higgins and Begoray (2012) offered a working definition of critical media health literacy:

> [C]ritical media health literacy (CMHL) is a right of citizenship and empowers individuals and groups, in a risky consumer society, to critically interpret and use media as a means to engage in decision-making processes and dialogues; exert control over their health and everyday events; and make healthy changes for themselves and their communities. (p. 142)

The principles and key questions presented in Table 7.8 can be a helpful exercise in developing media health literacy.

TABLE 7.8: UNDERSTANDING MEDIA CONSTRUCTION OF HEALTH MESSAGES

	Principle	Key question
1.	All media messages are carefully crafted constructions.	Who created this health message?
2.	Media messages represent reality and contain values and viewpoints.	What lifestyles, values, and viewpoints are represented in, or omitted from, this health message?
3.	Media messages are constructed using a unique set of rules.	What techniques are used to draw attention to this health message?
4.	Individuals interpret and make meaning of media messages based on their personal experiences.	How might different people interpret this health message?
5.	Most media messages are driven by profit within commercial, ideological, or political contexts.	Why was this health message communicated?

Source: Modified from Castellanos, L.M. (2007, p. 13). *Media literacy and health behaviour among children and adolescents.* WHO Technical Meeting on Building School Partnership for Health, Education Achievements and Development, Vancouver, Canada, June 5–8. Retrieved from http://www.jcsh-cces.ca/upload/Dr.%20Mantilla%20-%20Abstract%20Dr.%20Mantilla.pdf [accessed: 17 June 2013].

PROMOTING HEALTH LITERACY THROUGH ETHNIC MEDIA

Canada is experiencing an extraordinary increase in ethnocultural diversity (see Chapter 5 to review the concepts of culture and ethnicity). This increase in population diversity has been accompanied by a proliferation of online, radio, print, and television media actively created by ethnic and visible minority groups (Murray, Yu, & Ahadi, 2007; Ojo, 2006). Table 7.9 lists some examples of ethnic media outlets in Canada.

TABLE 7.9: SOME ETHNIC MEDIA OUTLETS IN CANADA

Newspapers	Canada China News (Chinese)
	Eco Latino (Spanish)
	Il Postino (Italian)
	Muslim Link
	The Ottawa Weekend (Chinese)
	Sada Almashrek (Arab)
	Canadian Courier (Russian)
	Al-Akhbar (Arabic)
	Akhbaar-e-Pakistan
	The Eastern News (Pakistani)
	First Nations Drum
Magazines	Ottawa Jewish Bulletin
	Egypt and the Arab World
	Canadian Immigrant
	Desi News (South Asian)
Radio	CHIN
	Radio Tibet
TV	The Aboriginal Peoples Television Network (APTN)

In today's communication-rich environment, these local, community, and ethnic media present untapped opportunities to close the health literacy gap among culturally and linguistically diverse groups in terms of communicating health information in trusted and linguistically appropriate ways. As argued by Amzel and Ghosh (2007), "Because of the general public's low rate of health literacy, the health world should collaborate with the media to present a consistent, simple message concerning gaps in care experienced by all racial/ethnic minority groups" (p. 1120). Furthermore, mainstream media and ethnic media outlets can partner to meet the health literacy needs of culturally, linguistically, and geographically isolated population groups.

Studies have found population subgroup differences in exposure to health information and source of health information used (Benjamin-Garner et al., 2002; Woodall et al., 2006). Although Stryker, Fishman, Emmons, and Viswanath (2009) found that both mainstream and ethnic newspapers rarely communicated numerically the magnitude of specific cancer risk factors, they did hold that "ethnic newspapers may have a stronger commitment to cancer prevention and education than do mainstream newspapers" (para. 39). Donelle and colleagues also raised important questions about the credibility of health information in newspapers. Considering the need for numeracy skills to understand genetic risks, Donelle, Hoffman-Goetz, and Clarke (2004) studied the portrayal of genetic risk for breast cancer in mass print ethnic (Ashkenazi Jews) and non-ethnic (general Canadian population) newspapers. The findings reveal inconsistent messaging about the value of genetic screening for breast cancer evenly across both ethnic and non-ethnic newspapers. Even the statistics were presented in complex and contradictory ways, making the decoding of the information likely incomprehensible.

In a Canadian context, mediated health information ought to be multilingual, culturally appropriate, and easy to read and understand. Relatively large gaps exist in the average level of health literacy among different subpopulation groups within Canada, especially between those who are employed and those who are unemployed and between immigrants and non-immigrants (CCL, 2008a). In addition, on average, seniors (aged 66 and older) have much lower levels of health literacy skills. The elderly, immigrants (especially those who do not speak either French or English), and the unemployed are at greater risk because of lower levels of health literacy skills (ibid.). Canadian consumers need to be taught how to evaluate and mediate health information sources and resources. In 2005, Alia and Bull called Canada "the world in indigenous broadcasting" with several hundred radio stations (p. 107). Launched in 1999, the Aboriginal Peoples Television Network (APTN) is the world's first broadcast network to have been produced by minority people and made available to all Canadians (Alia & Bull, 2005).

Ethnic media can provide important channels for producing tailored, culturally appropriate messages to address health literacy barriers (Canadian Public Health Association, 2006a). While culturally and linguistically diverse people in Canada may receive important health-related information, they may not be getting health information to help them become educated about their health and keep them engaged in promoting good health. Hoffman-Goetz, Shannon, and Clarke (2003) examined both the volume and focus of articles on four chronic diseases (cancer, cardiovascular disease, diabetes, and HIV/AIDS) in newspapers targeting First Nations, Métis, and Inuit in Canada. The study found more articles on HIV/AIDS and diabetes, and few articles on cancer and cardiovascular disease. Limited efforts had been made to provide mobilizing information to help readers take further health action, and more importantly, articles on cardiovascular disease and diabetes virtually did not have any mobilizing information. Considering the prevalence of tobacco-related cardiovascular disease and cancer among Aboriginal people in Canada, Hoffman-Goetz and colleagues (2003) called "the lack of coverage and limited mobilizing information in ethnic newspapers" as "a missed opportunity for health promotion" (p. 475).

Consuming health information and translating it into behaviour change requires the cultural tailoring of messages. For example, in their study of the presentation of cancer information in mass media that target ethnic minorities in Canada, Hoffman-Goetz and Friedman (2005) found that cancer coverage in 25 ethnic minority (Jewish, First Nations, Black/Caribbean, and East Indian) and 7 mainstream English-language newspapers did not accurately reflect the leading causes of cancer death in the country. In order to inform high-risk subgroups of ethnic minorities and appropriately tailor prevention and treatment programs, the researchers recommended mass print media disaggregate cancer statistics by ethnicity. In her study, Nimmon (2007) found that participatory photonovels can be used as an empowering functional health literacy tool with English-as-a-Second-Language Canadian immigrant women. Thus, ethnic media can be an integral part of effective health literacy media promotion efforts among culturally diverse immigrant communities in Canada. The following are some ways in which ethnic media can play this role:

- Serve as a public education tool in communicating general health information
- Debunk common health myths
- Provide an alternative viewpoint in commenting on health or health care–related issues

---

REVIEW AND REFLECT

With a growing immigrant population from all over the world, Canada has become more multicultural. In a Canadian context, what opportunities do ethnic media offer for bridging gaps in health literacy among culturally diverse groups? Do you perceive any potential barrier to these efforts?

KEY LEARNING POINTS

The mass media are important channels for the delivery of health-related information. These mediated channels have a key role in presenting growing information regarding different aspects of prevention, health promotion, and treatment for patients, their families, and health care providers, and thus can help in the pursuit of improved health literacy ability. Mass media offer both opportunities and challenges to the advancement of health literacy efforts. This chapter highlighted both positive and negative influences of existing mass media content on health literacy goals. Existing literature found positive effects of mass media influences on health outcomes, such as reproductive health behaviour and attitudes toward family planning. Negative effects of mass media influences on health outcomes include drinking, smoking, eating disorders, obesity, violence, and sexual risk behaviours. Given mass media's potential in advancing health literacy goals, there is an increased demand for collaboration among health care providers, practitioners, policy-makers, and consumers to realize these goals. What are the media strategies that promote health literacy? To what extent can mediated health messages positively influence health knowledge, attitude, and behaviour?

Canada has made great strides in integrating media literacy standards and curricula into its educational system. The increased availability of mediated health information comes with the responsibility to teach consumers how to evaluate the quality of that information. Accordingly, we need to become active consumers of mediated health information to leverage media's power in influencing behaviour change and public policy in ways that can help improve health literacy. In a multicultural society like Canada, ethnic media offers promising opportunities for bridging the health literacy gap among diverse population groups who are culturally, linguistically, and geographically isolated. Hence, Canada's growing ethnic media landscape has an important role to play in advancing health literacy efforts by reaching diverse population groups, and producing and disseminating culturally and linguistically appropriate health messages that may not be communicated through other media channels.

A CANADIAN MILESTONE

THE HEALTHY ABORIGINAL NETWORK

The Healthy Aboriginal Network is a non-profit organization that engages in the promotion of health, literacy, and wellness by creating comic books on youth health and social issues. The comic books cover a wide range of issues, such as maternal child health, sexual health, gang youth, youth in care, struggling in school, the importance of friendships, social support from friends and family, smoking prevention, team sports and culture, mental health, diabetes prevention, and gambling addiction. The stories and images are pilot-tested with youth and health professionals online and/or in person. The comic books are available in both English and French languages. Each comic book project is made possible through funding and support from different partners, such as the Canadian Council on Learning, Health Canada, British Columbia Ministry of Child and Family Development, Vancouver Coastal Health Authority, Aboriginal Health Services, and so on.

Sample rough videos of pilot focus group testing of the comic book stories can be accessed through the Healthy Aboriginal Network's YouTube channel at http://www.youtube.com/user/HealthyAboriginal.

Source: Healthy Aboriginal Network. (n.d.). *Home page.* Retrieved from http://www.thehealthyaboriginal. net/ [accessed: 19 June 2013].

ADDITIONAL RESOURCES OF INTEREST

MediaPulse: Measuring the Media in Kids' Lives, A Guide for Health Practitioners

http://mediasmarts.ca/sites/default/files/pdfs/MediaPulse-Guide.pdf

The Media Awareness Network and the Canadian Pediatric Society worked together to produce this guidebook. It provides physicians and parents with information that shows the association between media exposure and specific health issues such as obesity, body image, violence, and sexual behaviour and attitudes, among others. It also provides tools for assessing media use and offers practical tips to manage media use in the home.

Association for Media Literacy

http://www.aml.ca/

A voluntary non-profit organization, the Association for Media Literacy brings members together from across Canada, the U.S., and around the world. Teachers, librarians, consultants, parents, cultural workers, and media professionals in the Association are committed to promoting media education to help students understand the impact of the mass media on contemporary culture.

The British Columbia Association for Media Education

http://openmedia.ca/sites/openmedia.ca/files/BCAME%20Brochure_REV.pdf

The British Columbia Association for Media Education is a non-profit society that includes teachers and media professionals who aim to educate Canadians about the media, advance media education, and encourage Canadian cultural expression in the media.

Media Literacy Saskatchewan

http://www.quadrant.net/Media_Literacy/

A Special Subject Council of the Saskatchewan Teachers' Federation, Media Literacy Saskatchewan is mandated to assist teachers who wish to teach media literacy skills in the classroom.

Association for Media Literacy—Nova Scotia

http://www.chebucto.ns.ca/communitysupport/AMLNS/aml.html

The Association for Media Literacy—Nova Scotia, consisting of educators, parents, media professionals, and media consumers, promotes an understanding of the impact of media on modern life, culture, and education.

CHAPTER 8

RISK COMMUNICATION
AND HEALTH LITERACY

Three out of four of the 20,855 Canadians who took part in the Canadian Community Health Survey and who did not get the H1N1 vaccination in 2009 said they simply did not believe it was necessary. Another 13 per cent said they just didn't get around to it.... In the end, although 428 people died and more than 8,000 people were hospitalized, the H1N1 pandemic was not as bad as the worst-case scenarios had predicted.... This has left doctors wondering whether large numbers of Canadians will point to the pandemic experience of 2009 as justification for not getting vaccinated should a new strain of influenza develop in the future. Most experts believe that the next pandemic is likely a decade or more away, but they fear that when it occurs, people will accuse the health-care community of crying wolf. That's the challenge that we have—how to engage with the public and explain risk.

—GLORIA GALLOWAY, "CANADIANS BLASÉ ABOUT FLU SHOT, DOCTORS FEAR," 2010

CHAPTER LEARNING OBJECTIVES

- Introduce the importance of health literacy for public health risk communication
- Introduce the field of health risk communication and the concept of risk
- Introduce heuristics, biases, and message framing in health risk communication
- Introduce the role of numeracy in health risk communication
- Introduce the role of science literacy in health risk communication
- Describe the importance of numeracy and science literacy for health risk communication in Canada: the case of H1N1

INTRODUCTION

Every day Canadians are reminded of public health risks—at home and worldwide. As described in Chapters 2 and 3, low literacy has health consequences for individuals and for the population as a whole. However, nowhere does low literacy have such an immediate effect for great numbers of Canadians and Canadian society as in the case of a public health crisis. Often health risk situations require immediate action, as in the case of Severe Acute Respiratory Syndrome (SARS) or food contamination. Box 8.1 provides an example of a news report from the *Vancouver Sun* detailing the bacterial contamination of deli meats found in Canadian supermarkets (Baer & Liepins, 2008).

BOX 8.1: MEDIA REPORT: DEADLY LISTERIOSIS TRACED TO MAPLE LEAF MEATS

Nicole Baer and Larissa Liepins, Canwest News Service

OTTAWA—Maple Leaf Foods expanded a product recall Saturday after test results confirmed that an outbreak of listeriosis that has claimed four lives across Canada is linked to processed meats produced at one of the company's plants.

The expanded recall will include all products from the Toronto facility "as a precautionary measure," the company said. The Canadian Food Inspection Agency and the Public Health Agency of Canada have been testing samples of recalled meat for the past week to determine the source of a fatal outbreak of listeriosis.

At a news conference late Saturday night, Agriculture Minister Gerry Ritz and public health officials announced that results of genetic testing from three samples of the recalled products show that two tested positive for the outbreak strain of listeria. A third was a close match, but with a slight variance.

The results are "highly significant" and show the investigation is "on the right path," said the statement by the Public Health Agency of Canada. More test results are expected next week.[...]

Health authorities have been scrambling to determine how many deaths or illnesses can be confirmed as linked to ingestion of the particularly deadly strain of the Listeria monocytogenes bacterium carried in the contaminated food.

McCain called the fatal outbreak a "terrible tragedy" that has shaken confidence in Maple Leaf. "Tragically, our products have been linked to illness and loss of life," McCain continued. "To those people who are ill, and to the families who have lost loved ones, I offer my deepest and sincerest sympathies. Words cannot begin to express our sadness for their pain."

Earlier Saturday, the Public Health Agency of Canada upped to 21 the number of cases of the listeriosis outbreak that have been confirmed so far in four provinces.

The agency said 16 of the cases were found in Ontario, three in British Columbia, and one each in Saskatchewan and in Quebec.

Three deaths in Ontario—St. Catharines, Hamilton and Waterloo—have been officially tied to the deadly strain of the food-borne listeria bacterium, and a fourth death on Vancouver Island has also been attributed to the strain.

Source: Baer, N. & Liepins, L. (2008, August 23). Deadly listeriosis outbreak traced to Maple Leaf meats. *The Vancouver Sun.* Retrieved from http://199.71.40.195/vancouversun/story.html?id=222b628d-8dc8-46af-b1dd-540864db14b8 [accessed: 18 June 2013].

There is an assumption that readers of the "risk information" have a number of literacy skills: from being able to read the information (prose literacy), to understanding what the statistics and numbers mean (numeracy), to having a basic knowledge about what bacteria are (science literacy). Unfortunately, gaps in these skills are all too common, and affect comprehension and action by concerned citizens who need to respond to public health risk settings.

Canadians are warned of potential health risks from infectious diseases and are urged to take personal precautions by being vaccinated, covering exposed body parts, hand washing, avoiding certain travel destinations, and so on. The list of health threats is long and includes, to name only a few, influenza A/H1N1, West Nile Virus, Severe Acute Respiratory Syndrome (SARS), bovine spongiform encephalitis (mad cow disease), and food insecurity. Media headlines identifying threats can be confusing, anxiety producing, and frightening, even for those with excellent prose literacy, numeracy, and science literacy skills. Consider the following newspaper headlines about H1N1, warning of vaccine shortages and tragic deaths: from the *Winnipeg Free Press*, "H1N1 vaccine shortage looms. Province pleads for low-priority cases to wait" (Owen, 2009); and from *The Sault Star*, "Third person dies of H1N1 in Sudbury" (Mulligan, 2009).

Government alerts can directly affect the health decisions people make. A warning about one smoking cessation drug and its link to possible side effects might be perceived by someone who is trying to quit smoking as applying to all smoking cessation drugs (e.g., see www.champixinfo. co.uk/side-effects-contraindications.shtml). Women taking drugs for osteoporosis might inter-pret an extremely small risk of osteonecrosis of the jaw as a reason to stop taking these medications even before routine dental treatments (e.g., see American Dental Association, 2012). Product recalls of infant and children's pain killers (e.g., Infants' Tylenol) or warnings about baby formulas contaminated with melamine plastics raise intense concern for parents who need to understand what the information is about, how the warning or recall affects them, and what to do next. Be-cause public health risk information crosses international boundaries, people also may not know whether the health threat applies to them or their community. For example, despite international concerns about traces of melamine in some infant formulas manufactured in China, no contam inated infant formulas were actually sold in Canada (Rogers, 2008).

A person's understanding of health risk messages has far-reaching consequences for themselves, their families, and their communities. To provide context for the wider consequences of low health literacy consider childhood vaccination for polio. Polio is a very serious viral disease that damages nerves that control skeletal muscles. Polio has virtually been eliminated in Canada. This outcome has been due to successful childhood immunization programs and the development of herd immunity in communities. The Merriam-Webster dictionary (2012b) defines *herd immunity* as "a reduction in the probability of infection that is held to apply to susceptible members of a population in which a significant proportion of the individuals are immune because the chance of coming in contact with an infected individual is less." Most Canadian parents have never seen a case of polio, and they may want to know why they should have their child vaccinated. Polio vaccine information is complex and technical, and is often presented with statistics and numbers. The following is typical of information available for the public explaining the polio immunization program:

"Before a polio vaccine was available, there were epidemics of paralytic poliomyelitis (polio) in Canada causing up to 20,000 cases in some years. Following the introduction of the polio vaccine in 1955, the number of cases dropped by 99 per cent in 12 years. In Canada, the last case caused by a wild poliovirus was reported in 1988" (Government of Alberta, 2007). This information about polio is difficult to understand and requires that the reader have numeracy skills. Moreover, the polio information is written at a grade level of about 11 according to the Simplified Measure of Gobbledygook (SMOG) readability score. Health literacy needs to be viewed as a contributing factor in parental decisions about whether to vaccinate children. In fact, parents with low literacy skill (at or below IALS Level 2) reported better understanding the risks and benefits of polio vaccines when the information was given by animated cartoons as compared to text-based information (Leiner, Handal, & Williams, 2004). Although the researchers who conducted this study did not ask the parents whether they decided to vaccinate their children after seeing the animated cartoons, we learned in earlier chapters that higher health literacy skill is associated with better health decisions and health outcomes. In the polio vaccination example, we might expect that a greater understanding of a vaccine-preventable disease gained after watching the animated video (i.e., higher health literacy) would lead to better and more informed parental decisions about whether to vaccinate (i.e., better health outcome). Nonetheless, parental uptake of vaccines is influenced by other literacy skills, including an understanding of basic science concepts (e.g., what are bacteria, viruses). Cultural factors—beliefs, values, motivations, ways of knowing and interpreting information—are also important in shaping the public's understanding of science and perceptions of health risk. In the next two sections we will introduce the field of risk communication and define what is meant by the term *risk*.

WHAT IS RISK COMMUNICATION?

Risk communication is an approach to communicating with the public about issues that are a real, suspected, or potential threat to their health and safety, or to the environment. It involves shared communication flow between stakeholders (often the government) and the public. Much of what we know about risk communication comes from the lessons learned from "miscommunication" to the public about hazardous waste at Superfund sites in the United States. (Superfund refers to the Comprehensive Environmental Response, Compensation, and Liability Act of 1980 [CERCLA], a United States federal law mandating the cleanup of sites contaminated with hazardous substances) (United States Environmental Protection Agency, 2011). One of the most notorious Superfund sites is the Love Canal in New York; an "equivalent" site in Canada is the Sydney Tar Ponds in Nova Scotia.

Risk communication involves communicating with a large number of people, if not with the entire population. Many of the features of communication between two individuals apply to risk communication to the public (Bennett, Calman, Curtis, & Fischbacher-Smith, 2011). These features include how the risk information is presented, delivered, and understood. Problems develop when the information processes break down. As noted in Chapter 5 in our discussion on culture and health literacy, even simple words between two people can be perceived differently depending on culture, language, perceptions, assumptions, history, and social dynamics. Because risk communication involves many people with diverse cultural and language backgrounds, the consequences of miscommunication and misunderstanding can be enormous.

One of the most widely endorsed definitions of risk communication was developed by the United States National Research Council: risk communication is "an interactive process of exchange of information and opinion among individuals, groups, and institutions. It involves multiple meanings about the nature of the risk and other messages, not strictly about risk, that express concerns, opinions, or reaction to risk messages" (National Research Council, 1989, p. 21). The (Canadian) Network for Environmental Risk Assessment and Management indicates that risk communication is any two-way communication between stakeholders (e.g., the general public and various health agencies such as the Canadian Cancer Society) about the existence, nature, form, severity, or acceptability of risks (Shortreed, Hicks, & Craig, 2003). Leading Canadian researchers in the area of risk assessment and management define risk communication as a process involving exchanges among stakeholders about how best to assess and manage risk (Leiss & Powell, 2004). In other words, risk communication is a shared process involving feedback and back-and-forth communication between key stakeholders. This leads us to ask what is meant by the term *risk* in the risk communication exchange.

WHAT IS RISK?

Simply put, risk is "the possibility of an adverse outcome, and uncertainty over the occurrence, timing, or magnitude of that adverse outcome" (Covello & Merkhofer, 1993, p. 2). It is about a harm that may happen, the chance that the harm will happen, and how many people could be affected by the harm (Groth, 1991). Moreover, in risk communication, the information presented often has multiple meanings. To appreciate why there are multiple meanings for information about risk, consider the idea of uncertainty and the probability of harmful consequences occurring after some event or exposure. Risk always involves uncertainty. Risk is never zero—otherwise it wouldn't be a risk! This can be illustrated by the risk of lung cancer and cigarette smoking. Smokers are repeatedly warned that exposure to cigarette smoke has a very high probability of the later occurrence of lung cancer. Yet, the probability of lung cancer after a lifetime of heavy cigarette smoking is not 100 percent (although there are many reasons not to smoke, with higher risk of developing lung cancer being one of them). Because risk is based on calculations, statistics, probability, and their interpretation, most risk situations have multiple experts providing different risk estimates and messages, interpreting the calculations and statistics differently, and assessing potential outcomes through their own perception and background. These different messages often compete for acceptance with the public. Moreover, the uncertainty about the risk is often due to a lack of convincing scientific evidence and information. There is ambiguity in risk communication because the information available can be interpreted, debated, and contextualized in different ways (Sellnow, Ulmer, Seeger, & Littlefield, 2009). One expert might consider something to be a risk whereas another may not. And, as Sjöberg (1999) pointed out, what is perceived as a risk "is rarely equal for experts and the public, even if they may be, at times, in rough agreement" (p. 2). Not only do experts sometimes disagree about a risk, but the public may also disagree with the experts!

HEURISTICS AND BIASES IN HEALTH RISK COMMUNICATION

People use simple mental tools to deal with the ambiguity and probability tied up with risk. These informal rules-of-thumb are known as heuristics (Bennett et al., 2011). In some situations heuristics can help us to deal with the uncertainty of risk events. In other situations heuristics can lead to us to misinterpret and become confused about the results (Tversky & Kahneman, 1974). Our biases affect how and whether we view an exposure as a risk. There are many types of biases that affect people's risk perception. Four important ones are availability bias, confirmation bias, overconfidence bias, and optimism bias. *Availability bias* refers to the fact that we usually think of memorable events as being more common, even if they are actually uncommon. As a result, people tend to overestimate the likelihood of a rare event (or risk) when it is memorable and given a lot of media attention (e.g., a plane crash in Fort Simpson), and underestimate the likelihood of more common risks that are less memorable (e.g., a car accident on Highway 401). *Confirmation bias* involves our search for information that supports our position or orientation. In other words, our expectations tend to be self-fulfilling ("self-fulfilling prophecy"). As an example, imagine that you believe that more people see their family doctors on Mondays than on other days of the work or school week. Confirmation bias would lead you to pay more attention to how many people visit their family doctor on Mondays and less attention to the number of people who visit on other days of the week. Over time this tendency could reinforce your belief that visits to family doctors are linked to days of the week (more visits on Mondays at the beginning of the week, fewer visits on Fridays at the end of the week). *Overconfidence bias* suggests that people believe that their predictions are more likely to be correct than they actually are. In health care decisions, overconfidence bias can lead to disastrous outcomes, including misdiagnosis or mismanagement of patient treatment. Finally, *optimism bias* conditions people to expect "bad things to be more likely to happen to other people" and not to themselves (Bennett et al., 2011). An example of optimism bias is when someone believes that an allergic reaction to a medicine will be more likely to happen to someone else than to him or herself. You may want to read further (e.g., see Bornstein & Emler, 2001) about biases in the context of rationality in medical and health care decision making by physicians.

MESSAGE FRAMING AND FRIGHT FACTORS IN RISK COMMUNICATION

In Chapter 7, the concept of message framing was introduced—the presentation of the same information from different vantage points. Framing influences how we cognitively arrange and interpret information. Most of us are familiar with the framing metaphor of a glass as "half empty" (loss framing) or a glass as "half full" (gain framing). Do you think that how the risk is framed could lead to different outcomes in terms of public health decisions to prevent a potential emergency? To illustrate how framing could influence perception of a public health issue, interventions for "Disease X" are framed as loss or gain scenarios in Table 8.1. Although the outcomes for Disease X are the same regardless of the framing, the perception of its seriousness and its consequences may be different.

TABLE 8.1: LOSS AND GAIN FRAMING IN RISK COMMUNICATION

Loss framing	Gain framing
If no intervention is chosen, all of the 400 children will die from Disease X.	If no intervention is chosen, none of the 400 children will be saved from Disease X.
If intervention 1 is chosen, 100 children will die from Disease X.	If intervention 1 is chosen, 300 children will be saved from Disease X.
If intervention 2 is chosen, 10% of children will die from Disease X.	If intervention 2 is chosen, 90% of children will survive Disease X.

Source: Modified from Bennett, P., Calman, K., Curtis, S., & Fischbacher-Smith, D. (2011, p. 15). Understanding public responses to risk: Policy and practice. Boxes 1.4a and 1.4b. In P. Bennett, K. Calman, S. Curtis, & D. Fischbacker-Smith (Eds.), *Risk communication and public health* (2nd ed., pp. 2–22). Oxford, UK: Oxford University Press.

Framing also influences our understanding of numerical concepts in risk communication. Research in health numeracy suggests that numbers are often interpreted semantically in terms of vague relations, such as good versus bad, high versus low, some versus none, or more versus less (Mills, Reyna, & Estrada, 2008; Reyna, Nelson, Han, & Dieckmann, 2009). Verbal expressions of statistical information can be easily misunderstood; something that is presented verbally as extremely unlikely may be interpreted by one individual as unlikely to occur and by another as more likely to occur (Eiser, 1998).

Media, and primarily newspapers, are a powerful source of information about public health risks and help to set the agenda for the general public. Comparing print and televised news stories about the E. coli outbreak in Walkerton, Ontario, in May of 2000, Driedger (2007) suggests that "newspaper broadsheets may serve as a better measure of media coverage of a risk event [than does television]" and that "the media [newspapers] may influence the way in which people understand and/or interpret information about an event, by how it presents media messages and media content for the public to think about" (p. 784)—in other words, by the framing of an issue. At the beginning of this chapter, the example of food safety (Listeria contamination of deli meats) was presented to illustrate the public health information to which Canadians must respond. Consider the effect of newspaper framing on communication about the Listeria contamination of food. Gauthier (2011) conducted an interesting study of Ontario and Quebec newspaper framing of the deli meats (and cheese) Listeria outbreak. She identified four frames: "war against microbes," "collateral damage," "microbiological," and "lifestylism." Depending on which perspective on food security was presented, people could choose from a bewildering array of responses: "Avoid at all costs the recalled deli meat products or avoid the entire category of products [deli meats] on the basis of other risks? Do not buy fine cheeses because of microbial risks or buy them to show support for cheese makers or a gastronomic ideal considered above the risk? Leave it up to fate, in the view that only the weak are at risk?" (Gauthier, 2011, p. 283). Not surprisingly, people who turned to newspapers for clear and easy-to-understand direction about the outbreak and what they should do were likely to be left confused.

As described above, risk is essentially about the possibility that something will go wrong. Most people, however, do not think about risk in "statistical" terms (e.g., a 1 in 9 chance of developing breast cancer over the course of a woman's lifetime assuming a lifespan of 90 years); rather, they are more comfortable with broad, qualitative features (e.g., radiation exposure from repeated mammograms may be linked to breast cancer). These broad qualitative characteristics have been called fright factors (Bennett et al., 2011) and outrage factors (Sandman, 1987). We can also think of them as fear factors that trigger alarm, worry, and anxiety in people (Deignan, Harvey, & Hoffman-Goetz, 2013). Table 8.2 lists important fright, outrage, or fear factors. Table 8.3 gives some examples of how these factors can be applied to different risk scenarios.

TABLE 8.2: FRIGHT, OUTRAGE, OR FEAR FACTORS

Factor	Explanation
Voluntariness	Risk perceived as being forced upon people produces greater fright, outrage, or fear.
Fairness	Risk perceived as being inequitably distributed produces greater fright, outrage, or fear.
Inescapable	Risk perceived as being inescapable by taking personal precautions produces greater fright, outrage, or fear.
Unfamiliar or novel	Risk perceived as being novel or not familiar produces greater fright, outrage, or fear.
Hidden and irreversible	Risk perceived to cause harm through the onset of disease or disability years after the exposure produces greater fright, outrage, or fear.
Danger to future generations	Risk perceived to cause harm to children or future generations produces greater fright, outrage, or fear.
Causes dread	Risk perceived as more likely to cause illness, injury, or death produces greater fright, outrage, or fear.
Poorly understood by science	Risk perceived as not being well understood by science produces greater fright, outrage, or fear.
Contradictory statements and meanings	Risk information presented in a contradictory or ambiguous way produces greater fright, outrage, or fear.
Identifiable victims	Risk perceived as affecting specific, named people produces greater fright, outrage, or fear.
Memorability	Harmful event or accident that is highly memorable produces greater fright, outrage, or fear.

Source: Modified from Sandman, P.M. (1987). Risk communication: Facing public outrage. *EPA Journal, 13*(9), 21–22; and Bennett, P., Calman, K., Curtis, S., & Fischbacher-Smith, D. (2011, pp. 89). Understanding public responses to risk: Policy and practice. Box 1.1. In P. Bennett, K. Calman, S. Curtis, & D. Fischbacker-Smith (Eds.), *Risk communication and public health* (2nd ed., pp. 3–22). Oxford, UK: Oxford University Press.

TABLE 8.3: EXAMPLES OF LOW AND HIGH PERCEIVED RISKS

Lower perceived risk	
Voluntary	Cigarette smoking
Familiar	Household dust
Well understood by science	Landline telephones
Higher perceived risk	
Involuntary	Secondhand smoke
Unfamiliar	Fallout dust from World Trade Center
Poorly understood by science	Cellular telephones

Source: Modified from Aakko, E. (2004). Risk communication, risk perception, and public health. Table 2. *Wisconsin Medical Journal, 103*(1), 25–27.

Fright, outrage, or fear factors can lead people to exaggerate certain types of risks. A personal tendency to emphasize some risks over others reflects fundamental value judgments as well as heuristics and biases. One individual may perceive an event as particularly risky to their health, whereas another may consider the event to be well within their risk tolerance. Value judgments depend on context, beliefs, social interactions, attitudes, and culture. They help us to decide who to trust, what information is credible, and what particular factors are frightening. Trust refers to whether the risk message is seen as reliable, believable, open, and honest. If the risk message is considered untrustworthy, it will likely be disregarded, discounted, or ignored. Although it is beyond the scope of this chapter to review how trust is developed by the public with respect to government and expert authorities, one key factor is prior beliefs about a particular topic. People "choose to trust those who support their initial beliefs" (Bennett et al., 2011, p. 18). As new information becomes available, people filter what they hear, confirming what they already believe (confirmation bias). And, as described in Chapter 5, culture shapes the beliefs and values of people and the trust they have in specific sources and types of information.

REVIEW AND REFLECT

Think about a recent event that you considered to be a health risk. What fright, outrage, or fear factors contributed to your perception of that risk?

NUMERACY AND HEALTH RISK COMMUNICATION

In the mid-2000s, advertisements about Lipitor (a cholesterol-lowering drug belonging to a family of medicines known as statins) appeared in many newspapers. A *New York Times* ad featured Robert Jarvik, the inventor of the artificial heart, standing next to an image of a heart (to view this image, see www.mouseprint.org/2008/02/04/lipitor-reduces-bad-cholesterol-but/). The caption for the ad indicated a 36 percent reduction in heart attack risk for people taking Lipitor. The fine print stated that "in a large clinical study, 3% of patients taking a sugar pill or placebo had a heart attack compared to 2% of patients taking Lipitor" (Mouseprint.org, 2008). The manufacturer of Lipitor eventually withdrew the Jarvik ads (not because of the numeracy issues but rather due to misleading and false advertising; for more on this, see www.nytimes.com/2008/03/04/health/views/04essa.html?ref=science). Nevertheless, this example shows the striking degree of numerical skill that a person would need to understand the cost, benefit, and risks of taking this medication. What does a 36 percent reduction mean in the context of this medication? How does heart attack occurrence of 2 people in 100 compare with 3 people in 100? Are these numbers important for people to know in understanding their own risk for heart disease?

We have stressed that numeracy is a lifelong skill that is necessary for people to understand and use numbers. Applications may range from basic arithmetic operations to complex quantitative reasoning, including probability, statistics, and inference. Health numeracy is a broad concept within health literacy and involves the capacity to access, process, interpret, communicate, and act on numerical, quantitative, graphical, biostatistical, and probabilistic health information to make effective health decisions (Goldbeck, Ahlers-Schmidt, Paschal, & Dismuke, 2005). As noted in Chapter 3, the proportion of adult Canadians at or below International Adult Literacy Survey (IALS) proficiency Level 2 for numeracy is about 55 percent. Simple health numeracy problems can be challenging for low numerate adults. Consider the example in Box 8.2 as it relates to a public health risk scenario. Ask yourself how health numerate a person would have to be to determine the dosage of an antiviral medication.

BOX 8.2: VIGNETTE ABOUT TAMIFLU

To prepare for a potential flu pandemic, Tamiflu (an antiviral drug) is being offered to Canadians as a preventative measure. Tamiflu can be given safely to children two years and older. Tamiflu must be given twice daily for five days. For a family with three children who are 11 months old, 22 months old, and six years old, how many children in this family will be given Tamiflu? How many total doses of Tamiflu will be needed for the children in this family?

Low health numeracy distorts the perception of health risk whether in a clinical setting or in a public health context. Individuals with low health numeracy have greater susceptibility to extraneous or outside factors (namely, those that do not change the objective numerical information); low health numerate people are also more vulnerable to the effects of mood, how the information is presented, framing effects, and ratio bias (Reyna et al., 2009). To illustrate how low health numeracy affects individual risk perception, Brewer and colleagues (2009) found that women with low health numeracy had less precise or "fuzzy" mental representations of hypothetical risk of recurrence of early-stage breast cancer than did women with higher health numeracy. These researchers suggested that low numerate women were more likely to guess about risk estimates. Low health numeracy would also affect risk perception in an emergency situation. Using a narrative vignette of a potential terrorist attack, decision-makers with low numeracy skills reported greater perception of risk and recommended more security measures than those who were more numerate (Dieckmann, Slovic, & Peters, 2009). Although this study did not position the threat within a health setting, it would not be surprising if decision-makers' numeracy skills influenced risk perception responses to a public health threat. Zarcadoolas, Pleasant, and Greer (2006) reviewed the failures of risk communication with the 2001 anthrax threat in the United States. Difficult language, assumed knowledge, and scientific uncertainty characterized the complex communication challenges facing both risk communicators and the public during this threat. Further, "people with less education (linked to generally lower literacy and numeracy levels) were twice as likely to be worried about anthrax exposure" (Zarcadoolas, Pleasant, & Greer, 2006, p. 171). (For excellent analyses of health numeracy, bioterrorism, and risk communication, see Rudd, Comings, & Hyde, 2003; Gray & Ropeik, 2002.)

Numeracy is important for informed decision making during public health risk situations. Numerous surveys and research in the United States and Canada show that many people are unprepared to handle the quantitative activities of daily living. But, as Reyna and Brainerd (2007) point out, it may be unrealistic to expect people who are too uncomfortable or are unable to make rudimentary judgments about health-related tasks and probabilities to engage in decision making in a public health risk emergency. There are, however, some strategies that may be useful to encourage better understanding of quantitative information by people with lower numeracy skill. Among these are: (1) using verbal labels to describe situations where the probability of the risk is unknown or vague (because verbal labels are themselves vague); (2) using numerical representations of risk when the likelihood of the risk is well known (because of the precision and confidence associated with the risk estimate); and (3) using pictographs or pictograms to show the numerical representation of the risk, which is particularly useful for those with low numeracy and literacy (Burkell, 2004). Graphical representations (such as a circle or stick figure) are easier to understand than numerical risk frequencies (such as 1 in 500). An example of information presented as a pictograph for low numerate adults is shown in Figure 8.1. Nevertheless, even with the use of different visual formats such as pictographs, communicating health risks to the public that contain "deeper uncertainties resulting from incomplete or disputed knowledge … remains a challenge" (Spiegelhalter, Pearson, & Short, 2011, p. 1393).

To summarize the key points thus far, how numerical information is presented in a public health risk communiqué affects a person's understanding of the risk. Biases, heuristics, message framing, and health numeracy proficiency are critical to interpreting numbers, probabilities, and statistics for most individuals when faced with a health risk situation. As Gigerenzer and Edwards (2003) and Zarcadoolas and colleagues (2006) indicate, confusion also arises because of how the risk information is presented:

Statistical innumeracy is often attributed to problems inside our minds. We disagree: the problem is not simply internal but lies in the external representation of information, and hence a solution exists. Every piece of statistical information needs a representation—that is, a form. Some forms tend to cloud minds, while others foster insight. We know no medical institution that teaches the power of statistical representations; even worse, writers of information brochures for the public seem to prefer confusing representations. (Gigerenzer & Edwards, 2003, p. 741, cited in Zarcadoolas, Pleasant, & Greer, 2006, pp. 201–202)

FIGURE 8.1: PICTOGRAPH SHOWING NUMERIC INFORMATION

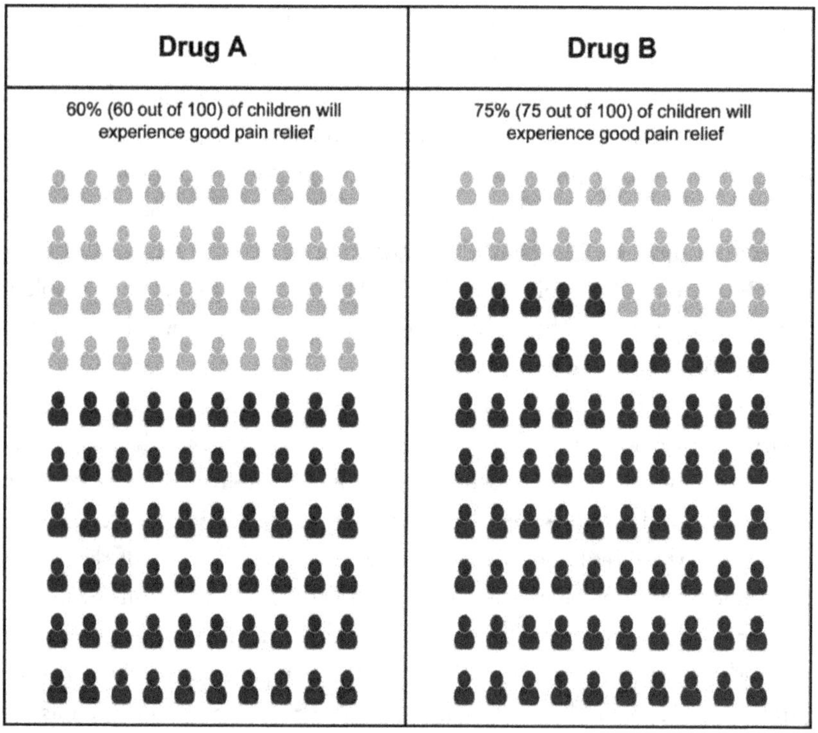

Drug A	Drug B
60% (60 out of 100) of children will experience good pain relief	75% (75 out of 100) of children will experience good pain relief

Source: Tait, A.R., Voepel-Lewis, T., Zikmund-Fisher, B.J., & Fagerlin, A. (2010, p. 719). Presenting research risk and benefits to parents: Does format matter? Figure 1. *Anesthesia & Analgesia, 111*(3), 718–723.

SCIENCE LITERACY AND HEALTH RISK COMMUNICATION

Another factor adding to difficulties in society's understanding of potential public health threats is a lack of familiarity and comfort with basic science concepts and terms (known as science literacy). Most Canadians recognize and appreciate the general benefits of science for health. An EKOS Research Associates (2004) poll reported that Canadians strongly believe that science and research contribute to an improved and sustainable health care system. About 70 percent of those surveyed indicated they were generally positive about the importance of science in societal (health) advancement. Science and technology play a role in the evaluation of food additives, the development of new vaccines, the manufacture of assistive devices, mobile apps that remind users about their unique health indicators, and so on.

Nevertheless, while Canadian adults are supportive of science and technology initiatives that have potentially beneficial health outcomes, public understanding of basic scientific facts and concepts or how science works is limited. The Canadian Council on Learning (CCL) points out that while Canadian schools do a good job of teaching science to young people, adults struggle with limited science literacy (CCL, 2007b, p. 2). If science literacy skills of Canadians mirror prose and numeracy skills, for many adults, scores would be in the marginal range. People with low science literacy cannot distinguish science from pseudoscience, voodoo science, or junk science (these latter two terms were coined in 2000 by Robert L. Park in his book *Voodoo Science: The Road from Foolishness to Fraud*). Understanding by the public of stem cell research, genetically modified foods, new cancer treatments, reproductive technologies, cloning, genomic mapping, "scientific" and health claims of advertisers, and a dizzying array of emerging issues assumes adequate science literacy skills.

The importance of science literacy for understanding public health issues and concepts cannot be overstated. To illustrate this concept, consider the following example from the U.S. National Science Board (NSB, 2004). The percentage of American adults who thought that antibiotics kill viruses as well as bacteria was close to 50 percent. About 60 percent of Americans surveyed thought that radioactive milk could be made safe by boiling it. Would low science literacy be relevant for communication about public health risks and the public's response? Absolutely! People might decide not to receive the H1N1 flu vaccine, justifying their decision on the belief that, if they get sick, an antibiotic would be an effective treatment against viruses. Or, consider the radiation leaking from the Fukushima nuclear power plant in Japan as a result of the 2011 tsunami. Boiling contaminated milk will most definitely not make it safe to drink.

Definitions of science literacy can be as confusing as definitions of health literacy. Generally, science literacy "encompasses knowledge of basic scientific concepts and processes … includes information management and problem solving skills … and enables us to understand and advance the links between science, technology, innovation, the economy and our society" (Knox & Schmidt, 2006, p. 74). Miller (2006) defines science literacy as "a level of understanding sufficient to read science and technology stories written at the level of the *New York Times* Science section" (as cited in Scearce, 2007, p. 2). Holbrook and Rannikmae (2009) provide a definition of science literacy that parallels that of health literacy: "Developing the ability to creatively utilise sound science knowledge in everyday life or in a career, to solve problems, make decisions and hence improve the quality of life" (p. 287).

Another example of why science literacy is essential for understanding risk is seen in the case of genetically modified (GM) foods. Genetically modified foods have been developed from genetically modified organisms. The World Health Organization (WHO) defines genetically modified organisms as "organisms in which the genetic material (DNA) has been altered in a way that does not occur naturally. The technology is often called 'modern biotechnology' or 'gene technology', sometimes also 'recombinant DNA technology' or 'genetic engineering'. It allows selected individual genes to be transferred from one organism to another, also between non-related species" (WHO, n.d.). How much genetically modified food is eaten annually by Canadians is not known. According to a 2011 CTV television report, about 70 percent of all processed foods in Canada have some genetic modifications (see www.ctvnews.ca/deal-reached-on-labels-for-genetically-modified-food-1.666410). Genetically modified foods have both ardent supporters and vocal critics. On the one hand, genetic modification can result in foods with potential health benefits, such as potential anti-cancer or anti-aging foods (e.g., high antioxidant levels in tomatoes) or edible bite-size delivery vehicles for vaccines to people in developing countries (e.g., banana-based vaccines for hepatitis B). Genetic modification can also produce greater disease resistance in plants (e.g., transgenic crops with improved fungal resistance), better yields (with the potential of reducing food shortages and famine), and other benefits. On the other hand, concerns about "Frankenfoods" and long-term effects on human health are pervasive. Public responses to genetically modified foods follow the fright and fear factors described earlier in this chapter. People are uncertain about what foods are genetically modified, how these foods are produced, and the strength of the evidence for human health effects, both short and long term.

In a 2006 Pew Opinion Poll on Americans' attitudes about food and biotechnology, public knowledge of genetically modified foods was reported to be very low. Consumers knew little about the extent to which their foods included genetically modified ingredients. Education influenced consumer attitudes about the safety of GM foods and especially animal cloning. But, perhaps not surprisingly, given the low science literacy, the educational effect was not as large as one might expect: 47 percent of those with high school or less education were uncomfortable with foods derived from cloned animals, compared with 40 percent of those with university or college degrees who felt such foods were unsafe (Pew Initiative on Food and Biotechnology, 2006). Even for respondents with high health literacy, as suggested by formal education, perceptions of risk were strong and may reflect factors other than science literacy. These may include the fact that products are not labelled (and the fierce resistance of producers to do so) and that there is little scientific evidence on the long-term health effects of these foods.

Is the situation different for Canadians in regard to science literacy and attitudes about GM foods? A 2008 Nielson survey of 5,000 Canadians on attitudes toward food, safety of meat products, and trust in food industry institutions suggests they might be similar to those of American adults. The Canadian survey found that 50 percent of respondents had relatively high levels of concern with GM feed used in livestock meat production. And, variation in education (as an indirect marker of science literacy) did not significantly affect respondents' concerns about GM feed (Komirenko, Veeman, & Unterschultz, 2010).

Many people obtain health risk information about public health (and environmental and technology) issues from newspapers. What level of science literacy would readers need to understand the following opinion-editorial piece by Nina Fedoroff (a former science and technology advisor to the U.S. Secretary of State) published in the *New York Times*?

> New molecular methods that add or modify genes can protect plants from diseases and pests and improve crops in ways that are both more environmentally benign and beyond the capability of older methods. This is because the gene

modifications are crafted based on knowledge of what genes do, in contrast to the shotgun approach of traditional breeding or using chemicals or radiation to induce mutations…. Crop modification by molecular methods is no more dangerous than crop modification by other methods. (Fedoroff, 2011)

Understanding of terms such as *mutation*, *molecular methods*, and *gene modification* requires considerable science and health literacy proficiencies.

REVIEW AND REFLECT

Find a recent newspaper article describing a public health emergency in Canada. Reflect on the numeracy and science literacy skills that the typical reader would need to understand the information.

NUMERACY AND SCIENCE LITERACY IN PUBLIC HEALTH RISK COMMUNICATION IN CANADA: THE CASE OF H1N1 INFLUENZA

Health numeracy and science literacy competencies are crucial for understanding public health risk information by the average adult. Yet, many people have insufficient skills in these domains to interpret health risk materials in ways that foster informed responses. The importance of these skills is illustrated using communication about the influenza H1N1 vaccine program in Canada.

On April 26, 2009, the first Canadian cases of influenza H1N1 were reported: four in Nova Scotia and two in British Columbia. By the end of May 2009, the number of laboratory-confirmed H1N1 influenza cases in Canada was over 1,000 (Cutler et al., 2009). In early June of 2009, the World Health Organization released a communiqué that a global pandemic of this new virus (influenza H1N1) was occurring. At that time, more than 70 countries reported cases of the novel virus infection. In Canada, the pandemic response lasted until December 2009, and by April 17, 2010, the cumulative number of people hospitalized with H1N1 flu was 8,678, and a total of 438 people had died. Canadians at greatest risk of having severe infection or of dying from the virus were pregnant women, children under five years of age, people with underlying chronic medical conditions, those who were severely obese, and First Nations people living in remote areas.

Despite intense media coverage of the H1N1 flu outbreak (e.g., Rachul, Ries, & Caulfield, 2011), and the conclusion of the Standing Senate Committee on Social Affairs, Science and Technology that Canada's response "effectively reduced the impact of the H1N1 influenza pandemic" (Eggleton & Ogilvie, 2010, p. vii), the public's uptake of the H1N1 vaccine was variable at best. According to the Canadian Community Health Survey, 11.6 million Canadians over the age of 12 received the H1N1 vaccine (or about 41 percent of the population) during the 2009 flu season. Self-reported vaccination rates ranged from a high of 69 percent in Newfoundland and Labrador to a low of 32 percent in Ontario (Statistics Canada, 2010a).

There were many reasons for the failure to achieve the vaccine coverage rates needed for herd immunity in all provinces. Laing (2011) reviewed a number of issues relating to communication about the H1N1 crisis from media, public, and government perspectives. As he pointed out, there was "a breakdown in the communications function during the H1N1 outbreak in the Fall of 2009 between public health communicators, the media, and the public, and that breakdown may have been a factor behind a shortfall in Ontarians immunized against the virus" (p. 142). Laing (2011) suggests,

> The public itself was not entirely blameless. Despite substantial information suggesting that H1N1 was a serious threat, and equally substantial quality of information available to the public to make an informed decision, two-thirds of Ontarians decided to ignore the warnings of public health experts and not get vaccinated. Analysis indicated that awareness of the topic was high. Whether their own experiences and biases, or some form of media-influencing effects, or both, were the cause, the result was that too few Ontarians did not think the threat was sufficiently credible to change their behaviour. (p. 144)

Of the many communication factors that contributed to poor vaccination rates by adult Ontarians (such as mixed and confusing messages and negative framing of media stories), the impact of numeracy and science literacy was not addressed. Prose literacy factors, such as whether the material was text heavy or the attention to visuals and layout, may also have influenced public perception of H1N1 flu information (Lagassé et al., 2011). To appreciate the literacy issues in the context of H1N1 reporting, read the Canadian newspaper report from 2009 in Box 8.3.

BOX 8.3: MEDIA REPORT: SINGLE DOSE OF H1N1 VACCINE ENOUGH FOR KIDS: WHO

One dose of swine flu vaccine appears to be enough for children, a vaccine committee that advises the World Health Organization reported Friday.

The committee, known as SAGE (Strategic Advisory Group of Experts on Immunization) said a single dose of vaccine is enough to immunize children over 10. It added that while more data on children between 6 months and 10 years are needed, countries should start by giving younger kids at least one dose.

"The SAGE recommendation (for children under 10) could change as more data come in," said WHO vaccine chief Marie-Paule Kieny.

For the time being, she said, "the priority should be to give them at least one dose of vaccine now, and to cover as many of them as possible."

Currently, Canada and many other countries are recommending children under 10 receive two doses of H1N1 vaccine, given at least 21 days apart. That could soon change.

Canada's Chief Medical Officer of Health, Dr. David Butler-Jones, said Friday that experts advising the Public Health Agency of Canada are considering moving to a one-dose recommendation for children, and have been studying the issue for a while.

SAGE also reversed its earlier recommendation that countries offer adjuvant-free vaccine to pregnant women because of a paucity of research on the adjuvanted vaccine in pregnant women.

The committee said animal studies of adjuvanted and non-adjuvanted vaccines found "no evidence of direct or indirect harmful effects on fertility, pregnancy, development of the embryo or fetus, birthing, or post-natal development."

Nor did studies using live-virus flu vaccines, which are not used in Canada; flu vaccines here use inactivated—i.e. dead—viruses. [...]

Source: CTV.ca News Staff. (2009, October 30). Single dose of H1N1 vaccine enough for kids: WHO. *CTV News.* Retrieved from http://www.ctv.ca/CTVNews/Health/20091030/vaccine_flow_091030/#ixzz1vEpQ0pYc [accessed: 18 June 2013].

Simple readability calculations (such as the SMOG index, the Gunning's Fog score, and others described in Chapter 2) show this media report to be at a grade 12 level, meaning that it is fairly difficult to read. People with low literacy may struggle when reading complex and technical words (e.g., "inactivated"). The complex words are strung together in long sentences, there are numerous distractors in many of the sentences, and multiple concepts or information points are presented per sentence. From a numeracy perspective, the reader would have to process information about different dosages and schedules for children under 10 years versus over 10 years and understand that those amounts could change as more data come in. The science literacy skill that an individual needs to understand this news report is high. In fact, it may be well beyond the basic science knowledge of many adult Ontarians. For a reader of this article, many basic science concepts are assumed. A reader would need to know about the following concepts, even before thinking about the issue of H1N1 vaccination for children:

- What is an adjuvant?
- What is a virus?
- How are viruses inactivated?

REVIEW AND REFLECT

Select a recent media report on an issue of public health interest in Canada (e.g., extreme heat alerts in Toronto or a boil water advisory for Montreal) and reflect on the numeracy, prose, and science literacy skills that a reader would need to understand the public health risk information.

KEY LEARNING POINTS

In this chapter, risk communication was defined as a shared communication approach involving stakeholders (often government) and the public to inform large numbers of people about issues that are real, suspected, or potential threats to their health. The term *risk* involves uncertainty, and people interpret ambiguity about health through their individual perceptions and biases (such as confirmation, availability, overconfidence, and optimism biases). The mental rules of thumb that people use to filter the public health information landscape and interpret potential health risks are known as heuristics. How a health risk message is framed, either positively (gain framing) or negatively (loss framing), influences people's responses to public health risk emergencies. Fright factors were shown to be potential triggers of anxiety, worry, and even outrage by the public. These fright factors are often subtle and embedded in media messages and communications about important public health situations. Adequate numeracy and science literacy were described as being essential for people's understanding of health risk information. Poor understanding of biostatistical, probability, and inferential concepts influence decision making; people with low numeracy skill often rely on "fuzzy" or vague descriptions of the public health risk. Pseudoscience is pervasive (including in media reports) and can influence people's responses to health situations. To illustrate the importance of health numeracy and science literacy, how the H1N1 flu outbreak in 2009 was communicated in the media and the required numeracy and science literacy skill set for understanding were reviewed. The failure of vaccine uptake by many communities in Ontario was presented as reflecting, in part, science literacy and health numeracy skills.

A CANADIAN MILESTONE

On 20 March 1996, British Health Secretary Stephen Dorrell rose in the House to inform colleagues that scientists had discovered a new variant of Creutzfeldt-Jacob disease (CJD) in 10 victims, and that they could not rule out a link with consumption of beef from cattle with bovine spongiform encephalopathy (BSE), also known as mad cow disease. Overnight, the British beef market collapsed and politicians quickly learned how to enunciate BSE and CJD. Within days, the European Union banned exports of British beef; consumption of beef fell throughout Europe, especially in France and Germany, and in Japan, where suspicion of foreign food runs high; and the tell-tale triumvirate of uncertain science, risk and politics was played out—and continues—in media headlines (p. 27).

The Canadian Cattlemen's Association began circulating an information memo on 27 March 1996, to grocery officials across Canada to inform consumers that "BSE is a British issue and does not affect the Canadian consumer. Canadian consumers can continue to be confident in the safety and wholesomeness of our product." But consumers have a much broader notion of risk. To say BSE was only a British issue was to ignore the numerous stories in Canadian media outlets criticizing the practice of using ruminant protein in feed, in Canada. Again, the message denies the legitimacy of a consumer concern, which usually makes things worse. (p. 57)

Source: Powell, D., & Leiss, W. (1997). *Mad cows and mother's milk: The perils of poor risk communication.* Montreal: McGill-Queen's University Press.

ADDITIONAL RESOURCES OF INTEREST

Campbell, A. (2000, July). *What You Don't Know Can Hurt You: Literacy's Impact on Workplace Health and Safety.* Conference Board of Canada Report.
http://abclifeliteracy.ca/files/11-019_WhatYouDon'tKnow_WEB.pdf.
This is important policy brief outlines the importance of literacy for occupational health and safety.

Drache, D., Feldman, S., & Clifton, D. (2003). *Media Coverage of the 2003 Toronto SARS Outbreak: A Report on the Role of the Press in a Public Crisis.* Roberts Centre Research Papers. Roberts Centre for Canadian Studies, York University.
This research study evaluated more than 1,600 SARS-related articles from three Canadian (*Toronto Star, The Globe and Mail, National Post*) and two U.S. (*USA Today* and *The New York Times*) newspapers. The report describes how the articles framed the SARS message.

Driedger, S.M. (2003). Different Frames, Different Fears: Communicating about Chlorinated Drinking Water and Cancer in the Canadian Media. *Social Science & Medicine, 56,* 1279–1293.
This research study provides an in-depth analysis of metaphors, framing, and presentation of risk fear/fright factors in the debate around chlorinated drinking water by-products in Canadian print media from 1977 to 2000.

Reynolds, B. (2002). *Crisis and Emergency Risk Communication.* Centers for Disease Control and Prevention.
http://www.bt.cdc.gov/cerc/pdf/CERC-SEPT02.pdf
This Web link provides an extensive "how to" manual and introductory course on risk communication, and crisis or disaster communication. The course contains 12 modules and includes illustrations, tables, and worksheets. Although prepared for the U.S. market, the basic information is applicable for Canadians involved in risk communication.

CHAPTER 9

HEALTH LITERACY IN THE
CLINICAL CONTEXT

Whatever the reasons, it is unfortunate that the Canadian medical community has not played a more active role in health literacy, since it is clearly an important issue in the practice of medicine. Moreover, it is an issue that can be addressed constructively by physicians and their professional organizations.

—IRVING ROOTMAN, "HEALTH LITERACY: WHERE ARE THE CANADIAN DOCTORS?" 2006

CHAPTER LEARNING OBJECTIVES
- Describe the importance of health literacy in the clinical context
- Describe and define the concept of patient-centred health care
- Describe the importance of health literacy skills training for all health care providers
- Describe how patient-centred health care can improve health literacy for Canadians

INTRODUCTION

In a clinical context, patients with low health literacy skills have difficulty with medication protocols and identifying medication taken (Persell, Osborn, Richard, Skripkauskas, & Wolf, 2007). Throughout this text we have emphasized that low health literacy is associated with poorer health outcomes as well as poorer use of health care services including "more hospitalizations; greater use of emergency care; lower receipt of mammography screening and influenza vaccine; poorer ability to demonstrate taking medications appropriately; poorer ability to interpret labels and health messages; and, among elderly persons, poorer overall health status and higher mortality rates" (Berkman, Sheridan, Donahue, Halpern, & Crotty, 2011, p. 97).

Imagine the following clinical scenarios. *Scenario One:* Mr. Butler is a 67-year-old male patient who is leaving his doctor's office. He is approached by his wife in the waiting room, who asks him about the doctor's diagnosis. Mr. Butler tells his wife that the doctor used a blood pressure test and found his numbers were high, and thus asked him to return for repeat tests to check his blood pressure over time. However, Mr. Butler did not think to tell his wife the two things the doctor asked him to do prior to his next blood pressure test: (1) not have coffee 30 minutes before the test, because it could result in a short-term rise in his blood pressure; and (2) to use the lavatory before the test, because having a full bladder may change his blood pressure reading.

Scenario Two: After examining Mrs. Akbar for episodic stomach pain, the doctor asks her if she has had a bladder infection before. Mrs. Akbar pauses for a minute or two and hesitantly says no. The doctor then explains that she does not think Mrs. Akbar has a bladder infection but that her abdominal pain may be caused by inflammation. The doctor tells Mrs. Akbar she needs to see a gastroenterologist, who will perform an upper gastrointestinal endoscopy for further examination. As she approaches the door, the doctor quickly asks Mrs. Akbar if she has any questions and then tells her to see the receptionist to make an appointment with a gastroenterologist. A confused Mrs. Akbar silently nods her head in compliance.

Scenario Three: Mr. Kusugak is in the emergency room for chronic complications of type 2 diabetes. The nurse asks him if he is taking his pills every day. Mr. Kusugak responds in the affirmative, emphasizing that he never forgets to take his pills. Mr. Kusugak also mentions that his family members are very supportive and remind him to take pills at the right time daily. The nurse checks his medical record and informs Mr. Kusugak of the doctor's recommendation to begin use of insulin immediately. Mr. Kusugak, however, refuses to accept this suggested move from oral medications to insulin therapy. The nurse reminds Mr. Kusugak that the use of insulin is the doctor-prescribed regimen for managing his diabetes-related complications. Thinking about how insulin therapy will restrict his daily life and in fear of using an insulin pump and blood glucose meter, Mr. Kusugak shrugs to reaffirm his resistance to switching to insulin therapy. The nurse gets frustrated and thinks that Mr. Kusugak is a difficult and non-compliant diabetic patient. Mr. Kusugak thinks that he may be better off talking with the Elders and members of the healing circle in his community about his pills.

The above three scenarios demonstrate how, in a clinical setting, patients with low health literacy skills can have difficulty making the next medical appointment, understanding medical terms and treatment recommendations, and using medical devices. While low health literacy may mean a patient's lack of ability to read, write, listen, speak, calculate, interact, communicate, and critically analyze information in a way to promote good health across the lifespan, in a clinical context, health care provider–patient communication is central to improving a patient's health literacy. From the three above scenarios, we can identify that Mr. Butler, an elderly patient, Mrs. Akbar, an immigrant patient, and Mr. Kusugak, an Aboriginal patient, are at risk for low health literacy in relation to their medical encounters with their health care providers. Hence, health literacy in the clinical context is a dynamic and communicative process. And, as such, improving patients' health literacy in the clinical context will require a patient-centred approach and medical education in health literacy.

In this chapter, we will examine the importance of health literacy in the clinical context. We will look at the patient-centred approach to health care and discuss the need to incorporate health literacy teaching into education programs for health care professionals. Finally, we will consider the role of patient-centred health care in improving health literacy for Canadians.

HEALTH LITERACY IN THE CLINICAL CONTEXT

In a clinical context, patients are often presented with information by their health professionals that is, to varying degrees, incomprehensible and frustrating. For example, patients may have problems with prescription directions, insurance applications, pre-surgery instructions, appointment slips, discharge instructions, informed consents, and health education materials. Or, as seen in Box 9.1, patients could find it difficult simply to navigate the hospital setting.

BOX 9.1: WHO DO PATIENTS ASK?

Dr. Rudd shared some findings from a research project with adult basic learners in the Boston area. Walking through a hospital with learners, researchers used a talk-aloud protocol to record the strategies the learners used to find their way. Apart from the difficulties posed by many of the signs, the study showed that when they need help, learners asked hospital personnel for information, and frequently chose to ask cleaners or housekeeping staff—"people who look like us." Dr. Rudd wondered how often hospitals have considered their housekeeping staff as potential "partners" in providing certain types of information to patients.

Source: Some current research on health and literacy (2000, p. 2). *Literacy Across the Curriculumedia Focus, 15*(1). Retrieved from http://centreforliteracy.qc.ca/sites/default/files/Some_current.pdf [accessed: 3 September 2013].

In such cases, the important health information perhaps falls short of its communicative function because: (1) the health professional used poor writing, difficult-to-understand concepts, or technical jargon; or (2) the patient has low health literacy, linguistic and cultural barriers, physical limitations, or cognitive impairment. Perhaps nowhere is this problem more important and pervasive than in health care. The consequences of health professionals not being able to communicate important health information clearly, in plain language, and of patients failing to understand health risks, follow health care recommendations, and engage in self-care disease management, can have serious, even fatal, consequences. Hence, clinicians' assumptions about the adequate health literacy skill of patients, poor communication skills on the part of health professionals, and poor health literacy skills on the part of patients contribute to a communication gap in the clinical context, especially between physicians and patients (Calkins et al., 1997; Weiss & Coyne, 1997). Research shows that contributing factors to low health literacy include low general literacy, inexperience with the health system, complexity of information, cultural and language factors, poor communicative practices (how information is communicated), and aging. Being unaware of the problem or lacking an understanding of health literacy issues, health professionals do not usually inquire into their patients' health literacy levels; instead, they tend to overestimate them. Health professionals may not know how to respond when faced with patients with low health literacy or be unable to identify patients with limited literacy skills (Bass, Wilson, Griffith, & Barnett, 2002; Powell & Kripalani, 2005; Seligman et al., 2005).

Thus, provider–patient communication in the clinical context is of great importance for improving patients' health literacy (Schillinger, Bindman, Wang, Stewart, & Piette, 2004; Makaryus & Friedman, 2005) and, in turn, improving public health. Effective provider–patient communication, that is, communicating "the right information, to the right people, in the right way, at the right time" (Berry, 2007, p. 4), can empower patients by facilitating their understanding of: (1) the health care system, which may involve making doctors' appointments and filling out health insurance forms; (2); medical instructions that may include medication use, and a diet and exercise plan; and (3) self-care skills that may include comprehension of food labels and nutrition facts. Not surprisingly, the processes that facilitate empowerment in the clinical communication exchange are not fundamentally different from the processes that facilitate empowerment as a feature of health promotion (see Chapter 4).

Achieving health literacy skills can help patients make informed decisions about their health and the health of their family. These decisions can include asking the physician or pharmacist about symptoms of hypoglycemia (low blood sugar) and proper action for hypoglycemic symptoms; asking whether or not to take antibiotics for acute bronchitis ("chest cold," a lung infection that is usually caused by a virus and lasts for a short time); and arriving with an empty stomach (e.g., no food or drink after midnight) to have an x-ray in the morning. Hence, effective communication in medical encounters "needs to be patient-centred, and informative and needs to promote trust and confidence" (Berry, 2007, p. 4) so that patients are able to discuss and make medical decisions with their health care providers. This "information trust" is especially critical to understanding the associated health risks and benefits of any medical decision and, in turn, improve an individual's health literacy. Research shows that improved health literacy can result in better understanding of medical conditions, health-related quality of life, use of preventive services, adherence to medical instructions, and self-management skills (Baker et al., 2007; DeWalt, Berkman, Sheridan, Lohr, & Pignone, 2004).

REVIEW AND REFLECT

What are the strengths and challenges of using new technology, such as the Internet, and social media platforms, such as Facebook and Twitter, to provide patient-centred health care to bridge the gap in health literacy among disadvantaged groups such as Aboriginal peoples?

PATIENT-CENTRED HEALTH CARE

In *Crossing the Quality Chasm* (IOM, 2001), the Institute of Medicine (IOM) outlined patient-centred care as one of the six domains for improving the quality of health care. The other five domains included providing health care that is safe, effective, timely, efficient, and equitable. The IOM defined patient-centred care as "care that is respectful and responsive to individual patient preferences, needs, and values, and ensuring that patient values guide all clinical decisions" (IOM, 2001, p. 3). Hence, patient-centred health care highlights "compassion, empathy, and responsiveness to the needs, values, and expressed preferences of the individual patient" (Betancourt, 2006, p. 9).

A Canadian researcher and strong advocate of patient-centred care, Dr. Moira Stewart and colleagues (1995) described patient-centred care along six dimensions, which include:

1. an exploration of the illness experience;
2. an understanding of the whole person;
3. a discovery of common ground regarding management issues;
4. an integration of prevention and health promotion;
5. an improvement of the doctor–patient relationship; and
6. an awareness of personal limitations of both doctor and patient.

The patient-centred approach to health care has also been equated with related concepts such as:

- Patient-centred medicine, which "seeks to focus medical attention on the individual patient's needs and concerns, rather than the doctor's" (Bardes, 2012, p. 782).

- Patient-centred interviewing, which "approaches the patient as a unique human being with his own story to tell, promotes trust and confidence, clarifies and characterizes the patient's symptoms and concerns, generates and tests many hypotheses that may include biological and psychosocial dimensions of illness, and creates the basis for an ongoing relationship" (Lipkin, Quill, & Napodano, 1984, p. 277).

- Patient-centred communication, which "is used to describe patient–practitioner interactions, but could include other modes of communication. For example, patients may experience patient-centred communication when interacting with the health system; when using e-mail to contact practitioners; when phone calls are answered by a pleasant and responsive receptionist, and when phone calls are returned in a timely manner. Similarly, written communication, such as signage and patient education materials, may be patient-centred to the extent that they meet patients' needs and are written in a way that enhances participation" (Beach, Saha, & Cooper, 2006, p. 3).

- Patient-centred medical communication, which is "an approach that seeks to place the patient and his or her understanding of health, healing, and illness at the center of the clinical communication encounter" (Bates & Ahmed, 2012, p. 3).
- Patient-centred access, which offers "patients secure appropriate and pre-ferred medical assistance when and where it is needed. Characteristics of patient-centred access include availability, appropriateness, preference, and timeliness" (Berry, Seiders, & Wilder, 2003, p. 568).

While various perspectives on patient-centred care have emerged over the years, the core fea-tures remain dedicated to providing and improving health care from the patient's perspective.

The Toronto Consensus Statement was prepared at a major conference on doctor–patient communication held in Toronto in 1991 (Simpson et al., 1991). The consensus statement identified the following elements of clinical communication that are considered essential in patient-centred communication:

1. Communication problems in medical practice are important and common.
2. Patient anxiety and dissatisfaction are related to uncertainty and lack of information, explanation and feedback.
3. Doctors often misperceive the amount and type of information that pa-tients want to receive.
4. Improved quality of clinical communication is related to positive health outcomes.
5. Explaining and understanding patients concerns, even when they cannot be resolved, results in a fall in anxiety.
6. Greater participation by the patient in the encounter improves satisfaction, compliance and treatment outcomes.
7. The level of psychological distress in patients with serious illness is less when they perceive themselves to have received adequate information.
8. Beneficial clinical communication is routinely possible in clinical practice and can be achieved during normal clinical encounters, without unduly prolonging them, provided that the clinician has learned the relevant tech-niques. (Berry, 2007, p. 3)

The Kalamazoo Consensus Statement resulted at a major conference on physician–patient communication held in Kalamzoo, Michigan, in 1999 (Makoul, 2001). Like the Toronto Consensus Statement, this consensus statement also identified elements of communication in clinical encounters deemed essential in patient-centred communication. Table 9.1 presents these essential elements and communication tasks.

TABLE 9.1: KALAMAZOO CONSENSUS STATEMENT: ESSENTIAL ELEMENTS AND TASKS OF CLINICAL COMMUNICATION

Essential element	Tasks
Establishes rapport	· Encourages a partnership between physician and patient · Respects patient's active participation in decision making
Opens discussion	· Allows patient to complete his/her opening statement · Elicits patient's full set of concerns · Establishes/maintains a personal connection
Gathers information	· Uses open-ended and closed-ended questions appropriately · Structures, clarifies, and summarizes information · Actively listens using non-verbal (e.g., eye contact, body position) and verbal (words of encouragement) techniques
Understands patient's perspective of illness	· Explores contextual factors (e.g., family, culture, gender, age, socio-economic status, spirituality) · Explores beliefs, concerns, and expectations about health and illness · Acknowledges and responds to patient's ideas, feelings, and values
Shares information	· Uses language patient can understand · Checks for understanding · Encourages questions
Reaches agreement on problems and plans	· Encourages patient to participate in decision to the extent he/she desires · Checks patient's willingness and ability to follow the plan · Identifies and enlists resources and supports
Provides closure	· Asks whether patient has other issues or concerns · Summarizes and affirms agreement with the plan of action · Discusses follow-up (e.g., next visit, plan for unexpected outcomes)

Source: Schirmer, J.M., Mauksch. L., Lang, F., Zoppi, K., Epstein, R.M., Brock, D., & Pryzbylski, M. (2005, p. 185). Assessing communication competence: A review of current tools. *Family Medicine, 37*(3), 184–192.

In summary, effective patient-centred care is a communicative practice, a collaboration between health care providers and receivers. Both parties should engage in information seeking and exchange, and rapport and relationship building to establish trust and facilitate shared decision making during the medical encounter. Of concern, research measuring the effect of health literacy skills on patient participation in health care decision making found that those with low or inadequate health literacy skills were less inclined to feel like a partner in their care or the care of their children, relied more on the doctor's knowledge, and preferred to leave decisions about their personal health care up to the doctor (Naik, Street, Castillo, & Abraham, 2011; Yin et al., 2012). These findings emphasize the importance of health literacy skill within the clinical setting and the need for health care providers to attend to issues of health literacy as predictive of patient engagement within their own care.

REVIEW AND REFLECT

Many popular movies and television shows display various aspects of patient-centred health care in the clinical context, for example, *ER*, *Grey's Anatomy*, *The Doctors*, and *House*. Pick two scenarios from a movie or a TV show that you have enjoyed watching and, drawing from the above discussion, examine how patient-centred health care can help improve health literacy in the clinical context.

THE IMPORTANCE OF HEALTH LITERACY FOR HEALTH PROFESSIONAL EDUCATION

The relationship between low health literacy and poor health outcomes highlights the need to educate all health professional students and providers about health literacy. Health literacy is one of the "knowledge features" highlighted in the Canadian Nurses Association "NurseOne" online education site (see www.nurseone.ca). As well, the Registered Nurses' Association of Ontario (n.d.), under the policy and political action section of their online site, positions health literacy as an important determinant of health and advocates for greater awareness and attention to health literacy as a significant component of health care (see www.RNAO.ca). The Canadian Medical Association (CMA) shares the concerns expressed by their American colleagues in the health literacy report of the Ad Hoc Committee on Health Literacy for the American Medical Association Council on Scientific Affairs (1999), which states:

> Patients with inadequate health literacy have a complex array of communications difficulties, which may interact to influence health outcome. These patients report worse health status and have less understanding about their medical conditions and treatment. Preliminary studies indicate inadequate health literacy may increase the risk of hospitalization. Professional and public awareness of the health literacy issue must be increased, beginning with education of medical students and physicians and improved patient-physician communication skills. (p. 552)

In response to these concerns, the CMA has established a continuing medical education course on health literacy (see www.cma.ca/health-literacy-course) as part of their Maintenance of Certification program of The Royal College of Physicians and Surgeons of Canada.

Among other issues, the health literacy report of the American Medical Association Council on Scientific Affairs (1999) underscored the importance of screening patients for low health literacy and effective health education methods.

Table 9.2 presents a list of possible indicators of low health literacy (Canadian Public Health Association, 2006b) that health care providers can use to screen patients for health literacy barriers.

TABLE 9.2: POSSIBLE SIGNS OF LOW HEALTH LITERACY

The patient may appear frustrated and angry about a treatment that has not worked.
The patient may not follow instructions or recommendations for self-care.
Incidence of high frequency of visits or not showing up at all for scheduled visits.
Despite repeating the same instructions over several visits, the condition may still not being managed. For example, high blood pressure or high blood sugar may persist, even with prescribed medication and instructions for self-management.
The patient may not look at pamphlets or information provided or may say no when they are offered.
When given forms to fill out or written information, the patient may say, "I left my reading glasses at home."
The patient may bring a caregiver or a family member along to the appointment and defer to them to answer questions. When taking the social history, the patient may say "I never was much good in school."
Noticeable language barriers.
Observing non-verbal signs of lack of understanding. For example, the patient may just nod and agree, so it goes undetected.

Source: Modified from the Canadian Public Health Association. (2006b, p. 4). *Low health literacy and chronic disease prevention and control: Perspectives from the health and public health sectors.* Table 3. Retrieved from http://www.cpha. ca/uploads/portals/h-l/kl_summary_e.pdf [accessed: 17 June 2013].

REVIEW AND REFLECT

What do you think is the strongest predictor of one's health? Is it age, income, employment status, education level, or race? (The correct answer is not included in these options!)

According to the Ad Hoc Committee on Health Literacy for the American Medical Association Council on Scientific Affairs (1999), poor health literacy is a stronger predictor of one's health than age, income, employment status, education level, or race.

Ask your family doctor if he/she knows this fact about health literacy!

PROVIDER AND PATIENT COMMUNICATION SKILLS TRAINING FOR IMPROVING HEALTH LITERACY

Human communication is central to the delivery of quality health care services. Research consistently shows that communication between health care providers and receivers (patients and their families) needs improvement (Ong, de Haes, Hoos, & Lammes, 1995; Street, 2003a, 2003b). The communicative dynamics of the medical encounter demand that health information be clear, comprehensible, credible, and accessible. Hence, communicative skills and skill development are of great importance to improving health literacy in the clinical context (Williams, Davis, Parker, & Weiss, 2002). While the significance of effective communication in the clinical context cannot be overemphasized, physicians do not always receive adequate communication skills training (Maguire, 1999), and patients too are not always effective communicators (Parrott, 1994; Street, 1991). There are a myriad of reasons why communication barriers occur in the clinical context, some of which were described in the chapter on culture and health literacy (see Chapter 5). Regardless of what causal pathway is leading to poor communication, the existing literature underscores the importance of communication skills training for both providers and patients to improve communication in clinical encounters (Cegala, 2006; Cegala & Broz, 2002, 2003; Cegala, McClure, Marinelli, & Post, 2000; Hulsman, Ross, Winnbust, & Bensing, 1999). When both health care providers and patients receive communication skills training, a positive impact on health outcomes follows, including physicians' display of patient-centred communication and patients' expression of greater involvement during the medical visit (Rao, Anderson, Inui, & Frankel, 2007). For example, studies showed that communication skills training for physicians resulted in their demonstration and maintenance of improved communication in clinical encounters (Fallowfield, Jenkins, Farewell, & Solis-Trapala, 2003; Jenkins & Fallowfield, 2002). During medical interviews with patients, "[d]octors continued to employ focused and open questions, valuable skills, particularly at the beginning of an interview, to enable collection of more reliable information and to help identify patient concerns. Efficient questioning was accompanied by a decrease in the number of times that patients were interrupted" (Fallowfield et al., 2003, p. 1448).

Other studies (Harrington, Noble, & Newman, 2004; Post, Cegala, & Miser, 2002) showed that communication skills training for patients also resulted in better dyadic communication in patient–health care provider participation in medical consultations. Patients were more directive in the medical interview, asking for clarification, recalling information, and adhering to recommendations.

Provider and patient communication skills training has important implications for health literacy. In his study about how physicians could educate patients to improve patient satisfaction with care and patients' experience with physician–patient communication, Terry (2000) found an increase in satisfaction with care for patients who received self-care information from their physicians as compared to patients who did not receive such information. While health care provider training in communication skills has received scholarly attention for some time (Thompson & Parrott, 2002), it is only recently that attention has been focused on communication skills training for patients (Cegala et al., 2000; Cegala & Broz, 2003; Cegala, Gade, Broz, & McClure, 2004). For example, Cegala et al. (2000) found that patient-centred communication is more often present in the medical encounter when the patient had received skills training than when the patient did not receive such training. These encounters also show a more active role on the part of the patient in information seeking and giving. Cegala and Broz (2003) argued that when both the provider and the patient receive communication skills training there is a strong positive effect for both participants. Therefore, physicians who have training in patient-centred communication can elicit pertinent health information from patients that would likely facilitate better patient understanding of diagnosis, test results, and self-care management plans. Correspondingly, trained patients can be more engaged in the medical visit and voice health care concerns to, ask questions of, and seek more information from physicians about their symptoms to make the best medical decisions for themselves. Thus, communication skills training in the clinical context is integral to health literacy issues and positive health outcomes.

Pharmaceutical company Pfizer has created a quiz on health literacy for health care providers (see www.pfizerhealthliteracy.com/physicians-providers/PolicyQuiz.aspx) as well as a checklist for health care providers on clear communication (see www.pfizerhealthliteracy.com/physicians-providers/Checklist.aspx).

REVIEW AND REFLECT

Drawing on the above discussion, work in groups of three to create communication guidelines for providers (e.g., doctors, nurses) and patients to improve the effectiveness of physician–patient communication for advancing health literacy. The guidelines should include "dos," "don'ts," and "to be researched and decided." Please provide literature support for each guideline that your group creates.

PROMOTING HEALTH LITERACY FOR CANADIANS THROUGH PATIENT-CENTRED HEALTH CARE

Rootman (2006) underscored the findings of the International Adult Literacy and Skills Survey (IALSS) report in 2005 (see Chapters 2 and 3 for details about the survey) on the Canadian adult population's rather low levels of prose and document literacy, numeracy, and problem solving skills. Research findings show an association between low health literacy and poor health outcomes (Rootman & Ronson, 2005), and how health information may be written at a higher than recommended reading level (Smith & Haggerty, 2003). In recognition of these findings, Rootman (2006) argued, "Little research has been conducted on health literacy by Canadian physicians," and "There are key reasons why Canadian physicians should be more concerned about health literacy" (p. 606). He offered suggestions as to how individual physicians can address the health literacy problem in Canada:

> Individual physicians could, for example, become more aware of the magnitude of the issue of low literacy and health literacy in the population and in their own practices. They also might become more sensitive to the signs of low literacy and health literacy among their patients and adjust their oral and written communication accordingly. (p. 607)

The importance of communication skills training for doctors is also apparent from the discussion found in Box 9.2.

BOX 9.2: ON DOCTORS' COMMUNICATION SKILLS

Dr. Hughes, a family doctor in Ottawa and Community Faculty Teacher at the University of Ottawa, who has done research and taught communications for 28 years, addressed the conference first. He is concerned that most doctors still do not get enough training in communication skills in medical school. According to research, Dr. Hughes says, their communication skills actually deteriorate as they progress through medical school. It has been documented that most doctors begin a response to the patient in 19 seconds, forgetting the basic principle, "Before you tell, ask."

This continues despite the knowledge that better consultation skills lead to better health outcomes, less frustration and more satisfaction for providers and patients. Dr. Hughes ended his opening remarks with a call to change medical training: "We need to convince medical schools that effective communication is essential to the practice of health care—it is no longer an option."

Source: Some current research on health and literacy. (2000, p. 1). *Literacy Across the Curriculummedia Focus, 15*(1). Retrieved from http://centreforliteracy.qc.ca/sites/default/files/Some_current.pdf [accessed: 3 September 2013].

Rootman (2006) also stressed the importance of screening patient education materials to ensure they are written at levels appropriate for the patients and of adopting effective communication approaches for dealing with patients with poor health literacy, such as the teach-back method.

Focusing on the management of chronic diseases with people with low health literacy, the Canadian Public Health Association presented good communication techniques to improve patient–provider interaction (see Table 9.3).

TABLE 9.3: COMMUNICATION TECHNIQUES TO IMPROVE PATIENT–PROVIDER INTERACTION IN MANAGING CHRONIC DISEASE WITH PEOPLE WITH LOW HEALTH LITERACY

Asking patients to explain what they know/understand about their chronic disease as a starting point for identifying level of health literacy and/or misconceptions that may present barriers to self-care
"Slowing things down completely" to allow adequate time for explanation and questions
Using simple terms in common use rather than complex medical terminology or jargon, e.g., high blood pressure rather than hypertension, or blood sugar rather than glucose
Asking patients how they learn best
Asking patients to teach-back what has been recommended to check for understanding of instructions and to identify areas for reinforcement or where barriers to learning exist
Reinforcing messages several times and explaining in several different ways during and at future appointments

Source: The Canadian Public Health Association. (2006b, p. 9). *Low health literacy and chronic disease prevention and control: Perspectives from the health and public health sectors.* Table 7. Retrieved from http://www.cpha.ca/uploads/portals/h-l/kl_summary_e.pdf [accessed: 17 June 2013].

Canada has made some important strides in health literacy interventions (Canadian Public Health Association [CPHA], 2006a) (see Chapter 10 for further information on health literacy interventions). For example, *Going to the Doctor* is a Yukon Learn resource produced to provide health information in plain language and guide health care receivers in experiencing a productive medical encounter (CPHA, 2006a). The Nova Scotia Heart Health Partnership prepared *It's Your Health*, a plain language health information resource to engage community groups and organizations in the western region of Nova Scotia in health promotion strategies (CPHA, 2006a). A partnership between Health Canada and the Canadian Diabetes Association and Dietitians of Canada resulted in the Healthy Eating is in Store for You strategy to help consumers better understand the nutrition information on the labels of packaged foods. By making nutrition information on food products easy to find and read, consumers can make healthy food choices (CPHA, 2006a). Health Canada has created an interactive nutrition label tool to help consumers learn how to use nutrition information for healthy eating (see http://www.hc-sc.gc.ca/fn-an/label-etiquet/nutrition/cons/inl_main-eng.php). It's Safe to Ask, a communication and health literacy initiative, was launched by the Manitoba Institute for Patient Safety to help promote the quality of health care for people in Manitoba (Byrd & Thompson, 2008). Modelled after the American Medical Association's Ask Me 3 programs, the It's Safe to Ask initiative also encourages patients to ask three simple questions of their health care providers:

• What is my health problem?
• What do I need to do?
• Why do I need to do this?

Although Canada is carrying out promising health literacy interventions to help improve the quality of health care for its people, gaps still exist in evaluating these health interventions in practice. For example, research is warranted to examine "how interventions affect the general health status of people with low literacy or whether they affect health care costs or health disparities based on race, ethnicity, culture, or age" (CPHA, 2006a, p. 1). There is also a need to design, implement, and evaluate more interventions for patient-centred health care and medical education in health literacy.

REVIEW AND REFLECT

Pair up with another student. One of you will role-play the doctor and the other, the patient. The "doctor" should try to use the different strategies discussed above for promoting patient health literacy through patient-centred care. The "patient" should reciprocate accordingly. You and your partner should switch roles in different rounds. Audio record each interaction and analyze the interactions. Then, discuss the various factors that influence the practice of the strategies, and how the strategies work in your role-play interactions.

KEY LEARNING POINTS

This chapter highlighted the importance of health literacy in the clinical context, especially in health care encounters. Low levels of health literacy are a significant problem for many Canadian adults because low levels of health literacy are associated with poorer health outcomes for both individuals and their families. Although individuals across all demographic groups may have low levels of health literacy, of particular concern is the prevalence of low literacy skill among seniors, immigrants, Aboriginal people, and those with limited income and education. Hence, patient-centred health care is paramount to help identify appropriate and preferred medical support to increase patient participation in care, collaborative goal setting, and planning of treatment.

Effective communication is an important consideration in improving health literacy in the clinical context. The chapter discussed some specific strategies for effective communication in provider–patient interaction to help increase health literacy. Recognizing the need for good communication skills for improving health literacy, communication skills training in medical schools should be coordinated at all levels—undergraduate, residency, and postgraduate. Although Canada is considered a global leader in its strides toward improving health literacy for the population, the Canadian health care community has only begun to recognize the significance of health literacy as a determinant of health. Indeed, given the importance of health literacy for enhancing patient decision making and health outcomes, it may be as much a priority area for Canadian undergraduate health professional education curricula as the other more traditional domains of medical education, professional practice, and knowledge development. The saliency and impact of health information literacy as part of regular Canadian health professional education has been suggested by those practitioners involved in information dissemination to patients and providers. Kloda (2008), a medical librarian, observed that "the majority of students in the health professions [in medical schools in Canada] are not learning how to find and convey the best information to their patients" (p. 322) and added that medical librarians can be involved in developing this critical component of medical curricula. Similarly, the Canadian Nurses Association document, *Toward 2020: Visions for Nursing* (Villeneuve & MacDonald, 2006), predicts a shift in the nurses' role to accommodate the increased information needs of individuals and patients. The document claims that nurses will take on the role of helping individuals and patients to navigate the information complexities within health care and our health care system. As Canadians we face mounting challenges in obtaining equitable, timely, and cost-responsible access to health care. Thus, health literacy training in the clinical encounter and for medical education takes on even greater urgency.

A CANADIAN MILESTONE

EASY DOES IT! PLAIN LANGUAGE AND CLEAR VERBAL COMMUNICATION: TRAINING MANUAL

This resource has been put together by the Canadian Public Health Association's (CPHA) National Literacy and Health Program. The aim is to advance awareness among health professionals about health information in plain language and clear verbal communication to help them serve clients with low literacy skills. The training manual offers health professionals effective communication tools, case studies, practical exercises, practical strategies, tips on office design, and samples of plain language information and consent forms. It also contains a list of provincial literacy coalitions and literacy-related health programs and activities. (See www.cpha.ca/uploads/portals/h-l/easy_does_it_e.pdf for an electronic version of this manual.)

Source: Canadian Public Health Association. (n.d.). *Health literacy resources.* Retrieved from http://www.cpha.ca/en/portals/h-l/resources.aspx [accessed: 19 June 2013].

ADDITIONAL RESOURCES OF INTEREST

Directory of Plain Language Health Information

http://www.cpha.ca/uploads/portals/h-l/directory_e.pdf

This website consists of a directory of plain language health resources from 49 North American organizations. It also lists tips on how to create and identify plain language health information.

Easy Does It! Plain Language and Clear Verbal Communication: Training Manual

http://www.cpha.ca/uploads/portals/h-l/easy_does_it_e.pdf

This online training manual features effective communication tools, case studies, and practical exercises for health professionals. It also includes samples of plain language information and consent forms, and a list of provincial literacy coalitions and literacy-related health programs and activities.

A Collection of Health Literacy Curricula
http://www.advancinghealthliteracy.com/curricula.html
A discussion on the National Institute for Literacy Health and Literacy listserv resulted in the creation of this resource. This site contains online health literacy curricula in easily accessible and downloadable format for educational purposes. In that same spirit, the site also welcomes submissions on an ongoing basis.

Health Canada
http://www.hc-sc.gc.ca/fn-an/label-etiquet/nutrition/educat/info-nutri-label-etiquet-eng.php
This Health Canada website contains information about how better to understand the nutritional value found on the labels of prepackaged foods. This interactive nutrition label tool is useful for making healthier food choices.

Picture Stories for Adult English-as-Second-Language (ESL) Health Literacy
http://www.cal.org/caela/esl_resources/health/healthindex.html#Emergency
This website contains picture stories for adult English-as-Second-Language (ESL) health literacy. The site includes educational resources designed to help both instructors and low-literacy students (also newcomers) to address and discuss topics related to health and well-being. Sample topics range from awareness of and access to health care services, to risks of more serious and chronic health outcomes. Stories about cartoon characters with minimum words and simple terms are used to promote speaking, listening, reading, and writing about health-related topics such as medication, doctor's appointments, depression, and so on.

CHAPTER 10

HEALTH LITERACY INTERVENTIONS
IN CANADA

Education is now going to be the buffalo of the future. It is our new means of survival.

—Chief Barry Ahenakew, *Ahtahkakoop*, 2000

CHAPTER LEARNING OBJECTIVES
- Introduce individual approaches to enhance health literacy
- Introduce health care provider approaches to enhance health literacy
- Consider system and organizational approaches to enhance health literacy

INTRODUCTION

In this text, we have addressed multiple aspects of health literacy. We have focused on the Canadian context but also moved beyond our borders to include health literacy within the global community. The previous chapters have provided an overview of health literacy within Canada and reported on the myriad factors that show how and why health literacy is a significant determinant of health. Scientific advances in medical knowledge and treatment have resulted in an increase in life longevity but also an increased prevalence of chronic disease. The expectation for self-health promotion and shared decision making between individuals and their health care provider is assumed within the disease-management model of health care. Increased access to health information, most noticeably within an online context, supports the management model of care, where the need for accurate and accessible health information exists. In contrast, we know from Chapters 2 and 3 of this book that the limited literacy and health literacy skill of Canadian adults challenges their ability to "access, understand, evaluate and communicate information as a way to promote, maintain and improve health in variety of settings across the life-course" (Rootman & Gordon-El-Bihbety, 2008, p. 11).

We have considered the multiple frameworks and definitions of health literacy and reviewed the research on the literacy and health literacy skills of Canadians. The importance of culture in understanding health literacy has been highlighted, and we have seen that health literacy contributes to issues of social justice and equity in the way that it creates inequitable health experiences and outcomes among Canadians. We hope that you are now convinced that adequate health literacy skills are crucial for effective health promotion and successfully navigating our health care system (Canadian Council on Learning, 2007a; Nielsen-Bohlman, Panzer, & Kindig, 2004; Nutbeam, 2000). Health decisions and behaviours taken by individuals are reflective of their health literacy skills and are significant in the prevention and management of chronic disease (Taggart et al., 2012). Literacy and health literacy skills are increasingly recognized as important social determinants of health (SDOH) (Public Health Agency of Canada, 2011). In fact, as with other SDOH, health literacy is considered both a contributor to poor health and an intervention for health promotion (Canadian Council on Learning, 2007a; Nutbeam, 2000).

In this final chapter, we will review individual-, provider-, and system-level interventions to enhance health literacy skill. These literacy and health literacy interventions focus on activities, programs, and exemplars that have relevance for Canadians. However, these interventions are only the first step toward enhancing the health literacy of Canadians. This final chapter will end with a consideration of the next steps we might consider as students, educators, and practitioners of health literacy.

HEALTH LITERACY INTERVENTIONS
INTERVENTIONS FOR INFANTS AND CHILDREN

Basic literacy skills are critical to health literacy skill development. The Canadian Council on Learning report on the health literacy of Canadians identified daily reading as one of the strategies in support of health literacy skill development (Canadian Council on Learning, 2008a). The importance of reading practice is greatest in the early years of childhood, when lifetime reading patterns are established. As an example of the importance of early reading programs, researchers in Nova Scotia investigated the effectiveness of an early literacy intervention program called Read to Me (see www.readtomeprogram.org) (Zanten, Coates, Hervas-Malo, & Mcgrath, 2012). The Read to Me program gives books and other literacy materials to new parents in hospital within 24–48 hours after giving birth. The Read to Me literacy package contains an assortment of material, including children's books, a book with nursery rhymes, a CD with nursery songs, information about libraries and other resources, and coupons for discounted book purchases in local bookstores. What the researchers showed was that mothers who received the literacy package tended to read more to their babies compared to mothers who did not receive it. The Read to Me program increased the amount of time family members engaged in literacy activities with children. In addition, giving the literacy package to parents highlights the importance of reading and literacy skill development from the time of birth. Importantly, the Read to Me program is an inexpensive and easily delivered intervention and has been made available in multiple languages including Mi'kmaq, Arabic, French, and English. Because children who begin school with poor literacy skill will experience chronic disadvantages throughout and beyond their academic years, early interventions that promote reading help to minimize the gap between poor and strong elementary school readers (Ogg, Sundman-Wheat, & Bateman, 2012).

A group of researchers in the United States reviewed the literature on early literacy interventions within pediatric health settings. In this review they concluded that physicians, and in particular, pediatricians, are influential and well positioned to advocate for enhanced literacy skill development among children. This is in part because of the regularity and frequency of physician contact with young families (e.g., well-child visits, early immunizations, illnesses). The literacy interventions reported in the research literature were intended to increase reading activities among preschool age children and especially among children at risk for reading failure. Specifically, the interventions included supplying children's books at well-child visits, physicians' advocacy for reading, and having volunteer readers or literacy resources in physicians' waiting rooms. In addition, physician-based early literacy interventions were very important in engaging low-income families at increased risk for deficits in early literacy development. Essentially, if parents have a positive attitude toward reading with their children, there is a greater likelihood that children will engage in reading at an early age and in this way improve literacy outcomes (Ogg et al., 2012).

REVIEW AND REFLECT

Consider the pros and cons of the use of electronic books or readers to develop literacy skill among preschool and elementary school age children. As a health educator, would you advocate for electronic readers and books for young children?

INTERVENTIONS FOR TEENS AND YOUNG ADULTS

A different strategy to build health literacy among young people was undertaken by U.S. educators. The Building Wellness program is a health literacy intervention based on a six-year curriculum (grades 3 to 8) designed to promote students' self-efficacy and sense of well-being through experiential learning with games, activities, and medical guest speakers (Diamond, Saintonge, August, & Azrack, 2011). All Building Wellness lessons are based on developing the literacy skills of reading, writing, numeracy, critical thinking, listening, and verbal fluency. The program focused on skill development that included students' understanding of food labels, making healthy choices, and understanding how their bodies function and develop. The students were "coached" to avoid peer pressure, provided with exercise tips, and given instruction in goal-setting skills and the development of communication skills—specifically with medical professionals. The success of the program was reflected in the evaluations of the Building Wellness curriculum, which demonstrated increased knowledge and retention of information within lessons and across years among the student participants (Diamond et al., 2011).

A similar participatory approach to health literacy development for Canadian teenagers has been strongly advocated by researchers from British Columbia who suggest "that collaboration with others builds knowledge.… [A]s a social process, learning lets individuals connect, interact and find meaning with others and their environment. Literacy educators now acknowledge that the development of knowledge, skills and attitudes occurs in relationships between and among students, teachers, family members and the broader community" (Wharf Higgins, Begoray, & MacDonald,

2009, p. 352). In Chapter 4 we introduced the key concept that enhancing health literacy skills includes "helping people to develop confidence to act on knowledge;… the ability to work with and support others will best be achieved through more personal forms of communication, and through community-based educational outreach" (Nutbeam, 2000, p. 267). Canadian researchers have used participatory approaches in developing interventions directed at enhancing the health literacy skill of health care providers as well as some of the most marginalized Canadians. As presented in Chapter 7, Vancouver's Healthy Aboriginal Network used a participatory approach to developing a health literacy intervention for youth. The project involved the development of an innovative community-based intervention—health-based comic books. It makes good sense that youth-determined health topics would be of greatest relevance to the adolescent population, and the Aboriginal Network organizers facilitated youth participation in the development of comic books that addressed issues of significance to Aboriginal youth (Maunder, 2007). The Healthy Aboriginal Network comic books address health and social issues for youth, including topics such as gambling, diabetes, smoking prevention, suicide and mental health, and youth gang issues (see www.thehealthyaboriginal.net). The comic books produced by the Healthy Aboriginal Network include storylines that offer alternative choices regarding behaviours about common but sometimes very difficult health situations facing Aboriginal youth. For example, *Droppin' the Flag* is based on conversations with incarcerated youth about their gang experiences.

FIGURE 10.1: *DROPPIN' THE FLAG*

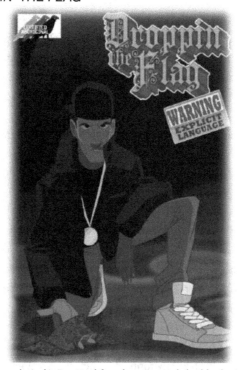

Source: Healthy Aboriginal Network. (n.d.). Retrieved from http://www.thehealthyaboriginal.net/ [accessed: 14 June 2013].

Droppin' the Flag discusses integrating gang youth back into communities. The comic book *An Invited Threat* focuses on diabetes care and prevention and is about a family's realization that certain foods and how they are consumed can cause ill health (see www.the-healthyaboriginal.net). The storyline in this comic book supports the development of health prevention in recognizing that making healthy decisions early on will decrease the risk of ill health (diabetes) later in life.

FIGURE 10.2: *AN INVITED THREAT*

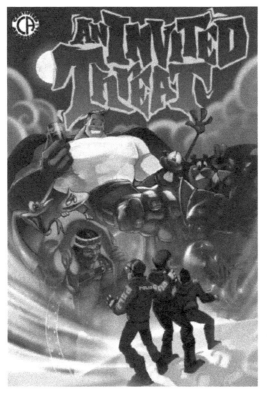

Source: Healthy Aboriginal Network. (n.d.). Retrieved from http://www.thehealthyaboriginal.net/ [accessed: 14 June 2013].

Instead of a comic book, a group of Canadian Indigenous students and their teachers developed an innovative health literacy intervention using videos. Through their video project, students were encouraged to develop a "critical consciousness about community, culture, confidence, and control" regarding health and health literacy within their culture (Stewart, Riecken, Scott, Tanaka, & Riecken, 2008, p. 181). In creating the videos, the students obtained information about health and wellness and in turn highlighted the cultural conceptions of health and wellness as an important component of health literacy (Stewart et al., 2008). Throughout the process of making the videos, students had the opportunity to interview community members and learn about their culture. Historically,

>Health policies and programmes designed by non-Indigenous individuals
>or institutions have been inappropriate for dealing with Indigenous prob-
>lems.... [U]tilizing video making ... provided students with opportunities
>for both expression and exploration of what it means to be healthy. As
>students explored this terrain, they developed a kind of health literacy that
>reflects their identities as Indigenous people. It is also a literacy that is
>grounded in the interests and concerns of their communities and cultures,
>and as such, it provided meaningful access to healthy ways of being. (Stew-
>art et al., 2008, p. 188)

As a final example of an innovative health literacy intervention aimed at reaching children
and youth, a "child-mediated stroke communication" was developed using hip hop music
to teach school-aged children about the signs and symptoms of stroke (Williams, DeSorbo,
Noble, & Gerin, 2012). Students ages 9 to 12 years "educated" their adult family members
about stroke symptoms, the correct course of action to take when strokes occur, and stroke
prevention measures (collectively termed "stroke literacy"). The Hip Hop Stroke intervention is easily delivered (e.g., three-day, one-hour-per-day multimedia classroom intervention)
and incorporates multiple strategies, such as hip hop songs, a 2- to 4-minute professionally
produced cartoon music video, and a comic book to teach stroke literacy. An evaluation of
the Hip Hop Stroke program concluded that the innovative health literacy intervention delivered by children can successfully enhance the health literacy (e.g., enhanced access to and
engagement with accurate health information) of the entire family (Williams et al., 2012).

These interventions are all seemingly different approaches (early reading, comic books,
videos, hip hop music) to enhancing health literacy. Yet, they share some important features.
First, they focus on young people. Second, they use delivery channels that resonate with
the target groups involved, Third, they take a participatory approach to enhancing health
literacy.

INTERVENTIONS FOR ADULTS

Establishing a shame-free environment was the guiding principle for a group of "street"
women, volunteers, community development workers, and literacy instructors who created a
"drop-in" literacy program for female sex-trade workers in Vancouver's Downtown Eastside
(Alderson & Twiss, 2003, 2006). Organizers of the drop-in learning centre recognized that
most women living and "working the streets" had nowhere to engage in personal development
and education. In creating a shame-free and comfortable space for learning, project organizers found that the women were eager and interested in learning and appreciated a place to
be creative, write poetry, and reflect on their lives. One of the early challenges in developing
the literacy program was finding learning materials that were applicable to the women participants. Based on their experiences working with street workers, the program developers
recommended the following strategies to engage women in literacy learning activities: (1)
hands-on activities for learning, such as word games, drawing, word searches, and journal

writing; (2) activities that are colourful and fairly quick to accomplish; and (3) activities that are relaxing and allow women to care for themselves or someone else. The hours of operation (early evenings from 7 to 11 p.m.) were also tailored to the needs of the female sex workers and enabled them to participate in the learning/literacy program. Through their attendance at the learning centre, some women began considering different possibilities for themselves. The women started organizing events, setting up meetings, publishing a monthly newsletter, using the computer for email, recommending policy changes to the host organization, and looking for opportunities for continued education. For some women, individual learning plans were created. "Many women were looking for a way to explore themselves as sex-trade workers, mothers, learners, junkies and artists outside of the relentless cycle of the street. The Learning Centre opened both a physical and a mental space for women" (Alderson & Twiss, 2003, p. 4).

Yet, to date, the majority of health literacy interventions for adults have focused predominantly on simplifying health information, with the aim of aligning the readability of health care materials and instructions with a population level approximating a grade 3–8 range of readability skill (Weiss, 2007; Xie, 2012). Beyond changes to health information readability, health educators are beginning to explore multiple information presentation formats, including the use of pictures and video. For example, U.S. researchers investigated cardiovascular health outcomes resulting from different health education interventions—an information booklet only, compared to both the booklet and an associated video component (Eckman et al., 2012). The booklet contained information on a variety of medical terms, common heart medications, supportive resources, and basic information about coronary artery disease. It discussed how to manage coronary artery disease through diet and exercise, blood pressure control, smoking cessation strategies, and long-term outcomes of health-enhancing behaviour change. Information in the booklet was written at a grade 5 reading level. The video component of the heart health intervention provided similar information but also included interview segments with patients of varying ethnicity and gender who were managing their own coronary artery disease. While knowledge about coronary disease and management strategies increased among all individuals, those people who had received both the information booklet and the video appeared to have a greater improvement in heart health knowledge. Individuals also experienced a positive impact on health behaviour change (e.g., diet and cigarette smoking), and among smokers who had access to the booklet and the video material, there was a significant decrease in the number of cigarettes smoked per day. Individuals who had received the booklet and video intervention also had a significant increase in exercise and greater weight loss. Importantly, those with lower health literacy relative to individuals with adequate health literacy had similar outcomes or changes in health behaviour following the interventions. What this study clearly suggests is that alternatives to conventional printed information are effective for improving health literacy among adults whose literacy skill levels are low.

An interactive pictorial educational intervention was designed to suit the learning patterns and psychomotor skills of older adults (Park, 2011). This educational intervention used a small group-based interactive intervention to address medication safety among U.S. seniors. Older adults residing in community senior centres were provided with: (a) an interactive group session using pictures/illustrations plus an information booklet; (b) a medication information booklet only; or (c) traditional treatment with no additional information about the safe use of medications. Again, the interactive pictorial education was most effective in increasing seniors' confidence and knowledge of safe medication use for self-health promotion. Older adults with low literacy comprise a population with special needs who are at higher risk of experiencing poor health. The small group interaction between the instructor and the participants allowed even older adults with less than optimal literacy levels to understand the medication information. Additional approaches focused on limited health numeracy skill include supplementing verbal instructions with written instructions, using simple graphs, pictures, or anecdotes, and removing unnecessary distractions (Apter et al., 2009).

Recall discussions from earlier chapters about the "knowledge gap" hypothesis, which proposes that individuals with limited access to the Internet and social media technology are significantly disenfranchised in terms of health information and service access. There is a great need for eHealth literacy interventions for older adults given that eHealth literacy is quickly becoming a basic rather than a specialized health literacy skill set (Xie, 2012). While the Internet holds great potential for supporting health literacy skills, older adults with limited computer skills are at greater risk for health information inequity (Xie, 2012). With this in mind, a health literacy intervention for seniors to enhance their aptitude and confidence in searching and assessing online health information was piloted in the United States. A 4-week-long curriculum was offered in two public libraries and included instruction on how to use the computer and search online for evidence-based health information. Surprisingly, over 75 percent of older adults reported greater participation in their own health based on the skills and knowledge gained from the 4-week program. Most importantly, older adults' knowledge about computers and the Internet improved, and their attitude toward (and self-efficacy with) computers increased. The intervention also provided older adults with the skills necessary to access and use the knowledge they had gained and the confidence to play a more active role in their own health care.

REVIEW AND REFLECT

Using the last conversation you had with your health care provider, illustrate (rather than verbally report) or write the instructions you were given regarding your health care.

INTERVENTIONS FOR HEALTH CARE PROVIDERS

As we have seen in both Chapter 5 and Chapter 9, limited health literacy can (and often does) lead to poor patient–health care provider communication and limited comprehension by patients of health care information. Research investigating the role of health literacy in patient–provider communication found that limited health literacy skills created a significant barrier to effective communication and that adequate health literacy skill may be an important facilitator for patients to effectively engage with and comprehend communication exchanges with their provider (Sudore et al., 2009). In fact, limited health literacy skills as well as limited proficiency in speaking and understanding English were associated with poor patient–provider communication. Physicians' use of plain language in their communication with patients and a decrease in the use of medical jargon supported patient comprehension of health information. Moreover, even for patients whose health care provider speaks the same language (remember how important language is in health literacy), effective communication interventions should include a focus on health literacy skill development. The challenge, however, is that limited health literacy skill and limited English proficiency are communication barriers that often co-exist. Therefore, designing interventions for vulnerable populations that focus solely on health literacy or language may not be sufficient to improve communication and comprehension.

Moreover, the suggestion to use clear communication and common non-medicalized terms applies to all health care consumers, no matter what their literacy level. Additional interventions to support effective communication include the use of techniques such as teach-back (Sudore et al., 2009; Weiss, 2007). Introduced in Chapter 2, Weiss (2007) advocates for patient safety as well as using a number of strategies, including the teach-back technique, to ensure patients' understanding of health care conversations and directions. The teach-back technique involves asking patients to explain or demonstrate instructions given to them within the patient–provider conversation. Weiss (2007) provides template statements that encourage information clarity among patients: "I want you to explain to me how you will take your medication, so I can be sure I have explained everything correctly," or "When you get home your spouse will ask you what the doctor said—what will you tell your spouse?" (p. 33).

To encourage effective communication with others, it is essential that health care providers and health care organizations and systems create a shame-free environment where individuals are made to feel comfortable asking questions about their care and, importantly, about what they do not understand. Even individuals with advanced literacy and health literacy skills may act as if they understand care instructions or health information to avoid seeming "stupid" or to avoid annoying their health care provider (Weiss, 2007). One simple strategy to encourage questions is to let patients know that "many people have difficulty reading and understanding medical information, so please feel comfortable asking questions if there's something you don't understand."

Moreover, a teach-back approach has been shown to be effective in aiding comprehension of health information even in a non-clinical setting. Older English-as-a-Second-Language (ESL) Chinese-speaking women living in the Greater Toronto Area were assessed for their understanding of colon cancer prevention information using both written and oral measures of health literacy. Using the teach-back method, almost 90 percent of the ESL seniors had adequate understanding of the information about preventative behaviours to reduce the risk of colon cancer; in contrast, fewer than 15 percent of the women had adequate understanding of the colon cancer prevention information when assessed with printed measures (McWhirter, Todd, & Hoffman-Goetz, 2011).

REVIEW AND REFLECT

As a health care provider, how would you ensure that your office and your organization present a shame-free environment to your patients? Are there strategies and/or policies that you could implement to create a safe space for patients?

Another example of a Canadian-initiated health literacy intervention for health care providers occurred in Ontario (Rukholm, Carter, & Newton-Mathur, 2009). This intervention involved an online course module that focused on Aboriginal health and healing practices. The online program was designed to improve the cultural competence and cultural humility of inter-professional groups of health care providers by enhancing their understanding of Aboriginal models of health and the role of Elders within Aboriginal health and wellness practices. Specifically, course participants learn how Western medicine intersects with Aboriginal health models and to appreciate the links between the physical, mental, spiritual, and emotional components of health as understood by Aboriginal people. According to Rukholm and colleagues (2009), "Healthcare professionals need to learn to recognize their own cultural beliefs and attitudes as well as the cultural beliefs and attitudes of the different populations they serve; understanding and respect develop through this recognition" (p. 139).

REVIEW AND REFLECT

Drawing on what you learned in earlier chapters, did the online inter-professional educational program for health care providers described above draw on a cultural awareness, cultural competence, or cultural safety focus to enhance the health literacy of their patients?

SYSTEM-LEVEL HEALTH LITERACY INTERVENTIONS

The contemporary model of health care requires accessible health information tailored to the individual and family. As stated by Barry (2012), "Fundamentally, patients need to want to be informed and involved in their healthcare decisions, clinicians need to see the value of informing patients and welcoming their participation, and both parties need to interact in a healthcare environment that makes it easy to do the right thing" (p. 96). Found within the *National Action Plan to Improve Health Literacy* (U.S. Department of Health and Human Services, 2010) and the *Calgary Charter on Health Literacy* (Coleman et al. 2008) is the call for system-level changes that support effective health communication (Coleman et al., 2008; Ridpath, Larson, & Greene, 2012). Health literacy experts are challenging the health care community to broaden their focus from the literacy skills of individuals to include health care providers and health care systems (Coleman et al., 2008; Ridpath, Larson, & Greene, 2012).

In taking on this challenge, some experts have begun to advocate for the systematic integration of health literacy knowledge and skills within the patient-centred medical home model of care (PCMH):

Integrating health literacy principles into the PCMH is a promising strategy for systematically implementing these improvements. The model's promise stems from features that address health literacy challenges across the continuum of care, increasing uptake that includes safety net clinics and community settings, incentives that help organizations prioritize communication improvement, and team-based solutions that better connect practitioners with each other and the patients they serve. (Ridpath, Larson, & Greene, 2012, p. 592)

The integration of health literacy within this model of care is shown in Figure 10.3.

FIGURE 10.3: THE PATIENT-CENTRED MEDICAL HOME (PCMH) MODEL OF CARE

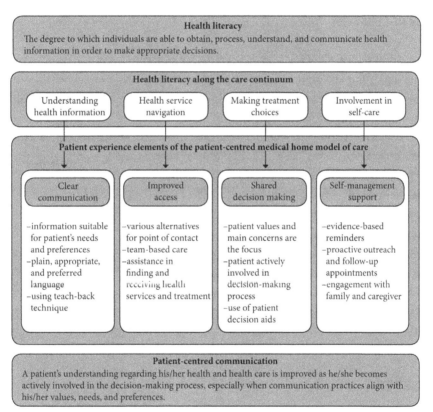

Source: Modified from Ridpath, J.R., Larson, E.B., & Greene, S.M. (2012). Can integrating health literacy into the patient-centered medical home help us weather the perfect storm? *Journal of General Internal Medicine, 27*(5), 588–594.

Researchers in British Columbia wanted to understand how the mandated provincial health education curricula "Planning 10" influenced the health literacy skill of high school students (Wharf Higgins et al., 2009). The "Planning 10" curriculum is intended to develop critical thinking about health issues and the social environment (e.g., impact of the media, online social media) within health care decision making. Within the "Planning 10" curriculum, teachers address the four main content areas of healthy living, health information, healthy relationships, and health decisions. They also address in depth adolescent health issues such as accident prevention (e.g., road safety), sexual health (e.g., sexual decision making), and mental health (e.g., bullying). As it turned out, the school system (e.g., high school) represents a relatively cost-free setting in which to learn about health and develop critical health literacy skills. At the same time that "health education is a necessary component of behavior change, [it] is insufficient without resources and supportive environments to facilitate change" (Wharf Higgins et al., 2009, p. 359). While "Planning 10" is a promising health education curriculum, the researchers caution that any health education program must consider the broader life context (e.g., home setting, neighbourhood, social norms, government policy) that influences peoples' health literacy skill (e.g., to access, understand, evaluate, and communicate health information) (Wharf Higgins et al., 2009).

KEY LEARNING POINTS

Developing and implementing effective communication strategies may be one of the most important interventions to reduce health disparities related to health literacy skill. In this chapter, we presented several exemplar literacy and health literacy interventions targeted to children, adolescents and young adults, adults, and seniors. The interventions described in this chapter have addressed health literacy development at the level of: (1) consumer and patient (e.g., accessing information and services, increasing health care knowledge, creating culturally tailored health information); (2) health care provider (e.g., patient-centred communication, plain language communication techniques, teach-back methods); and (3) health care systems and organizations (e.g., models of care informed by health literacy concepts, establishing health literacy modules for health professional education curricula, emphasizing cultural diversity within health professional education, and creating shame-free environments). In the words of Sudore and Schillinger (2009), "Because most of these strategies can benefit all patients regardless of health literacy level, clinicians, health system planners, and health policy leaders should promote the uptake of such strategies as part of routine health care" (p. 26).

NEXT STEPS

In this chapter we focused principally on health literacy interventions within the health care system. Yet we cannot end the chapter (and indeed the book) without offering a few concluding thoughts about some next steps for improving health literacy in Canada. Recognizing that health literacy is a critical social value, a fundamental right for health equity and social justice, and a significant outcome for the economic prosperity of Canadians, developing new and effective strategies will be a challenge for many decades. We suggest that the one-size-fits-all approach of using printed materials adapted for unique languages and tailored for specific culture groups will not be sufficient to meet health literacy needs in an increasingly linguistically and culturally diverse and technological Canada. We believe that improving health literacy for all Canadians will require multidisciplinary, multicultural, and inter-sectorial strategies. Whatever shape those strategies take, we are convinced they must: (1) foster reading and numeracy practice and self-efficacy across all socio-demographic segments of the population; (2) build health literacy skill through forward-looking and user-friendly technologies; (3) provide the knowledge and tools to enhance functional literacies, social networks and connections, and advocacy skills to empower people to make informed decisions for their health; and (4) engage Canadians in the commitment that health literacy and democracy are intertwined.

A CANADIAN MILESTONE

LEARNING IT TOGETHER (LiT)
Learning it Together—Learning about Healthy Living (LiT) is a student-run initiative sponsored by the Faculty of Health Sciences at Western University in Ontario. LiT focuses on a play-oriented curriculum for children that emphasizes the development of literacy and healthy lifestyle skills. These skills are influenced through participation in creative activities, science-related games, critical thinking, and physical activities. Using health promotion as the program basis, LiT focuses on three major health issues: physical health, health literacy, and self-esteem. By engaging children in creative play-learning activities, they will gain the skills and motivation to stay physically active, gain self-esteem, and to ultimately live a healthy life.

  LiT understands that each child is unique in their learning. Upon entry into the program, each child is paired with a Western University Health Sciences student mentor who works with the child to complete the planned program and play activities. The one-to-one pairing is intended to provide personalized interaction, timely feedback, and one-to-one guidance. In addition, healthy living skills will be encouraged by providing children with healthy snacks and juice during each session. Each of the eight program sessions features a "health" theme to further encourage a healthy/literacy lifestyle.

Source: University of Western Ontario. (2012). *Learning it Together (LiT)*. Retrieved from http://www. uwo.ca/fhs/LiT/ [accessed: 19 June 2013].

ADDITIONAL RESOURCES OF INTEREST
Read to Me: An Intergenerational Reading Program
http://www.readtomeprogram.org
The Read to Me program encourages parents to read books to their babies. The program offers an organized series of workshops to get young parents to appreciate, enjoy, and engage in literacy activities with their children.

WISH

http://wish-vancouver.net

Operated by women for the exclusive use of female sex workers, the WISH Drop-In Centre is a registered non-profit society that provides a number of services for sex workers within a nurturing and shame-free environment. Available services include: nutritious hot meals, showering facilities, makeup, hygiene items, and clothing. The drop-in centre also offers on-site nursing care, and referrals to detoxification centres, rehabilitation houses, and shelters. A literacy program has been established, and women have access to a learning centre that provides them with opportunities to engage in positive, empowering activities in a safe place.

Vancouver Youth

http://www.vancouveryouth.ca

Vancouver Youth is an online website created, and maintained by, youth and staff in the Social Policy Division of the City of Vancouver. The site has been online since 2003, with the goal of engaging Vancouver's young residents in municipal decision making and in their communities.

GLOSSARY

acculturation: The process of interaction between culture groups whereby aspects of two or more groups create a hybrid experience containing elements of both the dominant and non-dominant groups.

active communication channel: An avenue or means of communication that requires greater cognitive effort and engagement by individuals to seek out, understand, and ultimately make use of information. An example of an active communication channel is the Internet.

agenda setting: The ability of the mass media to provide information to the public, to determine what issues are important, and to present topics that are at the centre of public attention and action.

anglophone: In Canada, the word *anglophone* means an English-speaking person or someone whose mother tongue is English and who continues to speak English.

apomediation: People or applications that guide health information access.

Ask Me 3 technique: A technique trademarked by the U.S. National Patient Safety Foundation whereby an individual is encouraged to ask three basic questions during every health care encounter: What is my main problem? What do I need to do (about the problem)? Why is it important for me to do this?

assimilation: A gradual and irreversible change in the values, behaviours, and attitudes of one culture group to that of the host or dominant culture group.

availability bias: The psychological tendency to remember memorable events as being more common even if they are actually uncommon.

Canadian Council on Learning (CCL): A website hosted by the University of Ottawa featuring reports, research results, statistics, and tools for improving learning and conditions of learning in all regions and communities, and across all walks of life, in Canada.

Canadian Public Health Association (CPHA): A national not-for-profit voluntary association that is a chief proponent for public health and is at the forefront of health literacy efforts.

Centre for Literacy: Based in Quebec, the centre holds one of the largest and most comprehensive collections on literacy and related topics in Canada. Since 1995, the Centre has advocated for health literacy by holding workshops, producing newsletter articles, integrating evidence-based literacy research, and networking with local, national, and international partners.

Cloze procedure: The process of omitting words in sentences and having the reader choose the correct word to finish the sentence to measure his or her comprehension of printed information.

communication-vulnerable: People who have little or no proficiency in the main or dominant language of the country in which they live.

Composite Learning Index (CLI): A combination of statistical indicators on lifelong learning in the multiple ways and places Canadians learn (e.g., at work, in school, at home).

computer literacy: The ability to use a computer to solve problems or the ability to interact with information systems, such as computers, to perform basic tasks.

confirmation bias: The psychological tendency to look for information that supports one's own position or orientation.

contemporary model for intervention: Relating to health literacy, this approach involves creating accessible information tailored to the individual or family, rather than addressing the broader health care system.

critical health literacy: The advanced analytical, advocacy, empowerment, and social skills needed for positive change for health within communities and at the broader societal level.

crowdsourcing: A process whereby individuals can share their personal health experiences in an online site to help themselves, other individuals dealing with the same health or illness concerns, health care organizations caring for others with similar conditions, and researchers investigating health and illness.

cultivation: The extent to which media exposure shapes audience perception over a period of time.

cultural awareness: A perspective that entails observing how people carry out their lives, developing sensitivity toward another ethno-cultural group, and not assigning values to differences.

cultural competence: The effective integration and transformation of knowledge found in different cultural settings to improve health care delivery. The focus is on the skill set of the health care practitioner rather than the consumer or patient.

cultural mosaic: A concept that describes how each cultural group maintains its identity while contributing to the national cultural identity as a whole.

cultural safety: The mutual recognition and shared respect for individual cultural differences, and the understanding of differences in power relationships between the health care provider and the patient.

Cultural Sensitivity Assessment Tool (CSAT): An instrument that provides a quick checklist for assessing the cultural appropriateness of health information materials.

culture: A complex and multi-factorial concept used by anthropologists, psychologists, sociologists, public health practitioners, and other social scientists. Culture informs health literacy skill because it shapes what people believe, what people feel it is important to know, who they feel needs to know it, and what action follows from this knowledge.

determinants of health: Multiple social, economic, physical/environmental, and behavioural factors that influence the health of the population. These factors are often peripheral to the health care system.

digital divide: Differences in Internet access among demographic groups resulting in some populations being able to acquire new information at a faster rate than others.

eHealth: The intersection of medical informatics, public health, and business whereby health services and information can be delivered or enhanced through the Internet and related technologies.

eHealth literacy: The ability to seek, find, understand, and appraise health information from electronic sources and apply the knowledge gained to addressing or solving a health problem.

eHealth Literacy Scale (eHEALS): An instrument to assess a person's declared knowledge of eHealth skills, such as the ability to understand and make use of information found on the Internet.

emic: Refers to the analysis of cultural phenomena from the perspective of one who participates in the culture being studied. An emic account comes from a person within the culture.

endemic: Endemic refers to a disease or condition regularly found among a particular group of people or in a certain area.

equity: An ethical concept grounded in principles of distributive justice, which means social justice or fairness.

ethnicity: A socially sanctioned idea of shared ancestry and shared culture, including religion, language, politics, and history.

etic: Refers to the analysis of cultural phenomena from the perspective of one who does not participate in the culture being studied. Etic refers to objective or outsider accounts of cultural phenomena.

Expert Panel on Health Literacy: Formed in 2006 by the Canadian Public Health Association, this panel broadly evaluated health literacy in Canada and provided important recommendations for improvement.

Flesch Reading Ease Readability Formula (FRE): A readability assessment tool that uses words, syllables, and sentence length to calculate the minimum reading grade level required by an individual to read a piece of text. It was developed by Rudolph Flesch in 1948 and has been widely used to score school texts.

framing: The selection and increasing saliency of some aspects of an issue in communication. Framing promotes a particular problem definition, causal interpretation, moral evaluation, and/or treatment recommendation. Framing also refers to the presentation of the same information from different vantage points: gain framing uses a glass as "half full" reference point when describing an issue; loss framing uses a glass as "half empty" reference point when describing an issue.

francophone: In Canada, *francophone* means a French-speaking person or someone whose mother tongue is French and who continues to speaks French.

Freirian model of literacy education: A model of literacy that acknowledges the social dimensions of acquiring and applying literacy, and encourages individuals to question why things have to be the way they are and to collectively consider how to create change for the better. This approach originated with Paolo Freire, a Brazilian educator and philosopher, author of *Pedagogy of the Oppressed*.

functional health literacy: The ability of individuals to find, access, understand, and communicate health and health care system information.

functional literacy: A set of technical literacy skills including reading, writing, and numeracy for everyday use.

Gunning's Fog Index (FOG): A readability assessment tool that measures text difficulty, and supplies the number of years of education needed to understand a piece of text. It was developed by Robert Gunning in 1952 and has been widely used to score newspaper and business documents.

Health 2.0: A set of economic, social, and technology trends that together form the basis for the next generation of Internet users to create and generate health and medical content, share ideas, and connect with others.

health communication: A multifaceted field of study that overlaps with communication and health promotion, and focuses on any type of information exchange and information strategies about health.

health equity: The concept that all people should have equal opportunity to develop and maintain their health through fair and just access to resources for health.

health inequalities: Differences in the health status or in the distribution of health determinants of one population or group compared to another. An example of a health inequality is the difference in mobility between children and the elderly.

health inequities: Differences in health status or in the distribution of health determinants between groups that are unnecessary, avoidable, unfair, and unjust. Deciding whether an issue is one of health inequity requires making a value judgment. An example of a health inequity is the difference in access to mobility aids, such as wheelchairs, between people of different income classes.

health literacy: Ability to access, understand, evaluate, and communicate information as a way to promote, maintain, and improve health and to make appropriate health decisions in a variety of settings across the life course.

health numeracy: Degree to which individuals have the capacity to access, process, interpret, communicate, and act on numerical, quantitative, graphical, biostatistical, and inferential/probabilistic health information to make effective health decisions.

health promotion: The process of enabling people to increase control over and improve their health, and the health of their families and communities.

Healthy Aboriginal Network: A Canadian non-profit organization that engages in the promotion of health, literacy, and wellness by creating comic books on youth health and social justice issues.

heuristics: Simple mental tools used by individuals to deal with ambiguity and probability related to risk.

information literacy: The knowledge and skills necessary for searching and using information effectively.

information trust: Effective communication in medical encounters that promotes trust and confidence, and enables patients to discuss and make medical decisions with their health care provider.

interactive health literacy: The ability of individuals to use cognitive, social, and literacy skills to improve their health and that of their families and networks.

International Adult Literacy Survey (IALS): A cross-sectional, multi-year, multinational series of surveys that measure prose, document, and quantitative literacy in populations. The domains of problem solving and health literacy were added in the 2003 survey (also known as the International Adult Literacy and Skills Survey [IALSS]).

intersectionality theory: A theory that states that no one factor is more important than another; rather, it is at the intersection of many factors where an individual's health experience is defined and created. Intersectionality is concerned with the construction of social identity derived from the intersections between social characteristics (race/ethnicity, indigeneity, gender, class, sexuality, geography, age, disability/ability, migration status, religion) and forms of systemic oppression (racism, classism, sexism, ableism, ageism).

knowledge gap: The unequal distribution of information from the mass media, influenced by factors such as appeal, accessibility, and desirability of media content.

language: A system of codes and signals, with specific semantic rules that connect the signals and symbols to each other.

Learning it Together (LiT): A student-run initiative at the University of Western Ontario that involves a play-oriented curriculum emphasizing the development of literacy and healthy lifestyle skills.

literacy: The ability to understand and employ printed information in daily activities at home, at work, and in the community to achieve one's goals and to develop one's knowledge and potential.

mass media: Technological tools for the transmission of messages to a large group of mixed audiences.

media health literacy: Linked with both health literacy and media literacy, this concept is based on the premise that individuals have the capacity to control the determinants influencing their health through thought and action.

media literacy: The application of critical thinking in assessing information gained from the mass media.

mediated health information: A term used to describe the multiple sources of health information from the various forms of public mass media, such as news stories, specialized journals, health magazines, and the Internet.

multiculturalism: A perspective that identifies diversity within the demographics of a particular societal space and time and is built on sociological, ideological, process, and public policies aimed at maintaining discrete identities.

National Literacy and Health Program (NLHP): A program created by the Canadian Public Health Association to promote and educate health professionals about the relationship between literacy and health. It focuses on plain language and clear communication between health care professionals and the clients they serve.

Newest Vital Sign (NVS): A health literacy and numeracy assessment tool that screens individuals based on nutrition information from an ice-cream label. It is available in English and Spanish.

numeracy: Those abilities that people need to generally function around quantitative tasks, such as effectively budgeting and managing household finances, calculating a tip at a restaurant, or determining the timetable of a bus schedule.

optimism bias: The psychological tendency for people to expect that bad things are more likely to happen to other people and not to themselves.

Ottawa Charter for Health Promotion: An outcome of the first International Conference on Health Promotion that defines health as a positive rather than a deficit concept and emphasizes that health is determined by diverse prerequisite conditions and resources.

overconfidence bias: The psychological tendency to believe that one's own predictions are more likely to be correct than they actually are.

passive communication channel: An avenue or means of communication that typically involves little engagement and less personal effort by individuals to seek out, understand, and ultimately make use of, information. An example of a passive communication channel is television.

patient-centred care: Defined by the Institute of Medicine (IOM) as care that is respectful and responsive to individual patient preferences, needs, and values, ensuring that patient values guide all clinical decisions.

photonovel: A method for educating vulnerable and underserved people and groups about different health topics. Photographs taken by the participants to document important health issues in their lives are added to a storyline.

Planning 10: A health education curriculum, developed in British Columbia in 2004, intended to develop critical thinking skills about health issues and the social environment within health care decision making.

priming: Media messages that can stimulate recall of stored ideas, knowledge, opinions, or experience associated in some way with the message content.

Projections of Adult Literacy: Measuring Movement (PALMM): A tool developed by the Canadian Council on Learning to calculate literacy trends between 2011 and 2031.

provider–patient communication: Interactive communication between health care professionals and patients that can empower patients by facilitating their understanding of the health care system, medical instructions, and self-care skills.

Rapid Estimate of Adult Literacy in Medicine (REALM): An assessment tool used primarily in clinical situations that measures adults' ability to read common medical, anatomical, or illness terms by testing word recognition and pronunciation rather than text comprehension.

risk: The possibility of harm or an adverse outcome; the uncertainty about the timing of harm or occurrence of an adverse outcome; and the magnitude of the harm or adverse outcome (how many people could be affected by it).

risk communication: An approach to communicating with the public by stakeholders (such as government and non-governmental agencies) about issues that are real, suspected, or potential threats to their health, their safety, or the environment.

science literacy: The knowledge, skills, and abilities necessary for basic understanding of scientific concepts, ideas, and information.

shame-free environment: An atmosphere where individuals, especially those who are underserved or marginalized, are comfortable asking questions about their care and what they don't understand. This concept is related to cultural safety.

Short Assessment of Health Literacy for Spanish Adults (SAHLSA): A health literacy assessment instrument, based on REALM, which is designed to assess a Spanish-speaking adult's ability to read and understand common medical terms.

Simplified Measure of Gobbledygook (SMOG): A readability assessment tool that estimates the number of years of education needed to understand a piece of text. It was developed by G. Harry McLaughlin in 1969 and has been widely used to score health information.

social exclusion: Processes that deny citizens opportunities to participate in many aspects of cultural, economic, social, and political life.

social justice: The socially defined view in society about what is fair, just, and right. These views or judgments are dictated by the current moral beliefs and values of the society.

Suitability Assessment of Materials (SAM): A measurement instrument that focuses on readability, cultural appropriateness, and the self-efficacy of the reader.

system-level model for intervention: An approach that challenges the health care community to broaden the focus from the literacy skills of individuals to the communication skills of health care providers and a multi-system perspective on health literacy.

teach-back technique: A technique to avoid miscommunication and misunderstanding of health information between individuals and health care providers. The person receiving the instructions is asked to "teach back" or verbally explain the information or instructions they have been given.

Test of Functional Health Literacy of Adults (TOFHLA): A health literacy assessment tool, developed in the United States, which measures reading and numeracy skill using text passages based on real health care situations. A shortened version, known as the S-TOFHLA, and a Spanish version are available.

value judgments: Dependent on context, beliefs, social interactions, attitudes, and culture, these judgments help us decide who to trust, what information is credible, and what particular factors are most frightening.

Web 1.0: A term used to describe the static Hyper-Text Markup Language (HTML) of World Wide Web pages for information distribution and use. An example of Web 1.0 is a "read-only" Web page from Health Canada on consumer product safety or Canada's Food Guide.

Web 2.0: A term used to describe the functionality of the World Wide Web that allows people to collaborate and share information online. An example of Web 2.0 is a health blog.

Web 3.0: A term used to describe the potential of the World Wide Web to connect data, concepts, information, and people. An example of Web 3.0 is a smartphone app that reminds people to take their medication, monitors side effects of the medications they are taking, and digitally sends that information to health care providers.

REFERENCES

6S Marketing. (2012). *Mind-blowing Canadian Facebook usage statistics.* Retrieved from http:// www.6smarketing.com/canadian-facebook-statistics/

Aakko, E. (2004). Risk communication, risk perception, and public health. *Wisconsin Medical Journal, 103*(1), 25–27.

Adair, S.M. (2006). Media literacy and the Web: The good, the bad, and the ugly. *Pediatric Dentistry, 28*(3), 223.

Adelson, N. (2005). The embodiment of inequity health disparities in Aboriginal Canada. *Canadian Journal of Public Health, 96*(Supplement 2): S45–S61.

Advisory Council on Health Infostructure. (2000). *Canada Health Infoway: Paths to better health.* Final Report. Retrieved from http://publications.gc.ca/collections/Collection/H21-145-1999E.pdf

Agency for Healthcare Research and Quality. (2009). *Health literacy measurement tools.* U.S. Department of Health and Human Services, Rockville, MD. Retrieved from http://www.ahrq.gov/ populations/sahlsatool.htm

Alderson, L., & Twiss, D. (2003). *Literacy for women on the streets.* Vancouver: The British Columbia Adult Literacy Cost-Shared Program. Retrieved from http://www.nald.ca/library/research/ litforwm/litforwm.pdf

Alderson, L., & Twiss, D. (2006). *Dream soup ... and life stew: A collection of learning material for women on the street.* Vancouver: National Literacy Secretariat.

Alia, V., & Bull, S. (2005). *Media and ethnic minorities.* Edinburgh: University of Edinburgh Press.

Allen, D.G. (1999). Knowledge, politics, culture, and gender: A discourse perspective. *Canadian Journal of Nursing Research, 30*(4), 227–234.

Alvarez, R.C. (2002). The promise of e-Health—A Canadian perspective. *EHealth International, 1*(4).

American Academy of Pediatrics. (2010). Policy statement—Media education. *Pediatrics, 126*(5), 1012–1017. Retrieved from http://pediatrics.aappublications.org/content/126/5/1012.full.pdf

American Dental Association. (2012). *Oral health topics: Osteoporosis medications and oral health.* Retrieved from http://www.ada.org/2594.aspx

American Medical Association Council on Scientific Affairs. (1999). Health literacy: Report of the Council on Scientific Affairs. Ad Hoc Committee on Health Literacy. *Journal of American Medical Association, 281*(6), 552–557.

American Medical Association. (2006). *Improving communication—Improving care.* Retrieved from http://www.ama-assn.org/ama1/pub/upload/mm/369/ef_imp_comm.pdf

Amzel, A., & Ghosh, C. (2007). National newspaper coverage of minority health disparities. *Journal of the National Medical Association, 99*(10), 1120–1125.

Andrulis, D.P., & Brach, D. (2007). Integrating literacy, culture, and language to improve health care quality for diverse populations. *American Journal of Health Behavior, 31*(Supplement 1), S122–S133.

Annan, K. 1997. Message on occasion of International Literacy Day. United Nations. Press release, September 4, 1997. Retrieved from http://www.un.org/News/Press/docs/1997/19970904.SGSM6316.html

Apter, A.J., Wang, X., Bogen, D., Bennett, I.M., Jennings, R.M., Garcia, L., Sharpe, T., Frazier, C., & Ten Have, T. (2009). Linking numeracy and asthma-related quality of life. *Patient Education and Counseling, 75*(3), 386–91.

Association of Faculties of Medicine of Canada. (n.d.). *AFMC primer on population health.* Retrieved from http://phprimer.afmc.ca/Part1-TheoryThinkingAboutHealth/Chapter3CulturalCompetence-AndCommunication/Culturalawarenesssensitivityandsafety

Atkinson, N.L., & Gold, R.S. (2002). The promise and challenge of eHealth interventions. *American Journal of Health Behavior, 26*(6), 494–503.

Baer, N., & Liepins, L. (2008, August 23). Deadly listeriosis outbreak traced to Maple Leaf meats. *The Vancouver Sun.* Retrieved from http://199.71.40.195/vancouversun/story.html?id=222b628d-8dc8-46af-b1dd-540864db14b8

Baker, D.W. (2006). The meaning and the measure of health literacy. *Journal of General Internal Medicine, 21,* 878–883.

Baker, D.W., Wolf, M.S., Feinglass, J., Thompson, J.A., Gazmararian, J.A., & Huang, J. (2007). Health literacy and mortality among elderly persons. *Archives of Internal Medicine, 167*(14), 1503–1509.

Bardes, C.L. (2012). Defining "patient-centered medicine." *New England Journal of Medicine, 366,* 782–783.

Barnard, A., Nash, R., & O'Brien, M. (2005). Information literacy: Developing lifelong skills through nursing education. *Journal of Nursing Education, 44*(11), 505–510.

Barry, M.J. (2012). Shared decision making: Informing and involving patients to do the right thing in health care. *The Journal of Ambulatory Care Management, 35*(2), 90–98.

Barth, F. (1969). *Ethnic groups and boundaries: The social organization of culture difference.* Boston: Little, Brown, & Co.

Bass, L. (2005). Health literacy: Implications for teaching the adult patient. *Journal of Infusion Nursing, 28*(1), 15–22.

Bass, P.F. III, Wilson, J.F., Griffith, C.H., & Barnett, D.R. (2002). Residents' ability to identify patients with poor literacy skills. *Academic Medicine, 77*(10), 1039–1041.

Basu, A., & Dutta, M.J. (2008). The relationship between health information seeking and community participation: The roles of health information orientation and efficacy. *Health Communication, 23*(1), 70–79.

Bates, B.R., & Ahmed, R. (2012). Introduction: Medical communication in clinical contexts. In B.R. Bates & R. Ahmed (Eds.), *Medical communication in clinical contexts* (pp. 1–16). Dubuque, IA: Kendall Hunt Publishing Company.

Bateson, G. (1972). *Steps to an ecology of mind.* New York: Ballantine Books.

Bawden, D. (2001). Information and digital literacies: A review of concepts. *Journal of Documentation, 57*(2), 218–259.

Beach, M.C., Saha, S., & Cooper, L.A. (2006, October). *The role and relationship of cultural competence and patient-centredness in health care quality* (Vol. 36). New York: The Commonwealth Fund. Retrieved from http://www.commonwealthfund.org/~/media/Files/Publications/Fund%20Report/2006/Oct/The%20Role%20and%20Relationship%20of%20Cultural%20Competence%20and%20Patient%20Centeredness%20in%20Health%20Care%20Quality/Beach_rolerelationshipcultcomppatient%20cent_960%20pdf.pdf

Beacom, A.M., & Newman, S.J. (2010). Communicating health information to disadvantaged populations. *Family and Community Health, 33*(2), 152–162.

Beier, M.E., & Ackerman, P.L. (2005). Age, ability, and the role of prior knowledge on the acquisition of new domain knowledge: Promising results in a real-world learning environment. *Psychology and Aging, 20*(2), 341–355.

Benjamin-Garner, R., Oakes, J.M., Meischke, H., Meshack, A., Stone, E.J., Zapka, J., … & McGovern, P. (2002). Sociodemographic differences in exposure to health information. *Ethnicity & Disease, 12*(1), 124–134.

Bennett, P., Calman, K., Curtis, S., & Fischbacher-Smith, D. (2011). Understanding public responses to risk: Policy and practice. In P. Bennett, K. Calman, S. Curtis, & D. Fischbacher-Smith (Eds.), *Risk communication and public health* (2nd ed., pp. 3–22). Oxford: Oxford University Press.

Bergsma, L.J. (2004) Empowerment education: The link between media literacy and health promotion. *American Behavioral Scientist, 48*(2), 152–164.

Berkman, N.D., Sheridan, S.L., Donahue, K.E., Halpern, D.J., & Crotty, K. (2011). Low health literacy and health outcomes: An updated systematic review. *Annals of Internal Medicine, 155*(2), 97–107.

Berry, D. (2007). *Health communication: Theory and practice.* Maidenhead and New York: Open University Press.

Berry, J.W. (1997). Immigration, adaptation, and acculturation. *Applied Psychology: An International Review, 46*(1), 5–34.

Berry, L.L., Seiders, K., & Wilder, S.S. (2003). Innovations in access to care: A patient centered approach. *Annals of Internal Medicine, 139*(7), 568–574.

Betancourt, J.R. (2004). Cultural competence—marginal or mainstream movement? *New England Journal of Medicine, 351*(10), 953–955.

Betancourt, J.R. (2006, October). *Improving quality and achieving equity: The role of cultural competence in reducing racial and ethnic disparities in health care* (Vol. 37). New York: The Commonwealth Fund. Retrieved from http://www.cmwf.org/publications/publications_show.htm?doc_id=413825

Betancourt, J.R., Green, A.R., Carrillo, J.E., & Ananeh-Firempong, O. (2003). Defining cultural competence: A practical framework for addressing racial/ethnic disparities in health and health care. *Public Health Reports, 118*(4), 293–302.

Biswal, B. (2008). Literacy performance of working-age Aboriginal people in Canada: Findings based on the International Adult Literacy and Skills Survey (IALSS) 2003. *Human Resources and Social Development Canada.* Retrieved from http://publications.gc.ca/collections/collection_2008/hrsdc-rhdsc/HS28-147-2008E.pdf

Bornstein, B.H., & Emler, C. (2001). Rationality in medical decision making: A review of the litera-ture on doctors' decision-making biases. *Journal of Evaluation in Clinical Practice, 7*(2), 97–107.

Bow Valley College Centre. (n.d.). *ReadForward.* Retrieved from http://blogs.bowvalleycollegeweb.com/adultreadingassessment/readforward/#tests

Boyd, D.M., & Ellison, N.B. (2007). Social network sites: Definition, history, and scholarship. *Journal of Computer-Mediated Communication, 13*(1), 210–230.

Braveman, P. (2006). Health disparities and health equity: Concepts and measurement. *Annual Re-view of Public Health, 27,* 167–194.

Braveman, P., & Gruskin, S. (2003). Defining equity in health. *Journal of Epidemiology and Commun-ity Health, 57,* 254–258.

Braveman, P.A., Kumanyika, S., Fielding, J., Laveist, T., Borrell, L.N., Manderscheid, R., & Trout-man, A. (2011). Health disparities and health equity: The issue is justice. *American Journal of Public Health, 101*(Supplement 1), S149–S155.

Brewer, N.T., Tzeng, J.P., Lillie, S.E., Edwards, A.S., Peppercorn, J.M., & Rimer, B.K. (2009). Health literacy and cancer risk perception: Implications for genomic risk communication. *Medical Decision Making, 29*(2), 157–166.

Brodie, M., Flournoy, R.E., Altman, D.E., Blendon, R.J., Benson, J.M., & Rosenbaum, M.D. (2000). Health information, the Internet, and the digital divide. *Health Affairs, 19*(6), 255–265.

Brown, J.D., & Peuchaud, S.R. (2008). Media and breastfeeding: Friend or foe. *International Breastfeeding Journal, 3*(15). Retrieved from http://www.internationalbreastfeedingjournal.com/content/3/1/15

Browne, A.J., & Fiske, J. (2001). First Nations women's encounters with mainstream health care services. *Western Journal of Nursing Research, 23*(2), 126–147.

Brownell, K.D., & Napolitano, M.A. (1995). Distorting reality for children: Body size proportions of Barbie and Ken dolls. *International Journal of Eating Disorders, 18*(3), 295–298.

Buckingham, D. (2003). *Media education, literacy, learning and contemporary culture.* Cambridge: Polity Press.

Bullas, J. (n.d.). 35 mind numbing YouTube facts, figures and statistics—Infographic. *jeffbullas.com.* Retrieved from http://www.jeffbullas.com/2012/05/23/35-mind-numbing-youtube-facts-figures-and-statistics-infographic/

Bunker, J.P., Houghton, J., & Baum, M. (1998). Putting the risk of breast cancer in perspective. *Brit-ish Medical Journal, 317* (7168), 1307–1309.

Burkell, J. (2004). What are the chances? Evaluating risk and benefit information in consumer health materials. *Journal of the Medical Library Association, 92*(2), 200–208.

Bush, V. (1945). As we may think. *The Atlantic.* Retrieved from http://www.theatlantic.com/maga-zine/archive/1945/07/as-we-may-think/303881/

Byrd, J., & Thompson, L. (2008). "It's Safe to Ask": Promoting patient safety through health literacy. *Healthcare Quarterly, 11*(Special Issue), 91–94.

Calamai, P. (1987). *Broken words: Why five million Canadians are illiterate.* Toronto: Southam News-paper Group.

Calkins, D.R., Davis, R.B., Reiley, P., Phillips, R.S., Pineo, K.L., Delbanco, T.l., & Lezzoni, L.I. (1997). Patient-physician communication at hospital discharge and patients' understanding of the post-discharge treatment plan. *Archives of Internal Medicine, 157*(9), 1026–1030.

Canadian Council on Learning. (2007a). *Health literacy in Canada: Initial results from the International Adult Literacy and Skills Survey.* Retrieved from http://www.ccl-cca.ca/pdfs/HealthLiteracy/HealthLiteracyinCanada.pdf

Canadian Council on Learning. (2007b). *Lesson in learning: Informal science learning in Canada.* Retrieved from http://www.ccl-cca.ca/pdfs/LessonsInLearning/Apr-18-07-Informal-learning.pdf

Canadian Council on Learning. (2007c). *State of learning in Canada: No time for complacency.* Retrieved from http://www.ccl-cca.ca/ccl/reports/StateofLearning/StateofLearning2007.html

Canadian Council on Learning (2008a). *Health literacy in Canada: A healthy understanding.* Retrieved from http://www.ccl-cca.ca/pdfs/HealthLiteracy/HealthLiteracyReportFeb2008E.pdf

Canadian Council on Learning. (2008b). *Reading the future: Planning to meet Canada's future literacy needs.* Retrieved from www.ccl-cca.ca/pdfs/ReadingFuture/LiteracyReadingFutureReportE.pdf

Canadian Council on Learning. (2010a). Five years of measuring Canada's progress in lifelong learning. *Composite Learning Index.* Retrieved from http://www.cli-ica.ca/en/analysis/findings-year/2010.aspx

Canadian Council on Learning. (2010b). CLI interactive map. *Composite Learning Index.* Retrieved from http://www.cli-ica.ca/en/explore/interactives.aspx

Canadian Council on Learning. (2010c). *The future of literacy in Canada's largest cities.* Retrieved from http://www.ccl-cca.ca/pdfs/ReadingFuture/FutureLiteracyLargestCities2010_EN.pdf

Canadian Council on Learning. (n.d.). *Projections of adult literacy: Measuring movement (PALMM).* Retrieved from www.ccl-cca.ca/PALMM/projection.aspx

Canadian Heritage. (n.d.). Chapter 1: Mother tongue. Chart 1.2. Retrieved from http://www.pch.gc.ca/eng/1359983458549/1359983649745

Canadian Nurses' Association. (n.d.). *NurseOne.ca.* Retrieved from http://www.nurseone.ca

Canadian Public Health Association. (n.d.). *Health literacy resources.* Retrieved from http://www.cpha.ca/en/portals/h-l/resources.aspx

Canadian Public Health Association. (1998). *Easy does it! Plain language and clear verbal communication: Training manual.* Retrieved from http://www.cpha.ca/uploads/portals/h-l/easy_does_it_e.pdf

Canadian Public Health Association. (2001). *The captain's log.* Final report of the First Canadian Conference on Literacy and Health, "Charting the Course for Literacy and Health in the New Millennium," Ottawa, May 28–30, 2000. Retrieved from http://www.cpha.ca/uploads/portals/h-l/c_log_e.pdf

Canadian Public Health Association. (2006a). *Health literacy interventions.* Retrieved from http://www.cpha.ca/uploads/portals/h-l/interventions_e.pdf

Canadian Public Health Association. (2006b). *Low health literacy and chronic disease prevention and control: Perspectives from the health and public health sectors.* Retrieved from http://www.cpha.ca/uploads/portals/h-l/kl_summary_e.pdf

Canadian Public Health Association. (2007). *Perceptions of health literacy: Results of a questionnaire for practitioners, policy-makers and researchers. CPHA Report.* Retrieved from http://www.cpha.ca/uploads/portals/h-l/questionnaire_e.pdf

Canadian Radio-television and Telecommunications Commission. (2011). *Broadband report November 2011.* Retrieved from http://www.crtc.gc.ca/eng/publications/reports/broadband/bbreport1111.htm

Cegala, D.J. (2006). Emerging trends and future directions in patient communication skills training. *Health Communication, 20*(2), 123–129.

Cegala, D.J., & Broz, S.L. (2002). Physician communication skills training: A review of theoretical backgrounds, objectives, and skills. *Medical Education, 36*(11), 1004–1016.

Cegala, D.J., & Broz, S.L. (2003). Provider and patient communication skills training. In T.L. Thompson, A.M. Dorsey, K.I. Miller, & R. Parrott (Eds.), *Handbook of health communication* (pp. 95–119). Mahwah, NJ: Lawrence Erlbaum Associates.

Cegala, D.J., Gade, C., Broz, S.L., & McClure, L. (2004). Physicians' and patients' perceptions of patients' communication competence in a primary care medical interview. *Health Communication, 16*(3), 289–304.

Cegala, D.J., McClure, L., Marinelli, T.M., & Post, D.M. (2000). The effects of communication skills training on patients' participation during medical interviews. *Patient Education and Counseling, 41*(2), 209–222.

Center for Media Literacy. (2002–2011). *Home page.* Retrieved from http://www.medialit.org/

Central Intelligence Agency (CIA). (2012). *The World Factbook—South Asia: Pakistan.* Retrieved from http://www.cia.gov/library/publications/the-world-factbook/geos/pk.html

Centre for Literacy. (n.d.). *What is literacy?* Retrieved from http://www.champixinfo.co.uk/side-effects-contraindications.shtml

Champix. (n.d). *Champix side effects and contraindications.* Retrieved from http://www.champixinfo.co.uk/side-effects-contraindications.shtml

Chang, B.L., Bakken, S., Brown, S.S., Houston, T.K., Kreps, G.L., Kukafka, R., & Stavri, P.Z. (2004). Bridging the digital divide: Reaching vulnerable populations. *Journal of the American Medical Informatics Association, 11*(6), 448–457.

Chao, G.T., & Moon, H. (2005). The cultural mosaic: A metatheory for understanding the complexity of culture. *Journal of Applied Psychology, 90*(6), 1128–1140.

Chen, X., & Siu, L.L. (2001). Impact of the media and the Internet on oncology: Survey of cancer patients and oncologists in Canada. *Journal of Clinical Oncology, 19*(23), 4291–4297.

Christensen, D. (2000). *Ahtahkakoop: The epic account of a Plains Cree head chief, his people, and their struggle for survival, 1816–1896.* Shell Lake, SK: Ahtahkakoop Publishing.

Citizenship and Immigration Canada. (2010). *Canada facts and figures—Immigration Overview permanent and temporary residents.* Retrieved from http://www.cic.gc.ca/english/pdf/research-stats/facts2010.pdf

Citizenship and Immigration Canada. (2012). *Government of Canada's immigration planning story.* Retrieved from http:// www.cic.gc.ca/english/department/ips/index.asp

Cole, C.F. (2009). What difference does it make? Insights from research on the impact of international co-productions of *Sesame Street. NHK Broadcasting Studies, 7,* 157–177.

Coleman, C., Kurtz-Rossi, S., McKinney, J., Pleasant, A., Rootman, I., & Shohet, L. (2008). *The Calgary Charter on Health Literacy: Rationale and core principles for the development of health literacy curricula.* Montreal. Retrieved from http://centreforliteracy.qc.ca/health_literacy/calgary_charter

Coleman, R., & Thorson, E. (2002). The effects of news stories that put crime and violence into context: Testing the public health model of reporting. *Journal of Health Communication, 7*(5), 401–425.

Commission on the Social Determinants of Health. (2008). *Closing the gap in a generation: Health equity through action on the social determinants of health.* Geneva: World Health Organization. Retrieved from http://whqlibdoc.who.int/publications/2008/9789241563703_eng.pdf

Conference Board of Canada. (2012). *How Canada performs: Education and skills, adult literacy rate—low-level skills.* Retrieved from http://www.conferenceboard.ca/hcp/details/education/adult-literacy-rate-low-skills.aspx

Consortium for Media Literacy. (2012). *Health and media literacy.* Retrieved from http://www.consortiumformedialiteracy.org/index.php?option=com_content&view=article&id=4&Itemid=34

Costello, J.M., Patak, L., & Pritchard, J. (2010). Communication-vulnerable patients in the pediatric ICU: Enhancing care through augmentative and alternative communication. *Journal of Pediatric Rehabilitation Medicine: An Interdisciplinary Approach, 3*(4), 289–301.

Covello, V. (1992). Trust and credibility in risk communication. *Health & Environment Digest, 6*(1), 1–3.

Covello, V.T., & Merkhofer, M.W. (1993). *Risk assessment methods: Approaches for assessing health and environmental risks.* New York: Plenum Press.

Crockatt, K., & Symthe, S. (n.d.). Building culture and community: Family and community literacy partnerships in Canada's North. Retrieved from http://www.nunavutliteracy.ca/english/resource/reports/building/building.pdf

Crow, S., & Ondrusek, A. (2012). Video as a format in health information. *Medical Reference Services Quarterly, 21*(3), 21–34.

CTV.ca News Staff. (2009, October 30). Single dose of H1N1 vaccine enough for kids: WHO. *CTV News.* Retrieved from http://www.ctv.ca/CTVNews/Health/20091030/vaccine_flow_091030/#ixzz1vEpQ0pYc

CTV.ca News Staff. (2011, July 6). Deal reached on labels for genetically modified food. *CTV News.* Retrieved from http://www.ctvnews.ca/deal-reached-on-labels-for-genetically-modified-food-1.666410

Cuellar, I., Arnold, B., & Maldonado, R. (1995). Acculturation rating scale for Mexican Americans II: A revision of the original ARMSA scale. *Hispanic Journal of Behavioral Sciences, 17*, 275–304.

Cutler, J., Schleihauf, E., Hatchette, T.F., Billard, B., Watson-Creed, G., Davidson, R., … & Sarwal, S. (2009). Investigation of the first cases of human-to-human infection with the new swine-origin influenza A (H1N1) virus in Canada. *Canadian Medical Association Journal, 181*(34), 159–163.

Daghofer, D. (2011). *Communicating the social determinants of health scoping paper.* Rossland, BC. Retrieved from http://www.rrasp-phirn.ca/index.php?option=com_content&view=article&id=252%3Acommunicating-the-social-determinants-of-health&catid=6%3Alatest-news&Itemid=17&lang=en

Darville, R. (1992). *Adult literacy work in Canada.* Toronto: Canadian Association for Adult Education. Retrieved from http://www.nald.ca/library/research/work/adultlit.pdf

Davis, T.C., Long, S.W., Jackson, R.H., Mayeaux, E.J., George, R.B., Murphy, P.W., & Crouch, M.A. (1993). Rapid estimate of adult literacy in medicine: A shortened screening instrument. *Family Medicine, 25*(6), 391–395.

Davis, T.C., Michielutte, R., Askov, E.N., Williams, M.V., & Weiss, B.D. (1998). Practical assessment of adult literacy in healthcare. *Health Education & Behavior, 25*, 613–624.

Davis, T.C., & Wolf, M.S. (2004). Health literacy: Implications for family medicine. *Family Medicine, 36*(8), 595–598.

de Vreese, C.H., Boomgaarden, H.G., & Semetko, H.A. (2011). (In)direct framing effects: The effects of news media framing on public support for Turkish membership in the European Union. *Communication Research, 38*(2), 179–205.

Deignan, B., Harvey, E., & Hoffman-Goetz, L. (2013). Fright factors about wind turbines and health in Ontario newspapers before and after the Green Energy Act. *Health, Risk & Society, 15*(3), 234–250.

Derenne, J.L., & Beresin, E.V. (2006). Body image, media, and eating disorders. *Academic Psychiatry, 30*(3), 257–261.

DeWalt, D.A., Berkman, N.D., Sheridan, S., Lohr, K.N., & Pignone, M.P. (2004). Literacy and health outcomes: A systematic review of the literature. *Journal of General Internal Medicine, 19*(12), 1228–1239.

Dewing, M. (2009). *Canadian multiculturalism.* Parliamentary Information and Research Service, Library of Parliament. PRB 09-20E. Retrieved from www.parl.gc.ca/Content/LOP/ResearchPublications/2009-20-e.pdf

Diamond, C., Saintonge, S., August, P., & Azrack, A. (2011). The development of building wellness™, a youth health literacy program. *Journal of health communication, 16*(Supplement 3), 103–118.

Dieckmann, N.F., Slovic, P., & Peters, E.M. (2009). The use of narrative evidence and explicit likelihood by decisionmakers varying in numeracy. *Risk Analysis, 29*(10), 1473–1488.

Dingwall, J. (2000). *Improving numeracy in Canada: National Literacy Secretariat.* Retrieved from http://www.nald.ca/library/research/nls/inpub/numeracy/improve/improve.pdf

Doak, C., Doak, L., & Root, J. (1996). *Teaching patients with low literacy skills* (2nd ed.). Philadelphia: Lippincott.

Donelle, L., Arocha, J.F., & Hoffman-Goetz, L. (2008). Colorectal cancer risk comprehension of older Canadians: Impact of health literacy. *Chronic Diseases in Canada, 29*(1), 1–8.

Donelle, L., & Hoffman-Goetz, L. (2008). Health literacy and online health discussions of North American black women. *Women & Health, 47*(4), 71–90.

Donelle, L., Hoffman-Goetz, L., & Clarke, J.N. (2004). Portrayal of genetic risk for breast cancer in ethnic and non-ethnic newspapers. *Women & Health, 40*(4), 93–111.

Driedger, S.M. (2007). Risk and the media: A comparison of print and televised news stories of a Canadian drinking water risk event. *Risk Analysis, 27*(3), 775–786.

Dudo, A.D., Dahlstrom, M.F., & Brossard, D. (2007). Reporting a potential pandemic: A risk-related assessment of avian influenza coverage in U.S. newspapers. *Science Communication, 28*(4), 429–454.

Duffett-Leger, J., & Lumsden, J. (2008). Interactive online health promotion interventions: A "health check." *Proceedings of the 2008 IEEE International Symposium on Technology & Society* (pp. 26–28).

Dugas, A.F., Hsieh, Y.H., Levin, S.R., Pines, J.M., Mareiniss, D.P., Mohareb, A., & Rothman, R.E. (2012). Google flu trends: Correlation with emergency department influenza rates and crowding metrics. *Clinical Infectious Diseases, 54*(4), 463–469.

Dutta, M. (2007). Communicating about culture and health: Theorizing culture centered and cultural sensitivity approaches. *Communication Theory, 17*(3), 304–328.

Dutta, M.J. (2010). The critical cultural turn in health communication: Reflexivity, solidarity, and praxis. *Health Communication, 25*(67), 534–539.

Dutta-Bergman, M. (2004a). The unheard voices of Santalis: Communicating about health from the margins of India. *Communication Theory, 14*(3), 237–263.

Dutta-Bergman, M. (2004b). Reaching unhealthy eaters: Applying a strategic approach to media vehicle choice. *Health Communication, 16*(4), 493–506.

Dutta-Bergman, M. (2004c). Primary sources of health information: Comparison in the domain of health attitudes, health cognitions, and health behaviors. *Health Communication, 16*(3), 273–288.

Eckman, M.H., Wise, R., Leonard, A.C., Dixon, E., Burrows, C., Khan, F., & Warm, E. (2012). Impact of health literacy on outcomes and effectiveness of an educational intervention in patients with chronic diseases. *Patient Education and Counseling, 87,* 143–151.

Egede, L.E. (2006). Race, ethnicity, culture, and disparities in health care. *Journal of General Internal Medicine, 21*(6), 667–669.

Eggleton, A., & Ogilvie, K.K. (2010). Canada's response to the 2009 H1N1 influenza pandemic. Standing Senate Committee on Social Affairs, Science and Technology, Ottawa, Ontario. Retrieved from http://www.parl.gc.ca/content/sen/committee/403/soci/rep15dec10-e.pdf

Eiser, J.R. (1998). Communication and interpretation of risk. *British Medical Bulletin, 54*(4), 779–790.

EKOS Research Associates. (2004). Backgrounder: Rethinking science and society. *Public Survey by EKOS Research Associates.* Ottawa: Association of Universities and Colleges of Canada.

Entman, R.M. (1993). Framing: Towards clarification of a fractured paradigm. *Journal of Communication, 43,* 51–58.

Epperson, A. (2010). Computer literacy revisited: A comprehensive investigation of computer literacy. *ACM Inroads, 1*(2), 30–33.

Epstein, R.M., Alper, B.S., & Quill, T.E. (2004). Communicating evidence for participatory decision making. *Journal of the American Medical Association, 291*(19) 2359–2366.

Eriksen, T.H. (2001). Ethnic identity, national identity and intergroup conflict: The significance of personal experiences. In R.D. Ashmore, L. Jussim, & D. Wilder (Eds.), *Social identity, intergroup conflict and conflict reduction* (pp. 42–68). New York: Oxford University Press.

Eriksen, T.H. (2002). *Ethnicity and nationalism: Anthropological perspectives* (2nd ed.). London: Pluto Press.

Eysenbach, G. (2001). What is e-health? *Journal of Medical Internet Research, 3*(2), e20. Retrieved from http://www.jmir.org/2001/2/e20/

Eysenbach, G. (2008). Medicine 2.0: Social networking, collaboration, participation, apomediation, and openness. *Journal of Medical Internet Research, 10*(3), e22.

Faber, L. (2011). Canadian social media statistics 2011. *Webfuel.* Retrieved from http://www.webfuel.ca/canada-social-media-statistics-2011/

Fadiman, A. (1997). *The spirit catches you and you fall down.* New York: Farrar, Straus and Giroux.

Fallowfield, L., Jenkins, V., Farewell, V., & Solis-Trapala, I. (2003). Enduring impact of communication skills training: Results of a 12-month follow-up. *British Journal of Cancer, 89*(8), 145–149.

Federal, Provincial, and Territorial Advisory Committee on Population Health (ACPH), Health Canada, Statistics Canada, Canadian Institute for Health Information, and Centre for Health Promotion, University of Toronto. (1999). Backgrounder: The socioeconomic environment and health. *Toward a healthy future: Second report on the health of Canadians.* Retrieved from http://www.phac-aspc.gc.ca/ph-sp/report-rapport/toward/back/socio-eng.php

Fedoroff, N.V. (2011, August 18). Engineering food for all. *The New York Times*. Retrieved from http://www.nytimes.com/2011/08/19/opinion/genetically-engineered-food-for-all.html?_r=2

Feldman, M.D., Zhang, J., & Cummings, S.R. (1999). Chinese and U.S. internists adhere to different ethical standards. *Journal of General Internal Medicine, 14*(8), 469–473.

Finnegan, J.R., & Viswanath, K. (2008). Communication theory and health behavior change: The media studies framework. In K. Glantz, B.K. Rimer, & K. Viswanath (Eds.), *Health behavior and health education: Theory, research and practice* (4th ed., pp. 361–388). San Francisco: Jossey-Bass.

Fiske, S.T., & Taylor, S.E. (1991). *Social cognition* (2nd ed.). New York: McGraw-Hill.

Flesch, R. (1979). *How to write plain English: Let's start with the formula*. Retrieved from http://pages.stern.nyu.edu/~wstarbuc/Writing/Flesch.htm

Foster, C.H. (2006). What nurses should know when working in Aboriginal communities. *Canadian Nurse, 102*(4), 28–31.

Freire, P. (2000). *Pedagogy of the oppressed*. New York: Continuum.

Friedman, D., & Hoffman-Goetz, L. (2006). Assessment of cultural sensitivity of cancer information in ethnic print media. *Journal of Health Communication, 11*(4), 425–447.

Friedman, D.B., Hoffman-Goetz, L., & Arocha, J.F. (2004). Readability of cancer information on the Internet. *Journal of Cancer Education, 19*(2), 117–122.

Friedman, D.B., Hoffman-Goetz, L., & Arocha, J.F. (2006). Health literacy and the World Wide Web: Comparing the readability of leading incident cancers on the Internet. *Medical Informatics & the Internet in Medicine, 31*(1), 67–87.

Frontier College. (n.d.). *Literacy: Learning for life*. Retrieved from http://www.frontiercollege.ca/english_literacy.html

Galloway, G. (2010, December 28). Canadians blasé about flu shot, doctors fear. *The Globe and Mail*. Retrieved from http://www.theglobeandmail.com/life/health/canadians-blas-about-flu-shot-doctors-fear/article1850672/

Gasher, M., Hayes, M., Hackett, R., Gutstein, D., & Dunn, J. (2007). Spreading the news: Social determinants of health reportage in Canadian daily newspapers. *Canadian Journal of Communication, 32*(3–4), 557–574.

Gauthier, E. (2011). Foodborne microbial risks in the press: The framing of listeriosis in Canadian newspapers. *Public Understanding of Science, 20*(2), 270–286.

Gazmararian, J.A., Curran, J.W., Parker, R.M., Benhardt, J.M., & Debuono, B.A. (2005). Public health literacy in America: An ethical imperative. *American Journal of Preventive Medicine, 28*(3), 317–322.

Gazmararian, J.A., Williams, M.V., Peel, J., & Baker, D.W. (2003). Health literacy and knowledge of chronic disease. *Patient Education and Counselling, 51*(3), 267–275.

Geertz, C. (1973). Thick description: Toward an interpretive theory of culture. In *The interpretation of cultures: Selected essays* (pp. 3–30). New York: Basic Books.

Gerbner, G., Gross, L., Signorielli, N., & Morgan, M. (1980). Aging with television: Images on television drama and conceptions of social reality. *Journal of Communication, 30*(1), 37–47.

Gibbon, J.M. (1938). *Canadian mosaic: The making of a northern nation*. Toronto: McClelland & Stewart.

Gigerenzer, G., & Edwards, A. (2003). Simple tools for understanding risks: From innumeracy to insight. *British Medical Journal, 327*(7417), 741–744.

Gillis, D., Quigley, B., & MacIsaac, A. (2005). Responding to the challenge of literacy and health. *Literacies, 5*. Retrieved from http://www.literacyjournal.ca

Gillis, G., & Quigley, A. (2004). *Taking off the blindfold: Seeing how literacy affects health.* A report of the Health Literacy in Rural Nova Scotia Research Project. Retrieved from http://www.nald.ca/healthliteracystfx/pubs/takngoff/takngoff.pdf

Ginsberg, J., Mohebbi, M.H., Patel, R.S., Brammer, L., Smolinski, M.S., & Brilliant, L. (2009). Detecting influenza epidemics using search engine query data. *Nature, 457*(7232), 1012–1014.

Goffman, E. (1974). *Frame analysis: An essay on the organization of experience.* New York: Harper & Row.

Golbeck, A.L., Ahlers-Schmidt, C.R., Paschal, A.M., & Dismuke, S.E. (2005). A definition and operational framework for health numeracy. *American Journal of Preventive Medicine, 29*(4), 375–376.

Gonzales, R., Glik, D., Davoudi, M., & Ang, A. (2004). Media literacy and public health: Integrating theory, research, and practice for tobacco control. *American Behavioral Scientist, 48*(2), 189–201.

Google. (2012). *Doubleclick ad planner.* Retrieved from http://www.google.com/adwords/answer/3278806

Google.org. (2011). *Flu trends: Explore flu trends—Canada.* Retrieved from http://www.google.org/flutrends/ca/#CA

Gordon, M. (1964). *Assimilation in American life.* New York: Oxford University Press.

Government of Alberta. (2007). *Alberta's immunization strategy.* Retrieved from http:// www.health.alberta.ca/health-info/imm-program.html

Government of Canada. (1982). Constitution Act. Part I. Canadian Charter of Rights and Freedoms. Ottawa. Retrieved from http://laws-lois.justice.gc.ca/eng/Const/page-15.html

Government of Canada. (1985). Canadian Multiculturalism Act. Retrieved from http://laws-lois.justice.gc.ca/eng/acts/c-18.7/page-1.html#h-1

Government of Canada. (2004). *2003 report on Aboriginal community connectivity infrastructure.* Ottawa: Indian and Northern Affairs Canada.

Government of Canada. (n.d.). *Aboriginal languages: Native peoples and languages.* Retrieved from http:/www.salic-slmc.ca/showpage.asp?file=langues_en_presence/langues_autoch/peuples autoch &language=en&updatemenu=true11

Gray, G.M., & Ropeik, D.P. (2002). Dealing with the dangers of fear: The role of risk communication. *Health Affairs (Millwood), 21*(6), 106–116.

Griffiths, W., & Knutson, A. (1960). The role of mass media in public health. *American Journal of Public Health, 50*(5), 515–523.

Groth, E. (1991). Communicating with consumers about food safety and risk issues. *Food Technology, 45*(5), 248–252.

Gupta, G.K. (2006). Computer literacy: Essential in today's computer-centric world. *ACM SIGCSE Bulletin, 38*(2), 115–119.

Hankivsky, O., & Christoffersen, A. (2008). Intersectionality and the determinants of health: A Canadian perspective. *Critical Public Health, 18*(3), 271–283.

Hankivsky, O., & Cormier, R. (2010). Intersectionality and public policy: Some lessons from existing models. *Political Research Quarterly, 64*(1), 217–229.

Hanson, R.E. (2005). *Mass communication: Living in a media world.* Boston: McGraw-Hill.

Harmon, M.P., Castro, F.G., & Coe, K. (1996). Acculturation and cervical cancer: Knowledge, beliefs, and behaviors of Hispanic women. *Women & Health, 24*(3), 37–57.

Harrington, J., Noble, L., & Newman, S. (2004). Improving patients' communication with doctors: A systematic review of intervention studies. *Patient Education and Counseling, 52*(1), 7–16.

Hart, A. (1991). *Understanding the media: A practical guide.* New York: Routledge.

Hawn, C. (2009). Take two Aspirin and tweet me in the morning: How Twitter, Facebook, and other social media are reshaping health care. *Health Affairs, 28*(2), 361–368.

Hawthorne, K. (2001). Effects of culturally appropriate health education on glycaemic control and knowledge of diabetes in British Pakistani women with type 2 diabetes mellitus. *Health Education Research, 16*(3), 373–381.

Hayes, M., Ross, I.E., Gasher, M., Gutstein, D., Dunn, J.R., & Hackett, R.A. (2007). Telling stories: News media, health literacy and public policy in Canada. *Social Science & Medicine, 64*(9), 1842–1852.

Hayward, K., Pannozzo, L., & Colman, R. (2007). *Developing indicators for the educated populace domain of the Canadian Index of Wellbeing: Background information literature review.* Document 2, Parts IV–VI (of VI). Retrieved from http://uwaterloo.ca/canadian-index-wellbeing/sites/ca.canadian-index-wellbeing/files/uploads/files/Historical-Educated_Populace_Literature_Review_Doc2_August_2007.sflb_.pdf

Health Canada. (1997). *Health promotion and new information technologies, Section 4: Emergent issues, findings and specific recommendations.* Report submitted by NHN Consulting Group to Health Canada, Health Promotion Development Division. Retrieved from http://web.archive.org/web/20100606040545/http://www.phac-aspc.gc.ca/ph-sp/infotech-techinfo/infotech2-eng.php

Health Canada. (2003). How does literacy affect the health of Canadians? Retrieved from http://en.copian.ca/library/research/howdoes/howdoes.pdf

Health Canada. (2012). *Food and nutrition—Interactive nutrition label: Get the facts (HTML).* Retrieved from http://www.hc-sc.gc.ca/fn-an/label-etiquet/nutrition/educat/info-nutri-label-etiquet-eng.php

Health Disparities Task Group. (2005). *Reducing health disparities—Roles of the health sector: Discussion paper.* Retrieved from http://www.phac-aspc.gc.ca/ph-sp/disparities/ddp-eng.php

Healthy Aboriginal Network. (n.d.). *Home page.* Retrieved from http://www.thehealthyaboriginal.net/

Healthy Aboriginal Network. (2012). YouTube. Retrieved from http://www.youtube.com/user/HealthyAboriginal

Hiebert, R.E., & Gibbons, S.J. (2000). Impact: Effects of mass media. In R.E. Hiebert & S.J. Gibbons (Eds.), *Exploring mass media for a changing world* (pp. 124–140). Mahwah, NJ: Lawrence Erlbaum.

Higgins, J.W., & Begoray, D. (2012). Exploring the borderlands between media and health: Conceptualizing "critical media health literacy." *Journal of Media Literacy Education, 4*(2), 136–148.

Hines, K. (2011). Social media essentials for physicians. *Future Practice* (November), 31–34.

Hinnant, A., Oh, H.J., Caburnay, C.A., & Kreuter, M.W. (2011). What makes African American health disparities newsworthy? An experiment among journalists about story framing. *Health Education Research, 26*(6), 937–947.

Hirsch, E.D. (2003). *Reading comprehension requires knowledge of the words and the world.* Retrieved from http://www.aft.org/pdfs/americaneducator/spring2003/AE_SPRNG.pdf

Hoehndorf, R., Loebe, F., Kelso, J., & Herre, H. (2007). Representing default knowledge in bio-medical ontologies: Application to the integration of anatomy and phenotype ontologies. *BMC Bioinformatics, 8*, 377.

Hoffman, M., & Blake, J. (2003). Computer literacy: Today and tomorrow. *Journal of Computing Sciences in Colleges, 18*(5), 221–233.

Hoffman-Goetz, L., & Friedman, D.B. (2005). Disparities in the coverage of cancer information in ethnic minority and mainstream print media. *Ethnicity & Disease, 15*(2), 332–340.

Hoffman-Goetz, L., Shannon, C., & Clarke, J.N. (2003). Chronic disease coverage in Canadian Aboriginal newspapers. *Journal of Health Communication, 8*(5), 475–488.

Holbrook, J., & Rannikmae, M. (2009). The meaning of scientific literacy. *International Journal of Environmental & Science Education, 4*(3), 275–288.

Holton, A., Weberling, B., Clarke, C.E., & Smith, M.J. (2012). The blame frame: Media attribution of culpability about the MMR-autism vaccination scare. *Health Communication, 27*(7), 690–701.

Howard, P.N., & Busch, L. (2011). Comparing digital divides: Internet access and social inequality in Canada and the United States. *Canadian Journal of Communication, 35*, 109–128.

Howard, P.N., Busch, L., & Sheets, P. (2010). Comparing digital divides: Internet access and social inequality in Canada and the United States. *Canadian Journal of Communication, 35*(1), 109–128.

Hulsman, R.L., Ross, W.J., Winnbust, J.A., & Bensing, J.M. (1999). Teaching clinically experienced physicians communication skills: A review of evaluation studies. *Medical Education, 33*(9), 655–668.

Human Resources and Skills Development Canada (HRSDC) and Statistics Canada. (2005). *Building on our competencies: Canadian results of the International Adult Literacy and Skills Survey 2003.* Catalogue No. 89-617-XIE. Ottawa: Statistics Canada. Retrieved from http://www.statcan.gc.ca/pub/89-617-x/89-617-x2005001-eng.pdf

Human Resources and Skills Development Canada. (HRSDC). (n.d.-a). *Readers' guide to essential skills profiles.* Retrieved from http://www.hrsdc.gc.ca/eng/workplaceskills/LES/tools_resources/tools_audience/general/readers_guide_whole.shtml

Human Resources and Skills Development Canada (HRSDC). (n.d.-b). *Indicators of well-being in Canada: Learning—Adult numeracy.* Retrieved from http://www4.hrsdc.gc.ca/.3ndic.1t.4r@-eng.jsp?iid=79

Hunt, L.M., Schneider, S., & Comer, B. (2004). Should "acculturation" be a variable in health research? A critical review of research on US Hispanics. *Social Science & Medicine, 59*(5), 973–986.

Indigenous Physicians Association of Canada and the Royal College of Physicians and Surgeons of Canada. (2009). *First Nations, Inuit and Métis health core competencies.* Winnipeg & Ottawa. Retrieved from http://www.afmc.ca/pdf/CoreCompetenciesEng.pdf

Industry Canada. (2012). *Broadband Canada: Connecting rural Canadians.* Retrieved from http://www.ic.gc.ca/eic/site/719.nsf/eng/home

Institute of Medicine. (2001). *Crossing the quality chasm: A new health system for the 21st century.* Washington, DC: National Academies Press.

Institute of Medicine. (2004). *Health literacy: A prescription to end confusion.* Washington, DC: The National Academies Press.

Institute of Medicine. (2012). *How can health care organizations become more health literate? Workshop summary.* Roundtable of Health Literacy Board on Population Health and Public Health Practice, Institute of Medicine of the National Academies. Washington, DC. Retrieved from http://download.nap.edu/cart/download.cgi?&record_id=13402&free=1

Jenkins, V., & Fallowfield, L. (2002). Can communication skills training alter physicians' beliefs and behavior in clinics? *Journal of Clinical Oncology, 20*(3), 765–769.

Jiang, W. (2000). The relationship between culture and language. *ELT Journal, 54*(4), 328–334.

Jibaja-Weiss, M.L., & Volk, R.J. (2007). Utilizing computerized entertainment education in the development of decision aids for lower literate and naïve computer users. *Journal of Health Communication, 12*(7), 681–697.

Johnson, T. (1998). Shattuck Lecture—Medicine and the media. *New England Journal of Medicine, 339*(2), 87–92.

Jones, C.A., Mawani, S., King, K.M., Allu, S.O., Smith, M., Mohan, S., & Campbell, N.R.C. (2011). Tackling health literacy: Adaptation of public hypertension educational materials for an Indo-Asian population in Canada. *BMC Public Health, 11*, 24.

Jordan-Bychkov, T.G., Domosh, M., Neumann, R.P., & Price, P. (2006). *The human mosaic* (10th ed., pp. 2–3). New York: W.H. Freeman Company.

Karpf, A. (1988). *Doctoring the media: The reporting of health and medicine.* London: Routledge.

Kaufert, J.M., & Putsch, R.W. (1997). Communication through interpreters in healthcare: Ethical dilemmas arising from differences in class, culture, language, and power. *Journal of Clinical Ethics, 81*(1), 71–87.

Kessels, R.P. (2003). Patients' memory for medical information. *Journal of the Royal Society of Medicine, 96* (5), 219–222.

Kickbusch, I. (2004). *Improving health literacy in the European Union: Towards a Europe of informed and active health citizens* [Background paper]. Retrieved from http://old.ilonakickbusch.com/health-literacy/health-literacy-gastein.pdf

Kickbusch, I., & Maag, D. (2008). Health literacy. In K. Heggenhougen & S. Quah (Eds.), *International encyclopedia of public health* (Vol. 3, pp. 204–211). San Diego: Academic Press.

Kickbusch, I., Wait, S., & Maag, D. (2005). *Navigating health: The role of health literacy.* Alliance for Health and the Future, International Longevity Centre. Retrieved from http://www.emhf.org/resource_images/NavigatingHealth_FINAL.pdf

Kickbusch, I.S. (2001). Health literacy: Addressing the health and education divide. *Health Promotion International, 16*(3), 289–297.

King, J., & Taylor, M.C. (2010). Adults living with limited literacy and chronic illness: Patient education experiences. *Adult Basic Education and Literacy Journal, 4*(1), 24–33. Retrieved from http://www.nald.ca/library/research/mtaylor/patient/patient.pdf

Kleinman, A. (1980). *Patients and healers in the context of culture: An exploration of the borderland between anthropology, medicine, and psychiatry.* Berkeley: University of California Press.

Kleinman, A., & Benson, P. (2006a). Culture, moral experience and medicine. *Mount Sinai Journal of Medicine, 73*(6), 834–839.

Kleinman, A., & Benson, P. (2006b). Anthropology in the clinic: The problem of cultural competency and how to fix it. *PLoS Medicine, 3*(10), e294.

Kloda, L.A. (2008). Health information literacy in Canadian medical curricula: An opportunity for librarians? *Journal of Hospital Librarianship, 8*(3), 314–322.

Knox, K., & Schmidt, B. (2006). *A wake-up call on science literacy: Canada's future depends on it.* Policy Options Dossier, November. Retrieved from http://www.letstalkscience.ca/our-research/publications.html

Koch-Weser, S., Ruud, R.E., & DeJong, W. (2010). Quantifying word use to study health literacy in doctor-patient communication. *Journal of Health Communication, 15*(6), 590–602.

Kohring, M., & Matthes, J. (2002). The face(t)s of biotech in the nineties: How the German press framed modern biotechnology. *Public Understanding of Science, 11*(2), 143–154.

Komirenko, Z., Veeman, M.M., & Unterschultz, J.R. (2010). Do Canadian consumers have concerns about genetically modified animal feeds? *AgBioForum, 13*(3), 242–250.

Krahn, H., & Lowe, G.S. (1999). Literacy in the workplace. *Perspectives on Labour and Income, 11* (Summer 1999), 38–44. Cat. No. 75-001-XPE. Ottawa: Statistics Canada. Retrieved from http://www.statcan.gc.ca/studies-etudes/75-001/archive/1999/5023030-eng.pdf

Kramsch, C. (1998). *Language and culture.* Oxford: Oxford University Press.

Kreps, G.L., Bonaguro, E.W., & Query, J.L. (1998). The history and development of the field of health communication. In L.D. Jackson & B.K. Duffy (Eds.), *Health communication research: Guide to developments and directions* (pp. 1–15). Westport, CT: Greenwood Press.

Kreuter, M., & McClure, S. (2004). The role of culture in health communication. *Annual Review of Public Health, 25*, 439–455.

Kreuter, M.W., Caburnay, C.A., Chen, J.J., & Donlin, M.J. (2004). Effectiveness of individually tailored calendars in promoting childhood immunization in urban public health centers. *American Journal of Public Health, 94*(1), 122–127.

Kripalani, S., Jacobson, T.A., Mugalla, I.C., Cawthon, C.R., Niesner, K.J., & Vaccarino, V. (2010). Health literacy and the quality of physician-patient communication during hospitalization. *Journal of Hospital Medicine, 5*(5), 269–275.

Kroeber, A.L., Kluckhohn, C., & Untereiner, W. (1952). *Culture: A critical review of concepts and definitions.* New York: Vintage Books.

Krotz, L., Martin, E., & Fernandez, P. (1999). *Frontier College letters: One hundred years of teaching, learning and nation building.* Toronto: Frontier College Press. Retrieved from http://www.nald.ca/library/learning/frontier/letters/letters.pdf

Kunz, J.L., & Sykes, S. (2007). *From mosaic to harmony—Multicultural Canada in the 21st century:* Results of regional roundtables. Ottawa: Policy Research Initiative. Retrieved from http://www.horizons.gc.ca/eng/content/mosaic-harmony-multicultural-canada-21st-century

Kutner, M., Greenberg, E., Jin, Y., Paulsen, C., & White, S. (2006). *The health literacy of America's adults: Results from the 2003 National Assessment of Adult Literacy (NCES 2006-483).* Washington, DC: National Center for Education Statistics. Retrieved from http://nces.ed.gov/pubs2006/2006483.pdf

Lachapelle, R., & Lepage, J.-F. (n.d.). *Languages in Canada: 2006 Census.* New Canadian Perspectives. Cat. No. CH3-2/8-2010. Ottawa: Department of Canadian Heritage & Statistics Canada. Retrieved from http://www.pch.gc.ca/pgm/lo-ol/pubs/npc/index-eng.cfm

Lagassé, L.P., Rimal, R.N., Smith, K.C., Storey, J.D., Rhoades, E., Barnett, D.J., ... & Links, J. (2011). How accessible was information about H1N1 flu? Literacy assessments of CDC guidance documents for different audiences. *PloS One, 6*(10), e23583. doi:10.1371/journal.pone.0023583

Laing, A. (2011). The H1N1 crisis: Roles played by government communicators, the public and the media. *Journal of Professional Communication, 1*(1), 123–149.

Lalonde, M. (1974). *A new perspective on the health of Canadians—A working document.* Retrieved from http://www.phac-aspc.gc.ca/ph-sp/pdf/perspect-eng.pdf

Laugksch, R.C. (2000). Scientific literacy: A conceptual overview. *Science Education, 84*(1), 71–94.

Laverack, G. (2005). Power and empowerment. In G. Laverack (Ed.), *Public health: Power, empowerment and professional practice* (pp. 27–36). New York: Palgrave MacMillan.

Laverack, G. (2006). Improving health outcomes through community empowerment: A review of the literature. *Journal of Health, Population, and Nutrition, 24*(1), 113–120. Retrieved from http://www.ncbi.nlm.nih.gov/pubmed/16796158

Leary, V.A. (2009). Health care in Canada: Does a health care system based on shared values ensure respect for the right to health? In A. Clapham & M. Robinson (Eds.), *Realizing the right to health.* Swiss Human Rights Book (Vol. 3, pp. 472–481). Zurich: Rüffer & Rub.

Leiner, B.M., Cerf, V.G., Clark, D.D., Kahn, R.E., Kleinrock, L., Lynch, D.C., & Wolff, S. (2009). A brief history of the Internet. *SIGCOMM Computer Communication Review, 39*(5), 22–31.

Leiner, M., Handal, G., & Williams, D. (2004). Patient communication: A multidisciplinary approach using animated cartoons. *Health Education Research, 19*(5), 591–595.

Leiss, W., & Powell, D. (2004). *Mad cows and mother's milk: The perils of poor risk communication* (2nd ed.). Montreal: McGill-Queen's University Press.

Levin-Zamir, D., Lemish, D., & Gofin, R. (2011). Media Health Literacy (MHL): Development and measurement of the concept among adolescents. *Health Education Research, 26*(2), 323–335.

Liira, H. (2011). Patient information for better health outcomes in primary care. *Scandinavian Journal of Primary Health Care, 29*(2), 65–66.

Lipkin, M. Jr., Quill, T.E., & Napodano, R.J. (1984). The medical interview: A core curriculum for residencies in internal medicine. *Annals of Internal Medicine, 100*(2), 277–284.

Lister, P. (1999). A taxonomy for developing cultural competence. *Nurse Education Today, 19*(4), 313–318.

Literacy and Health Research Workshop: Setting priorities in Canada. (2002). Ottawa, October 27–28. Retrieved from http://www.nald.ca/library/research/wrkshp_e/wrkshpre.pdf

Looker, E., & Thiessen, V. (2003). *The digital divide in Canadian schools: Factors affecting student access to and use of information technology.* Ottawa: Statistics Canada. Retrieved from http://www.statcan.gc.ca/pub/81-597-x/81-597-x2003001-eng.pdf

Lorence, D.P., Park, H., & Fox, S. (2006). Racial disparities in health information access: Resilience of the digital divide. *Journal of Medical Systems, 30*(4), 241–249.

MacDonald, M. (2002). Health promotion: Historical, philosophical, theoretical perspectives. In L. Young & V. Haynes (Eds.), *Transforming health promotion practice: Concepts, issues and applications* (pp. 22–48). Philadelphia: F.A. Davis Co.

MacDonald, M., & Hoffman-Goetz, L. (2002). A retrospective study of the accuracy of cancer information in Ontario daily newspapers. *Canadian Journal of Public Health, 93*(2), 142–145.

Maguire, P. (1999). Improving communication with cancer patients. *European Journal of Cancer, 35*(10), 2058–2065.

Maibach, E., & Parrott, R. (1995). *Designing health messages*. Thousand Oaks, CA: Sage.

Makaryus, A.N., & Friedman, E.A. (2005). Patients' understanding of their treatment plans and diagnosis at discharge. *Mayo Clinic Proceedings, 80*(8), 991–994.

Makoul, G. (2001). Essential elements of communication in medical encounters: The Kalamazoo Consensus Statement. *Academic Medicine, 76*(4), 390–393.

Manafo, E., & Wong, S. (2012). Exploring older adults' health information seeking behaviors. *Journal of Nutrition Education and Behavior, 44*(1), 85–89.

Mancuso, J.M. (2009). Assessment and measurement of health literacy: An integrative review of the literature. *Nursing and Health Sciences, 11* (1), 77–89.

Manganello, J.A. (2008). Health literacy and adolescents: A framework and agenda for future research. *Health Education Research, 23*(5), 840–847.

Marin, G., & Gamba, R.J. (1996). A new measurement of acculturation for Hispanics: The bidimensional acculturation scale for Hispanics (BAS). *Hispanic Journal of Behavioral Sciences, 18*(3), 297–316.

Marlow, I., & McNish, J. (2010, April 3). Canada's digital divide. *The Globe and Mail*. Retrieved from http://www.theglobeandmail.com/report-on-business/canadas-digital-divide/article4313761/?page=all

Martin, P., & Midgley, E. (2006). Immigration: Shaping and reshaping America (2nd ed.). *Population Bulletin, 61*(4). Washington, DC: Population Reference Bureau. Retrieved from http://www.prb.org/pdf06/61.4USMigration.pdf

Maunder, S. (2007). Comic books tackle Aboriginal youth health issues. *CrossCurrents, 10*(2), 2.

McCombs, M., & Shaw, D. (1972). The agenda-setting function of mass media. *Public Opinion Quarterly, 36*, 176–187.

McCombs, M.E. (2004). *Setting the agenda: The mass media and public opinion*. Malden, MA: Blackwell Publishing Inc.

McLaughlin, G.H. (2008). *SMOG: Simple Measure of Gobbledygook*. Retrieved from http://www.harrymclaughlin.com/SMOG.htm

McLuhan, M. (1973). *Understanding media*. London: Abacus.

McNeil-Mulak, S. (2004). *Literacy and health environmental scan summary: Examining the level of awareness, programs and policies in Nova Scotia's health care sector*. Retrieved from http://www.nald.ca/healthliteracystfx/pubs/literacy/literacy.pdf

McWhirter, J., Todd, L., & Hoffman-Goetz, L. (2011). Comparing written and oral measures of comprehension of cancer information by English-as-a-second-language Chinese immigrant women. *Journal of Cancer Education, 26*(3), 484–489.

Merchant, R.M., Elmer, S., & Lurie, N. (2011). Integrating social media into emergency-preparedness efforts. *New England Journal of Medicine, 365*(4), 289–291.

Merriam-Webster Dictionary. (2012a). *Frame of reference*. Retrieved from http://www.merriam-webster.com/dictionary/frame+of+reference?show=0&t=1378572220

Merriam-Webster Dictionary. (2012b). *Herd immunity*. Retrieved from http://www.merriam-webster.com/medical/herd%20immunity

Mikkonen, J., & Raphael, D. (2010). *Social determinants of health: The Canadian facts*. Toronto: York University School of Health Policy and Management.

Mills, B.A., Reyna, V.F., & Estrada, S. (2008). Explaining contradictory relations between risk perception and risk taking. *Psychological Science, 19*(5), 429–434.

Misra-Hebert, A.D., & Isaacson, J.H. (2012). Overcoming health care disparities via better cross-cultural communication and health literacy. *Cleveland Clinic Journal of Medicine, 79*(2), 127–133.

Mitic, W., & Rootman, I. (2012). *An inter-sectoral approach for improving health literacy for Canadians: A discussion paper*. Victoria, BC: Public Health Association of BC. Retrieved from http://www.phabc.org/modules.php?name=Contentpub+pa=showpage+pid=182

Moggridge, B. (2008). *Here to stay: Interviews with Paul Saffo, James Truman, Chris Anderson, Neil Stevenson, & DJ Spooky*. Retrieved from http://www.designing-media.com/pdf/Chapter01.pdf

Morrison, J.H. (n.d.). *Albert Fitzpatrick*. Retrieved from http://www.frontiercollege.ca/english/learn/alfred_fitzpatrick.html

Mouseprint.org. (2008). *Lipitor: Reduces bad cholesterol, but...* Retrieved from http://www.mouse-print.org/2008/02/04/lipitor-reduces-bad-cholesterol-but/

Moynihan, R., Bero, L., Ross-Degnan, D., Henry, D., Lee, K., Watkins, J., ... & Soumerai, S.B. (2000). Coverage by the news media of the benefits and risks of medications. *New England Journal of Medicine, 342*, 1645–1650.

Mulligan, C. (2009, December 1). Third person dies of H1N1 in Sudbury. *The Sault Star*. Retrieved from http://www.saultstar.com/ArticleDisplay.aspx?e=2200545&archive=true

Murray, C., Yu, S., & Ahadi, D. (2007). *Cultural Diversity and Ethnic Media in BC*. A report to the Department of Canadian Heritage, Western Region. Vancouver: SFU Centre for Policy Studies on Culture and Communities.

Murray, E., Lo, B., Pollack, L., Donelan, K., Catania, J., Lee, K. ... & Turner, R. (2003a). The impact of health information on the Internet on health care and the physician-patient relationship: National U.S. survey among 1,050 U.S. physicians. *Journal of Medical Internet Research, 5*(3), e17. Retrieved from http://www.jmir.org/2003/3/e17/

Murray, E., Lo, B., Pollack, L., Donelan, K., Catania, J., White, M., ... & Turner, R. (2003b). The impact of health information on the Internet on the physician-patient relationship: Patient perceptions. *Archives of Internal Medicine, 163*(14), 1727–1734.

Murray, J.P. (2008). Media violence: The effects are both real and strong. *American Behavioral Science, 51*(8), 1212–1230.

Murray, S. (2008). Health literacy in Canada: Highlighting library initiatives. In M. Kars, L.M. Baker, & F.L. Wilson (Eds.), *The Medical Library Association guide to health literacy* (pp. 209–216). New York: Neal-Schuman Publishers, Inc.

Murthy, P. (2009). Health literacy and sustainable development. *UN Chronicle Online*. Retrieved from http://unchronicle.un.org/article/health-literacy-and-sustainable-development/index.html

Naik, A.D., Street, R.L. Jr., Castillo, D., & Abraham, N.S. (2011). Health literacy and decision making styles for complex antithrombotic therapy among older multimorbid adults. *Patient Education and Counseling, 85*(3), 499–504.

Natharius, D. (2004). The more we know, the more we see: The role of visuality in media literacy. *American Behavioral Scientist, 48*(2), 238–247.

National Aboriginal Health Organization (NAHO). (2008). *Cultural competency and safety: A guide for health care administrators, providers and educators.* Ottawa: National Aboriginal Health Organization. Retrieved from www.naho.ca/documents/naho/publications/culturalCompetency.pdf

National Adult Literacy Database (NALD). (n.d.). *Home page.* Retrieved from http://www.nald.ca

National Cancer Institute (NCI). (2004). *Making health communication programs work.* Bethesda, MD: Office of Communications of the National Cancer Institute. Retrieved from http://www.cancer.gov/cancertopics/cancerlibrary/pinkbook/Pink_Book.pdf

National Patient Safety Foundation (n.d.). *Ask Me 3.* Retrieved from http://www.npsf.org/for-health-care-professionals/programs/ask-me-3/

National Research Council. (1989). *Improving risk communication.* Washington, DC: National Academies Press.

National Research Council. (2012). *Improving adult literacy instruction: Options for practice and research.* Committee on Learning Sciences: Foundations and Applications to Adolescent and Adult Literacy, A.M. Lesgold and M. Welch-Ross (Eds). Division of Behavioral and Social Sciences and Education. Washington, DC: National Academies Press.

National Science Board. (2004). Science and technology: Public attitudes and understanding. In *Science and Engineering Indictors 2004* (Chapter 7). Arlington, VA: National Science Foundation. Retrieved from http://www.nsf.gov/statistics/seind04/c7/c7s2.htm

Nerlich, B., & Halliday, C. (2007). Avian flu: The creation of expectations in the interplay between science and the media. *Sociology of Health & Illness, 29*(1), 46–65.

Netcraft. (2012). *December 2012 Web server survey.* Retrieved from http://news.netcraft.com/archives/2012/

Neuliep, J.W. (2012). *Intercultural communication: A contextual approach.* California: Sage Publishing.

Niederdeppe, J., & Frosch, D. (2009). News coverage and sales of products with trans fats: Effects before and after changes in federal labeling policy. *American Journal of Preventive Medicine, 36*(5), 395–401.

Nielsen-Bohlman, L., Panzer, A.M., & Kindig, D.A. (Eds.). (2004). *Health literacy: A prescription to end confusion.* Washington, DC: National Academies Press.

Nimmon, L. (2007). Within the eyes of the people: Using a photonovel as a consciousness-raising health literacy tool with ESL-speaking immigrant women. *Canadian Journal of Public Health, 98*(4), 337–340.

Noar, S. (2006). A 10-year retrospective of research in health mass media campaigns: Where do we go from here? *Journal of Health Communication, 11*(1), 21–42.

Norman, C.D., & Skinner, H.A. (2006). eHealth literacy: Essential skills for consumer health in a networked world. *Journal of Medical Internet Research, 8*(2), e9. Retrieved from http://www.jmir.org/2006/2/e9/

Norris, M.J. (2007). *Aboriginal languages in Canada: Emerging trends and perspectives on second language acquisition*. Cat. No. 11008. Ottawa: Statistics Canada. Retrieved from http://www.statcan.gc.ca/pub/11-008-x/2007001/pdf/9628-eng.pdf

Nova Scotia Department of Health and Wellness, Primary Health Care. (2011). *An introduction to cultural competence in health care—Session I: Culture in health & care participant materials*. Retrieved from http://www.chd.ubc.ca/dhcc/sites/default/files/documents/Introduction%20to%20Cultural%20Competence.pdf

Nunavut Literacy Council. (n.d.). *Home page*. Retrieved from http://www.nunavutliteracy.ca/home.htm

Nutbeam, D. (2000). Health literacy as a public health goal: A challenge for contemporary health education and communication strategies into the 21st century. *Health Promotion International, 15*(3), 259–267.

Ogg, J.A., Sundman-Wheat, A.N., & Bateman, L.P. (2012). A primary approach to reading: Review of early literacy interventions implemented in pediatric settings. *Journal of Applied School Psychology, 28*(2), 111–132.

Oh, H., Rizo, C., Enkin, M., Jadad, A., Powell, J., & Pagliari, C. (2005). What is eHealth (3): A systematic review of published definitions. *Journal of Medical Internet Research, 7*(1), e1. Retrieved from http://www.jmir.org/2005/1/e1/

Ojo, T. (2006). Ethnic print media in the multicultural nation of Canada. *Journalism, 7*(3), 343–361.

Olson, S R., & Pollard, T. (2004). The muse pixeliope: Digitalization and media literacy education. *American Behavioral Scientist, 48*(2), 248–255.

Ong, L.M.L., de Haes, C.J.M., Hoos, A.M., & Lammes, F.B. (1995). Doctor-patient communication: A review of the literature. *Social Science & Medicine, 40*(7), 903–918.

Oppenheimer, G.M. (2001). Paradigm lost: Race, ethnicity, and the search for a new population taxonomy. *American Journal of Public Health, 91*(7), 1049–1055.

Organisation for Economic Co-operation and Development (OECD). (2001). *Education policy analysis 2001*. Centre for Educational Research and Innovation. Paris, France: OECD Publishing. Retrieved from http://www.oecd-ilibrary.org/education/education-policy-analysis-2001_epa-2001-en

Owen, B. (2009, October 30). H1N1 vaccine shortage looms, Province pleads for low-priority cases to wait. *Winnipeg Free Press*. Retrieved from http://www.winnipegfreepress.com/local/h1n1-vaccine-shortage-looms-67497797.html

Oxford English Dictionary. (2012). *Mosaic*. Retrieved from http://oxforddictionaries.com/definition/mosaic?region=us

Papps, E., & Ramsden, I. (1996). Cultural safety in nursing: The New Zealand experience. *International Journal for Quality in Health Care, 8*(5), 491–497.

Park, M. (2011). Effects of interactive pictorial education on community dwelling older adult's self-efficacy and knowledge for safe medication. *Journal of Korean Academic Nursing, 41*(6), 795–804.

Park, R.L. (2000). *Voodoo science: The road from foolishness to fraud*. New York: Oxford University Press.

Parker, R.M., Baker, D.W., Williams, M.V., & Nurss, J.R. (1995). The test of functional health literacy in adults: A new instrument for measuring patients' literacy skills. *Journal of General Internal Medicine, 10*(10), 537–541.

Parrott, R. (1994). Exploring family practitioners' and patients' information exchange about pre-scribed medications: Implications for practitioners' interviewing and patients' understanding. *Health Communication, 6*(4), 267–280.

Parrott, R. (1996). Advocate or adversary?: The self-reflexive roles of media messages for health. *Critical Studies in Mass Communication, 13*(3), 266–278.

Partnerships in Learning. (n.d.). *Fostering partnership development: An historical look at the National Literacy Secretariat Business and Labour Partnership Program.* Retrieved from http://www.partner-shipsinlearning.ca/Fostering/doc/FPD_Report.pdf

PatientsLikeMe®. (2012). *Home page.* Retrieved from http://www.patientslikeme.com/

Patterson, O. (2000). Taking culture seriously: A framework and an Afro-American illustration. In L.E. Harrison & S.P. Huntington (Eds.), *Culture matters* (pp. 202–218). New York: Basic Books.

Payne, J.G., & Schulte, S.K. (2003). Mass media, public health, and achieving health literacy. *Journal of Health Communication, 8*(Supplement 1), 124–125.

Perrin, B. (1989). *The Literacy and Health Project, Phase One: Making the world healthier and safer for people who can't read.* Research Report. Toronto: Ontario Public Health Association (OPHA) and Frontier College. Retrieved from http://www.opha.on.ca/OPHA/media/Resources/Resource%20 Documents/literacy1summary.pdf?ext=.pdf

Perrin, B. (1998). *How does literacy affect the health of Canadians? A profile paper presented to Health Canada.* Ottawa: Health Canada. Retrieved from http://en.copian.ca/library/research/howdoes/ howdoes.pdf

Persell, S.D., Osborn, C.Y., Richard, R., Skripkauskas, S., & Wolf, M.S. (2007). Limited health literacy is a barrier to medication reconciliation in ambulatory care. *Journal of General Internal Medicine, 22*(11), 1523–1526.

Petch, E., Ronson, B., & and Rootman, I. (2004). *Literacy and health in Canada: What have we learned and what can help in the future?* A Research Report. Clear language edition. Ottawa: Canadian In-stitutes of Health Research. Retrieved from http://www.cpha.ca/uploads/portals/h-l/literacy_e.pdf

Pew Initiative on Food and Biotechnology. (2006). *Review of public opinion research.* Washington, DC: The Mellman Group. Retrieved from http://www.pewtrusts.org/uploadedFiles/wwwpewtrustsorg/ Public_Opinion/Food_and_Biotechnology/2006summary.pdf

Pfizer. (2002–2012a). *Clear health communication checklist for providers.* Retrieved from http://www. pfizerhealthliteracy.com/physicians-providers/Checklist.aspx

Pfizer. (2002–2012b). *Provider quiz on health literacy.* Retrieved from http://www.pfizerhealthliteracy. com/physicians-providers/PolicyQuiz.aspx

Pomerantz, K., Muhammad, A., Downey, S., & Kind, T. (2010). Connecting for health literacy: Health information partners. *Health Promotion Practice, 11*(1), 79–88.

Porter, J. (1965). *The vertical mosaic: An analysis of social class and power in Canada.* Toronto: Univer-sity of Toronto Press.

Post, E.M., Cegala, D.J., & Miser, W.F. (2002). The other half of the whole: Teaching patients to communicate with physicians. *Family Medicine, 34*(5), 344–352.

Potter, L., & Martin, C. (2005). *Health literacy fact sheets.* Hamilton, NJ: Center for Health Care Strategies. Retrieved from http://www.chcs.org/publications3960/publications_show.htm?doc_id=291711

Potter, W.J. (2004). *Theory of media literacy: A cognitive approach.* Thousand Oaks, CA: Sage Publications.

Pottie, K. (2007). Misinterpretation: Language proficiency, recent immigrants, and global health disparities. *Canadian Family Physician, 53*(11), 1899–1901.

Potvin, L., Mantoura, P., & Ridde, V. (2007). Evaluating equity in health promotion. In C.M. McQueen & D.V. Jones (Eds.), *Global perspectives on health promotion effectiveness* (pp. 367–384). New York: Springer Science. Retrieved from http://www.springerlink.com/index/x305728727l23335.pdf

Poureslami, I., Rootman, I., Doyle-Waters, M.M., Nimmon, L., & Fitzgerald, J.M. (2011). Health literacy, language, and ethnicity-related factors in newcomer asthma patients to Canada: A qualitative study. *Journal of Immigrant and Minority Health, 13*(2), 315–322.

Powell, C.K., & Kripalani, S. (2005). Resident recognition of low literacy as a risk factor in hospital re-admission. *Journal of General Internal Medicine, 20*(11), 1042–1044.

Powell, D., & Leiss, W. (1997). *Mad cows and mother's milk: The perils of poor risk communication.* Montreal: McGill-Queen's University Press.

Price, V., Tewksbury, D., & Powers, E. (1997). Switching trains of thought: The impact of news frames on readers' cognitive responses. *Communication Research, 24*(5), 481–506.

Prime Minister of Canada Stephen Harper. (2006, June 19). *Address by the Prime Minister to the World Urban Forum.* Vancouver, BC. Retrieved from http://www.pm.gc.ca/eng/media.asp?id=1212

Public Health Agency of Canada (PHAC). (2003). *What makes Canadians healthy or unhealthy?* Retrieved from http://www.phac-aspc.gc.ca/ph-sp/determinants/index-eng.php

Public Health Agency of Canada (PHAC). (2008). *Priorities for action: Outcomes from the National Symposium on Health Literacy.* Ottawa: Canadian Public Health Association. Retrieved from http://www.cpha.ca/uploads/portals/h-l/priorities_e.pdf

Public Health Agency of Canada. (2011). *What determines health?* Retrieved from http://www.phac-aspc.gc.ca/ph-sp/determinants/index-eng.php

Pungente, J.J. (1993). The second spring: Media education in Canada's secondary schools. *Canadian Journal of Educational Communication, 22*(1), 47–60.

Pungente, J.J. (2002–2011). *Canada's key concepts of media literacy.* Center for Media Literacy. Retrieved from http://www.medialit.org/reading-room/canadas-key-concepts-media-literacy

Rachul, C.M., Ries, N.M., & Caulfield, T. (2011). Canadian newspaper coverage of the A/H1N1 vaccine program. *Canadian Journal of Public Health, 102*(3), 200–203.

Radford, T. (1996). Influence and power in the media. *Lancet, 347*(9014), 1533–1535.

Ramanadhan, S., & Viswanath, K. (2009). Health and the information nonseeker: A profile. *Health Communication, 20*(2), 131–139.

Rao, J.K., Anderson, L.A., Inui, T.S., & Frankel, R.M. (2007). Communication interventions make a difference in conversations between physicians and patients: A systematic review of the evidence. *Medical Care, 45*(4), 340–349.

Raphael, D., Bryant, T., & Curry-Stevens, A. (2004). Toronto charter outlines future health policy directions for Canada and elsewhere. *Health Promotion International, 19*(2), 269–273.

Raphael, D., & Curry-Stevens, A. (2004). Addressing and surmounting the political and social barriers to health. In D. Raphael (Ed.), *Social determinants of health: Canadian perspectives* (pp. 345–359). Toronto: Canadian Scholars' Press.

Raphael, D., Curry-Stevens, A., & Bryant, T. (2008). Barriers to addressing the social determinants of health: Insights from the Canadian experience. *Health Policy, 88*(2–3), 222–235.

Read to Me. (n.d.) *Home page.* Retrieved from http://www.readtomeprogram.org/

Readability Formulas. (n.d.). *The Gunning's Fog Index (or FOG) Readability Formula.* Retrieved from http://www.readabilityformulas.com/gunning-fog-readability-formula.php

Redfield, R. (1936). Memorandum for the study of acculturation. *American Anthropologist, 38*(1), 149–152.

Reese, S.D. (2001). Prologue—Framing public life: A bridging model for media research. In S.D. Reese, J. Oscar, H. Gandy, & A.E. Grant (Eds.), *Framing public life* (pp. 7–32). Mahwah, NJ: Lawrence Erlbaum.

Registered Nurses' Association of Ontario. (n.d.). *Home page.* Retrieved from http://www.RNAO.ca

Reid, J.C., Kardash, C.M., & Robinson, R.D. (1994). Comprehension in patient literature: The importance of text and reader characteristics. *Health Communication, 6*, 327–335.

Resnicow, K., Baranowski, T., Ahluwalia, J.S., & Braithwaite, R.L. (1999). Cultural sensitivity in public health: Defined and demystified. *Ethnicity and Disease, 9*(1), 10–21.

Reyna, V.F., & Brainerd, C.J. (2007). The importance of mathematics in health and human judgment: Numeracy, risk communication, and medical decision making. *Learning and Individual Differences, 17*(2), 147–159.

Reyna, V.F., Nelson, W.L., Han, P.K., & Dieckmann, N.F. (2009). How numeracy influences risk comprehension and medical decision making. *Psychological Bulletin, 135*(6), 943–973.

Rich, P. (2011a). Social media make inroads into Canadian medicine. *Future Practice,* (November), 15–18.

Rich, P. (2011b). Doctors use social media to share medical information. *Future Practice,* (November), 22–23.

Rick Wilson Consulting Inc. (for the National Literacy and Health Research Project Team). (2004, August). *Retrospective evaluation of the national literacy and health program—Final report.* Retrieved from http://www.cpha.ca/uploads/portals/h-l/nlahp-final_e.pdf

Ridpath, J.R., Larson, E.B., & Greene, S.M. (2012). Can integrating health literacy into the patient-centered medical home help us weather the perfect storm? *Journal of General Internal Medicine, 27*(5), 588–594.

Robu, I., Robu, V., & Thirion, B. (2006). An introduction to the semantic Web for health sciences librarians. *Journal of the Medical Library Association, 94*(2), 198–205.

Rogers, B. (2008, September 16). Vancouver dodges contaminated Chinese infant milk-powder scandal. *Straight.com: Et Cetera* (blog). Retrieved from http://straight.com/blogra/vancouver-dodges-contaminated-chinese-infant-milk-powder-scandal

Romanow, R.J. (2002). *Building on Values: The Future of Health Care in Canada—Final Report.* Ottawa: Commission on the Future of Health Care in Canada. Retrieved from http://publications.gc.ca/site/eng/237274/publication.html

Rootman, I. (2006). Health literacy: Where are the Canadian doctors? *Canadian Medical Association Journal, 175*(6), 606–607.

Rootman, I. (2009). Relation between literacy skills and the health of Canadians. *Encyclopedia of language and literacy development.* Retrieved from http://www.literacyencyclopedia.ca/index.php?fa=items.show&topicId=264

Rootman, I., & Gordon-El-Bihbety, D. (2008). *A vision for a health literate Canada: Report of the Expert Panel on Health Literacy.* Ottawa: Canadian Public Health Association. Retrieved from http://www.cpha.ca/uploads/portals/h-l/report_e.pdf

Rootman, I., Gordon-El-Bihbety, D., Frankish, J., Hemming, H., Kaszap, M., Langille, L., ... & Ronson, B. (2002). *National Literacy and Health Research Program needs assessment and environmental scan.* Retrieved from http://www.nlhp.cpha.ca/clhrp/needs_e/needs_e.pdf

Rootman, I., & Ronson, B. (2005). Literacy and health research in Canada: Where have we been and where should we go? *Canadian Journal of Public Health, 96*(Supplement 2), S62–S77.

Rosenkoetter, L.I., Rosenkoetter, S.E., & Acock, A.C. (2009). Television violence: An intervention to reduce its impact on children. *Journal of Applied Developmental Psychology, 30*(4), 381–397.

Rowell, L. (2008). In search of Web 3.0. *netWorker, 12*(3), 18–24.

Rubenson, K., Desjardins R., & Yoon, E.-S., International Adult Literacy Survey, & Statistics Canada. (2007). *Adult learning: A comparative perspective: Results from the adult literacy and life skills survey.* International Adult Literacy Survey Series. Cat. No. 89-552-XIE, no. 17. Ottawa: Statistics Canada. Retrieved from http://www.statcan.gc.ca/pub/89-552-m/89-552-m2007017-eng.pdf

Rubenson, K., & Walker, J. (2011). *An examination of IALS and its influence on adult literacy in Canada.* Fall Institute 2011. IALS (International Adult Literacy Survey): Its Meaning and Impact for Policy and Practice, Banff, AB, October 23–25. Retrieved from http://www.centreforliteracy.qc.ca/sites/default/files/Rubenson_Canada.pdf

Rudd, R. (2007). Health literacy skills of U.S. adults. *American Journal of Health Behavior, 31*(Supplement 1), S8–S18.

Rudd, R.E. (2010). *Assessing health materials: Eliminating barriers—Increasing access.* Boston: Health Literacy Studies, Harvard School of Public Health. Retrieved from http://www.hsph.harvard.edu/healthliteracy/files/2012/09/eliminating_barriers_assessing.pdf

Rudd, R.E., Comings, J.P., & Hyde, J.N. (2003). Leave no one behind: Improving health and risk communication through attention to literacy. *Journal of Health Communication, 8*(Supplement 1), 104–115.

Rudd, R.E., Kirsch, I., & Yamamoto, K. (2004). *Literacy and health in America.* Princeton, NJ: Educational Testing Service.

Rukholm, E., Carter, L., & Newton-Mathur, D. (2009). Interprofessional collaboration and culturally-safe Aboriginal health care. *Journal of Distance Education, 23*(2), 137–146.

Saisana, M., & Cartwright, F. (2007). Measuring lifelong learning and its impact on happiness—The Canadian paradigm. International Conference on Policies for Happiness, Siena, June 14–17. Retrieved from http://www3.unisi.it/eventi/happiness/curriculum/saisana.pdf

Salant, T., & Lauderdale, D.S. (2003). Measuring culture: A critical review of acculturation and health in Asian immigrant populations. *Social Science & Medicine, 57*(1), 71–90.

Samuelstuen, M.S., & Braten, I. (2005). Decoding, knowledge, and strategies in comprehension of expository text. *Scandinavian Journal of Psychology, 46* (2), 107–117.

Sandman, P.M. (1987). Risk communication: Facing public outrage. *EPA Journal, 13*(9), 21–22.

Saranto, K., & Hovenga, E. (2004). Information literacy—What it is about? Literature review of the concept and the context. *International Journal of Medical Informatics, 73*(6), 503–513.

Saul, S. (2008, February 26). Pfizer to end Lipitor ads by Jarvik. *The New York Times*. Retrieved from http://www.nytimes.com/2008/02/26/business/26pfizer.html?_r=0

Sawada, M., Cossette, D., Wellar, B., & Kurt, T. (2006). Analysis of the urban/rural broadband divide in Canada: Using GIS in planning terrestrial wireless deployment. *Government Information Quarterly, 23*(34), 454–479.

Scearce, C. (2007). Scientific literacy. *ProQuest Discovery Guides*. Retrieved from http://www.csa.com/discoveryguides/discoveryguides-main.php

Schaefer, C.T. (2008). Integrated review of health literacy interventions. *Orthopedic Nursing, 27*(5), 302–317.

Scheufele, D.A. (1999). Framing as a theory of media effects. *Journal of Communication, 19*(1), 103–122.

Schillinger, D., Bindman, A.B., Wang, F., Stewart, A.L., & Piette, J. (2004). Functional health literacy and the quality of physician-patient communication among diabetes patients. *Patient Education and Counseling, 52*(3), 315–323.

Schirmer, J.M., Mauksch, L., Lang, F., Zoppi, K., Epstein, R.M., Brock, D., & Pryzbylski, M. (2005). Assessing communication competence: A review of current tools. *Family Medicine, 37*(3), 184–192.

Sciadas, G. (2002). *The digital divide in Canada*. Ottawa: Science, Innovation and Electronic Information Division, Statistics Canada.

Segall, M.H., Lonner, W.J., & Berry, J.W. (1998). Cross-cultural psychology as a scholarly discipline. *American Psychologist, 53*(10), 1101–1110.

Seligman, H.K., Wang, F.F., Palacios, J.L., Wilson, C.C., Daher, C., Piette, J.D., & Schillinger, D. (2005). Physician notification of their diabetes patients' limited health literacy: A randomized, controlled trial. *Journal of General Internal Medicine, 20*(11), 1001–1007.

Sellnow, T.L., Ulmer, R.R., Seeger, M.W., & Littlefield, R.S. (2009). *Effective risk communication—A message-centered approach*. New York: Springer Science & Business Media.

Sen, A. (2003). Reflections on literacy. In *Literacy as Freedom: A UNESCO Roundtable* (pp. 20–30). Paris, France: United Nations Educational, Scientific and Cultural Organization. Retrieved from http://unesco.org.pk/education/life/files/literacy_as_freedom.pdf

Shah, D.V., Domke, D., & Wackman, D.B. (1996). "To thine own self be true": Values, framing and voter decision-making strategies. *Communication Research, 23*(5), 509–560.

Shah, D.V., McLeod, D.M., Gotlieb, M.R., & Lee, N-J. (2009). Framing and agenda setting. In R.L. Nabi & M.B. Oliver (Eds.), *The Sage handbook of media processes and effects* (pp. 83–98). Thousand Oaks, CA: Sage Publications.

Shields, M. (2005). Measured obesity: Overweight Canadian children and adolescents. *Nutrition: Findings from the Canadian Community Health Survey.* Cat. No. 82-620-MWE. Ottawa: Statistics Canada. Retrieved from http://s3.amazonaws.com/zanran_storage/www.calgaryhealthregion.ca/ContentPages/18451313.pdf

Shields, M. (2006). Overweight and obesity among children and youth. *Health Reports, 17*(3), 27–42.

Shortreed, J., Hicks, J., & Craig, L. (2003). *Basic frameworks for risk management. Final report to the Ontario Ministry of the Environment.* NERAM Report 7. Retrieved from http://www.irr-neram.ca/pdf_files/basicFrameworkMar2003.pdf

Shuchman, M., & Wilkes, M.S. (1997). Medical scientists and health news reporting: A case of miscommunication. *Annals of Internal Medicine, 126*(12), 976–982.

Silverblatt, A. (2001). *Media literacy: Keys to interpreting media messages* (2nd ed.). Westport, CT: Praeger Publishers.

Silverblatt, A. (2004). Media as social institution. *American Behavioral Scientist, 48*(35), 35–41.

Simich, L. (2009). *Health literacy and immigrant populations.* Policy brief for the Public Health Agency of Canada and Metropolis Canada. Ottawa: Public Health Agency of Canada. Retrieved from http://canada.metropolis.net/pdfs/health_literacy_policy_brief_jun15_e.pdf

Simpson, M., Buckman, R., Stewart, M., Maguire, P., Lipkin, M., Novack, D., & Till, J. (1991). Doctor–patient communication: The Toronto consensus statement. *British Medical Journal, 303*, 1385–1387.

Singleton, K., & Krause, E.M.S. (2009). Understanding cultural and linguistic barriers to health literacy. *Online Journal of Issues in Nursing, 14*(3), 2.

Sjöberg, L. (1999). Risk perception by the public and by experts: A dilemma in risk management. *Human Ecology Review, 6*(2), 1–9.

Skinner, H., Biscope, S., & Poland, B. (2003). Quality of Internet access: Barrier behind Internet use statistics. *Social Science & Medicine, 57*(5), 875–880.

Sloat, E., & Willms, J.D. (2000). The International Adult Literacy Survey: Implications for Canadian social policy. *Canadian Journal of Education, 25*(3), 218–233.

Smith, J.L., & Haggerty, J. (2003). Literacy in primary care populations: Is it a problem? *Canadian Journal of Public Health, 94*, 408–412.

Smylie, J., Williams, L., & Cooper, N. (2007). Culture-based literacy and Aboriginal health. *Canadian Journal of Public Health, 97*(Supplement 2), S21–S25.

Snyder, L.B., Milici, F.F., Slater, M., Sun, H., & Strizhakova, Y. (2006). Effects of alcohol advertising exposure on drinking among youth. *Archives of Pediatrics and Adolescent Medicine, 160*, 18–24.

Some current research on health and literacy. (2000). *Literacy Across the Curriculumedia Focus, 15*(1). Retrieved from http://centreforliteracy.qc.ca/sites/default/files/Some_current.pdf

Sorensen, K., Van den Broucke, S., Fullam, J., Doyle, G., Pelikan, J., Slonska, Z., & Brand, H. (2012). Health literacy and public health: A systematic review and integration of definitions and models. *BMC Public Health, 12*, 80. Retrieved from http://www.biomedcentral.com/1471-2458/12/80

Soumerai, S.B., Ross-Degnan, D., & Kahn, J.S. (1992). Effects of professional and media warnings about the association between Aspirin use in children and Reye's syndrome. *Milbank Quarterly, 70*(1), 155–182.

Speros, C. (2005). Health literacy: Concept analysis. *Journal of Advanced Nursing, 50*(6), 633–640.

Spiegelhalter, D., Pearson, M., & Short, I. (2011). Visualizing uncertainty about the future. *Science, 333*(6048), 1393–1400.

Spires, H.A., & Donley, J. (1998). Prior knowledge activation: Inducing engagement with informal texts. *Journal of Educational Psychology, 90*(2), 249–260.

St. John, B., Pitts, M., & Tufts, K.A. (2010). Disconnects between news framing and parental discourse concerning the state-mandated HPV vaccine: Implications for dialogic health communication and health literacy. *Communication & Medicine, 7*(1), 75–84.

Statistics Canada. (1997). *Reading the future: A portrait of literacy in Canada—Highlights*: National Literacy Secretariat. Retrieved from http://www.statcan.gc.ca/pub/89f0093x/4198665-eng.pdf

Statistics Canada. (2000). *Literacy in the information age: Final report of the International Adult Literacy Survey*. Retrieved from http://www.oecd.org/education/educationeconomyandsociety/39437980.pdf

Statistics Canada. (2002). *Section A: General information—Canada IALLS*. Retrieved from http://www23.statcan.gc.ca/imdb-bmdi/pub/instrument/4406_Q1_V1-eng.pdf

Statistics Canada. (2005). *Building on our competencies: Canadian results of the International Adult Literacy and Skills Survey*. Cat. No. 89-617-XIE. Ottawa: Human Resources and Skills Development Canada. Retrieved from http://www.statcan.ca/pub/89-617-x/89-617-x2005001-eng.pdf

Statistics Canada. (2006). *Census snapshot—Immigration in Canada: A portrait of the foreign-born population, 2006 census*. Retrieved from http://www.statcan.gc.ca/pub/11-008-x/2008001/article/10556-eng.htm#3

Statistics Canada. (2008). *Canada's ethnocultural mosaic, 2006 Census*. Cat. No. 97-562-X. Ottawa: Minister of Industry.

Statistics Canada. (2009a). *2006 Census: Immigration in Canada: A portrait of the foreign-born population*. Retrieved from http://www12.statcan.ca/census-recensement/2006/as-sa/97-557/p1-eng.cfm

Statistics Canada. (2009b). *Language spoken most often at home by immigrant status and broad age groups, 2006 counts, for Canada, provinces and territories*. Retrieved from http://www12.statcan.ca/census-recensement/2006/dp-pd/hlt/97-557/T405-eng.cfm?Lang=E&T=405&GH=4&GF=1&SC=1&S=1&O=D

Statistics Canada. (2010a). *Canadian community health survey: H1N1 vaccinations*. Retrieved from http://www.statcan.gc.ca/daily-quotidien/100719/dq100719b-eng.htm

Statistics Canada. (2010b). *Table 3580124—Canadian Internet Use Survey, Internet use, by location of access, sex and age group, every 2 years (percent), CANSIM (database)*. Retrieved from http://www5.statcan.gc.ca/cansim/pick-choisir?lang=eng&id=3580124&pattern=3580124&searchTypeByValue=1

Statistics Canada. (2011a). Canadian Internet Use Survey 2010. *The Daily*, May 25, 5–6. Retrieved from http://www.statcan.gc.ca/daily-quotidien/110525/dq110525-eng.pdf

Statistics Canada. (2011b). Individual Internet use and E-commerce, 2010. *The Daily*, October 12, 18. Retrieved from http://www.statcan.gc.ca/daily-quotidien/111012/dq111012-eng.pdf

Statistics Canada. (2013). Skills in Canada: First results from the Programme for the International Assessment of Adult Competencies (PIAAC). Cat. No. 89-555-X. Ottawa: Minister of Industry.

Statistics Canada and OECD. (2005). Learning a living. First results of the Adult Literacy and Life Skills Survey. Annex A: A construct-centered approach to understanding what was measured in the Adult Literacy and Life Skills (ALL) Survey, 275–333. Retrieved from http://www.oecd.org/education/country-studies/34867438.pdf

Stephenson, P.H. (1995). Vietnamese refugees in Victoria, BC: An overview of immigrant and refugee health care in a medium-sized Canadian urban centre. *Social Science & Medicine, 40*(12), 1631–1642.

Stewart, M., Brown, J., Weston, W., McWhinney, I., McWilliam, C., & Freeman, T. (1995). *Patient-centered medicine: Transforming the clinical method*. London: Sage.

Stewart, S., Riecken, T., Scott, T., Tanaka, M., & Riecken, J. (2008). Expanding health literacy: Indigenous youth creating videos. *Journal of Health Psychology, 13*(2), 180–189.

Strasburger, V.C. (2005). Adolescents, sex, and the media: Ooooo, baby, baby—A Q & A. *Adolescent Medicine Clinics, 16*(2), 269–288.

Street, R.L. Jr. (1991). Information-giving in medical consultations: The influence of patients' communicative styles and personal characteristics. *Social Science & Medicine, 32*(5), 541–548.

Street, R.L. Jr. (2003a). Communicating in medical encounters: An ecological perspective. In T.L. Thomson, A.M. Dorsely, K.I. Miller, & R. Parrott (Eds.), *Handbook of health communication* (pp. 63–89). London: Lawrence Erlbaum.

Street, R.L. Jr. (2003b). Interpersonal communication skills in health care contexts. In J.O. Greene & B.R. Burleson (Eds.), *Handbook of communication and social interaction skills* (pp. 909–934). Mahwah, NJ: Lawrence Erlbaum.

Stryker, J.E., Fishman, J., Emmons, K.M., & Viswanath, K. (2009). Cancer risk communication in mainstream and ethnic newspapers. *Preventing Chronic Disease, 6*(1), A23. Retrieved from http://www.cdc.gov/pcd/issues/2009/jan/08_0006.htm

Subramanian, S.V., & Kawachi, I. (2004). Income inequality and health: What have we learned so far? *Epidemiologic Reviews, 26*, 78–91.

Sudore, R.L., Landefeld, C.S., Pérez-Stable, E.J., Bibbins-Domingo, K., Williams, B.A., & Schillinger, D. (2009). Unraveling the relationship between literacy, language proficiency, and patient-physician communication. *Patient Education and Counseling, 75*(3), 398–402.

Sudore, R.L., & Schillinger, D. (2009). Interventions to improve care for patients with limited health literacy. *Journal of Clinical Outcomes Management, 16*(1), 20–29.

Suinn, R., Ahuna, C., & Khoo, G. (1992). The Suinn-Lew Asian self-identity acculturation scale: Concurrent and factorial validation. *Education and Psychological Measurement, 52*, 1041–1046.

Sunnybrook Health Sciences Centre. (2012). *Home page.* Retrieved from http://www.sunnybrook.ca/

Surbone, A. (2006). Telling the truth to patients with cancer: What is the truth? *Lancet Oncology, 7*(11), 944–950.

Taggart, J., Williams, A., Dennis, S., Newall, A., Shortus, T., Zwar, N., … & Harris, M.F. (2012). A systematic review of interventions in primary care to improve health literacy for chronic disease behavioral risk factors. *BMC Family Practice, 13*(1), 49. Retrieved from htttp://www.ncbi.nlm.nih.gov/pubmed/22656188

Tait, A.R., Voepel-Lewis, T., Zikmund-Fisher, B.J., & Fagerlin, A. (2010). Presenting research risk and benefits to parents: Does format matter? *Anesthesia & Analgesia, 2010, 11*(3), 718–723.

Terry, P.E. (2000). The physician's role in educating patients. *Journal of Family Practice, 49*(4), 314–318.

Thoman, E. (2004). Media literacy: A national priority for a changing world. *American Behavioral Scientist, 48*(1), 18–29.

Thoman, E., & Jolls, T. (2003) *MediaLit kit—Literacy for the 21st century: An overview and orientation guide to media literacy education.* Retrieved from http://www.medialit.org/sites/default/files/01_MLKorientation.pdf

Thompson, T.L., Dorsey, A.M., Miller, K.I., & Parrott, R. (2003). *Handbook of health communication.* Mahwah, NJ: Lawrence Erlbaum.

Thompson, T.L., & Parrott, R. (2002). Interpersonal communication and healthcare. In M.L. Knapp & J.A. Daly (Eds.), *Handbook of interpersonal communication* (3rd ed., pp. 680–725). Thousand Oaks, CA: Sage Publications.

Thomson, M.D., & Hoffman-Goetz, L. (2009). Defining and measuring acculturation: A systematic review of public health studies with Hispanic populations in the United States. *Social Sciences & Medicine, 69*(7), 218–244.

Thomson, M.D., & Hoffman-Goetz, L. (2011). Cancer information comprehension by English-as-a-second-language immigrant women. *Journal of Health Communication, 16*(1), 17–33.

Thomson, M.D., & Hoffman-Goetz, L. (2012). Application of the health literacy framework to diet-related cancer prevention conversations of older immigrant women to Canada. *Health Promotion International, 27*(1), 33–44.

Todd, L., & Hoffman-Goetz, L. (2011). Predicting health literacy among English-as-a-second-language older Chinese immigrant women to Canada: Comprehension of colon cancer prevention information. *Journal of Cancer Education, 26*(2), 326–332.

Tong, A., Chapman, S., Sainsbury, P., & Craig, J.C. (2008). An analysis of media coverage on the prevention and early detection of CKD in Australia. *American Journal of Kidney Diseases, 52*(1), 159–170.

Triandis, H.C. (1993). Collectivism and individualism as cultural syndromes. *Cross Cultural Research, 27*(3–4), 155–180.

Tuijnman, A. (2001). *Benchmarking adult literacy in North America: An international comparative study.* International Adult Literacy Survey. Cat. No. 89-572-XPE. Ottawa: Statistics Canada. Retrieved from http://www.statcan.gc.ca/pub/89-572-x/89-572-x1998001-eng.pdf

Tversky, A., & Kahneman, D. (1974). Judgement under uncertainty: Heuristics and biases. *Science, 185*(4157), 1124–1131.

Tyner, K.R. (2010). Introduction: Agendas for media literacy. In K.R. Tyner (Ed.), *New media literacy: New agendas in communication* (pp. 1–7). New York: Routledge.

U.S. Department of Health and Human Services (DHHS). (n.d.). *Quick guide to health literacy: Fact sheets, strategies, resources.* Washington, DC: U.S. Department of Health and Human Services, Office of Disease Prevention and Health Promotion. Retrieved from http://www.health.gov/communication/literacy/quickguide/quickguide.pdf

U.S. Department of Health and Human Services, Office of Disease Prevention and Health Promotion. (2010). *National Action Plan to Improve Health Literacy.* Washington, DC: Author. Retrieved from http://www.health.gov/communication/hlactionplan/pdf/Health_Literacy_Action_Plan.pdf

U.S. Department of Health and Human Services, Office of Minority Health. (2005). *What is cultural competency?* Retrieved from http://minorityhealth.hhs.gov/templates/browse.aspx?lvl=2&lvlID=11

United Nations. (1948). Universal Declaration of Human Rights. Paris, France. Retrieved from www.un.org/en/documents/udhr/index.shtml

United Nations Economic and Social Council. (2009). *Economic and Social Council* (Vol. 2., pp. 1–18). Geneva: United Nations.

United Nations Educational, Scientific and Cultural Organization (UNESCO). (2004). *The Plurality of literacy and its implications for policy and programmes.* Paris, France: UNESCO Publishing.

United Nations Educational, Scientific and Cultural Organization (UNESCO). (2005). *Education for all global monitoring report: Literacy for life 2006*. Paris, France: UNESCO Publishing.

United States Environmental Protection Agency. (2011). *CERCLA overview*. Retrieved from http://www.epa.gov/superfund/policy/cercla.htm

University of Western Ontario. (2012). *Learning it Together (LiT)*. Retrieved from http://www.uwo.ca/fhs/LiT/

Van den Berg, P., Neumark-Sztainer, D., Hannan, P.J., & Haines, J. (2007). Is dieting advice from magazines helpful or harmful? Five-year associations with weight-control behaviors and psychological outcomes in adolescents. *Pediatrics, 19*, 30e–7e.

Villeneuve, M., and MacDonald, J. (2006). *Toward 2020: Visions for nursing*. Ottawa: Canadian Nurses' Association. Retrieved from http://www.canadian-nurse.com/images/pdf/2006/cnj-may-2006/files/assets/downloads/page0024.pdf

Viswanath, K., & Ackerson, L.K. (2011). Race, ethnicity, language, social class, and health communication inequalities: A nationally-representative cross-sectional study. *PLoS ONE, 6*(1), e145–150. doi:10.1371/journal.phone.0014550

Viswanath, K., & Bond, K. (2007). Social determinants and nutrition: Reflections on the role of communication. *Journal of Nutrition Education and Behavior, 39*(Supplement 2), S20–S24.

Viswanath, K., Breen, N., Meissner, H., Moser, R.P., Hesse, B., Steele, W.R., & Rakowski, W. (2006). Cancer knowledge and disparities in the information age. *Journal of Health Communication, 11*(Supplement 001), 1–17.

Warschauer, M. (2003). Demystifying the digital divide. *Scientific American, 289*(2), 42–47.

Weiss, B. (2007). *Health literacy and patient safety: Help patients understand. Manual for clinicians* (2nd ed.). Chicago: American Medical Association Foundation and American Medical Association. Retrieved from: http://www.ama-assn.org/ama1/pub/upload/mm/367/hl_monograph.pdf

Weiss, B.D., & Coyne, C. (1997). Communicating with patients who cannot read. *New England Journal of Medicine, 337*(4), 272–274.

Weiss, B.D., Mays, M.Z., Martz, W., Castro, K.M., DeWalt, D.A., Pignone, M.P., ... & Hale, F.A. (2005). Quick assessment of literacy in primary care: The newest vital sign. *The Annals of Family Medicine, 3*(6), 514–522.

Welinrich, S., Viajayakumar, S., Powell, I.J., Priest, J., Hamner, C.A., McCloud, L., & Pettaway, C. (2007). Knowledge of hereditary prostate cancer among high-risk African American men. *Oncology Nursing Forum, 34*(4), 854–860.

Wharf Higgins, J., Begoray, D., & MacDonald, M. (2009). A social ecological conceptual framework for understanding adolescent health literacy in the health education classroom. *American Journal of Community Psychology, 44*(3-4), 350–362.

Whitehead, M. (1990). *The concepts and principles of equity in health*. Copenhagen, Denmark: WHO Regional Office for Europe. Retrieved from http://salud.ciee.flacso.org.ar/flacso/optativas/equity_and_health.pdf

Whitehead, M. (1991). The concepts and principles of equity and health. *Health Promotion International, 6*(3), 217–228.

Whitehead, M. (1992). The concepts and principles of equity and health. *International Journal of Health Services: Planning, Administration, Evaluation, 22*(3), 429–445

Whitehead, M. (1996). Working towards social justice in health (conference paper). *Journal of the Royal Society of Health, 116*(4), 256–263.

Wicks, P., Massagli, M., Frost, J., Brownstein, C., Okun, S., Vaughan, T., … & Heywood, R. (2010). Sharing health data for better outcomes on PatientsLikeMe. *Journal of Medical Internet Research, 12*(2), e19. doi:10.2196/jmir.1549

Wikibooks. (2012). *Internet technologies*. Retrieved from http://en.wikibooks.org/wiki/Internet_Technologies

Wilkinson, R., & Marmot, M. (Eds.). (2003). Introduction. In R.G. Wilkinson & M.G. Marmot (Eds.), *Social determinants of health: The solid facts* (pp. 7–9). Copenhagen, Denmark: WHO Regional Office for Europe. Retrieved from http://www.euro.who.int/__data/assets/pdf_file/0005/98438/e81384.pdf

Williams, M.V., Davis, T.C., Parker, R.M., & Weiss, B.D. (2002).The role of health literacy in patient-physician communication. *Family Medicine, 34*(5), 383–389.

Williams, O., DeSorbo, A., Noble, J., & Gerin, W. (2012). Child-mediated stroke communication: Findings from Hip Hop Stroke. *Stroke: A Journal of Cerebral Circulation, 43*(1), 163–169.

Willms, J.D. (1997). *Literacy skills of Canadian youth*. Cat. No. 89-552-MPE, no. 1. Ottawa: Statistics Canada. Retrieved from http://publications.gc.ca/collections/Collection/CS89-552-1E.pdf

Willms, J.D., & Watson, B. (2008). Literacy, numeracy and problem-solving skills of Canadian youth. Human Resources and Social Development Canada. Cat. No. HS28-145/2008E-PDF. Retrieved from http://publications.gc.ca/collection_2008/hrsdc-rhdsc/HS28-145-2008E.pdf

Wister, A.V., Malloy-Weir, L., Rootman, I., & Desjardins, R. (2010). Lifelong educational practices and resources: Enabling health literacy among older adults. *Journal of Aging and Health, 22*(6), 827–854.

Wizowski, L., Harper, T., & Hutchings, T. (2008). *Writing health information for patients and families* (3rd ed.). Hamilton, ON: Hamilton Health Sciences. Retrieved from http://www.hamiltonhealthsciences.ca/workfiles/PATIENT_ED/Writing%20health%20information%20Sept%203%2008%20With%20hyperlinks.pdf

Wolfe, B., & Haveman, R. (2001). Accounting for the social and non-market benefits of education. In J.F. Helliwell (Ed.), *The contribution of human and social capital to sustained economic growth and well-being*. International symposium report, OCED/Human Resources and Development Canada. Vancouver: University of British Columbia Press.

Wood, F.G. (2005). Health literacy in a rural clinic. *Online Journal of Rural Nursing and Health Care, 5*(1). http://rnojournal.binghamton.edu/index.php/RNO/article/view/187/

Woodall, E.D., Taylor, V.M., Yasui, Y., Ngo-Metzger, Q., Burke, N., Thai, H., & Jackson, J.C. (2006). Sources of health information among Vietnamese American men. *Journal of Immigrant and Minority Health, 8*(3), 263–271.

World Factbook. (2011). Washington, DC: Central Intelligence Agency. Retrieved from: http://www.cia.gov/library/publications/the-world-factbook/index.html

World Health Organization. (n.d.). *Food safety: 20 questions on genetically modified foods.* Retrieved from http://www.who.int/foodsafety/publications/biotech/20questions/en/

World Health Organization. (1978). *Declaration of Alma-Ata.* International Conference on Primary Health Care, Alma-Ata, U.S.S.R., September 6–12. Retrieved from http://www.who.int/publications/almaata_declaration_en.pdf

World Health Organization. (1981). *Global strategy for health for all by the year 2000.* Geneva: WHO. Retrieved from http://whqlibdoc.who.int/publications/9241800038.pdf

World Health Organization. (1997). *Intersectoral action for health: A cornerstone for health-for-all in the twenty-first century.* Report of the International Conference, Halifax, Nova Scotia, April 20–23. Retrieved from http://whqlibdoc.who.int/hq/1997/WHO_PPE_PAC_97.6.pdf

World Health Organization. (1998). *Health promotion glossary.* WHO/HPR/HEP/98.1 Retrieved from http://www.who.int/healthpromotion/about/HPG/en/

World Health Organization. (2002). *25 questions & answers on health and human rights.* Publication series, issue no. 1. Geneva: World Health Organization. Retrieved from http://whqlibdoc.who.int/hq/2002/9241545690.pdf

World Health Organization. (2012). *Social determinants of health.* Retrieved from http://www.who.int/social_determinants/en/

World Health Organization, Health and Welfare Canada, and the Canadian Public Health Association. (1986). *Ottawa Charter for Health Promotion.* International Conference on Health Promotion, Ottawa, November 21. Retrieved from http://www.phac-aspc.gc.ca/ph-sp/docs/charter-chartre/pdf/charter.pdf

Wyatt, S., Henwood, F., Hart, A., & Smith, J. (2005). The digital divide, health information and everyday life. *New Media & Society, 7*(2), 199–218.

Xie, B. (2012). Library & information science research improving older adults' e-health literacy through computer training using NIH online resources. *Library and Information Science Research, 34*(1), 63–71.

Yin, H.S., Dreyer, B.P., Vivar, K.L., MacFarland, S., Van Schaick, L., & Mendelsohn, A.L. (2012). Perceived barriers to care and attitudes towards shared decision-making among low socioeconomic status parents: Role of health literacy. *Academic Pediatrics, 12*(2), 117–124.

Zach, L., Dalrymple, P.W., Rogers, M.L., & Williver-Farr, H. (2011). Assessing Internet access and use in a medically underserved population: Implications for providing enhanced health information services. *Health Information & Libraries Journal, 29*(1), 61–71.

Zanchetta, M., & Poureslami, I.M. (2006). Health literacy within the reality of immigrants' culture and language. *Canadian Journal of Public Health, 97*(Supplement 2), S26–S30.

Zanten, S.V.V., Coates, C., Hervas-Malo, M., & Mcgrath, P.J. (2012). Newborn literacy program effective in increasing maternal engagement in literacy activities: An observational cohort study. *Pediatrics, 12*(100), 7. Retrieved from http://www.biomedcentral.com/content/pdf/1471-2431-12-100.pdf

Zarcadoolas, C. (2011). The simplicity complex: Exploring simplified health messages in a complex world. *Health Promotion International, 26*(3), 338–350.

Zarcadoolas, C., Pleasant, A., & Greer, D.S. (2005). Understanding health literacy: An expanded model. *Health Promotion International, 20*(2), 195–203.

Zarcadoolas, C., Pleasant, A., & Greer, D. (2006). *Advancing health literacy: A framework for understanding and action.* San Francisco: Jossey Bass.

Zrinyi, M., & Balogh, Z. (2004). Student nurse attitudes towards homeless clients: A challenge for education and practice. *Nursing Ethics, 11*(4), 334–348.

COPYRIGHT ACKNOWLEDGEMENTS

INDEX

A

Aboriginal peoples
 acculturation and assimilation, 86
 culture and health literacy, 94–95
 health as human right, 69
 health literacy interventions, 186–188, 192
 Healthy Aboriginal Network, 145, 186
 inequities in health system, 71–72
 intersectionality theory application, 73
 literacy statistics, 48
 mass media and health literacy, 143–144
 medical education framework for, 99
 numeracy, 50
 social inequity and inequality, 62
acculturation and assimilation, 84–86
adolescents. *See* youth and young adults
adults, health literacy interventions, 188–190
advertising, and youth health, 129
age, 45–46, 110, 118–119
agenda setting, in mass media, 128
alcohol, 130
alternative medical models, in Canada, 85–86
apomediation and apomediaries, 104
Ask Me 3 technique, 35
aspirin, 125–126
Australia, IALS results, 57

B

Begoray, D., 141
best practices for health literacy, 72
bias, in risk perception, 152
body shape and weight, and mass media, 129–131
breastfeeding, 140
British Columbia, health literacy interventions, 185–186, 188–189
BSE (bovine spongiform encephalopathy), 164–165
Building Wellness program, 185

C

Calgary Charter on Health Literacy, 3, 28, 192
Canada Health Infoway, 120

Canadian Charter of Rights and Freedoms, 68–69
Canadian Conference on Literacy and Health, 8–9
Canadian Council on Learning (CCL)
 Composite Learning Index, 54
 definition of health literacy, 13
 definition of literacy, 17
 development of health literacy, 9, 184
 health literacy factors, 54–55
 low literacy and health outcomes, 5
 map of health literacy in Canada, 53–54
Canadian Medical Association (CMA), health literacy training, 174–175
Canadian Public Health Association (CPHA), 7–9, 77, 178–179, 181
cancer, in mass media, 143–144
cardiovascular health, health literacy interventions, 189
CCL. *See* Canadian Council on Learning (CCL)
Centre for Literacy, 8, 17–18
Charter of Rights and Freedoms, 68–69
children
 effects of media on, 130–133
 health literacy interventions, 184–185, 195
 See also youth and young adults
Christoffersen, A., 72–73
chronic disease, 21, 36, 80, 178–179
clinical context
 communications in, 169–170, 171–173, 175–176, 190–191
 health literacy, 169–170, 177–180
 low literacy patients, 168–169, 180
 patient-centred health care, 171–174, 177–180
clinical encounters, health literacy examples, 96–98
Colman, R., 138
comic books, 145, 186–188
communication, provider–patient
 barriers and challenges, 191
 in clinical context, 169–170, 190–191

health literacy interventions, 190–191
patient-centred, 171–173, 175–176, 178–179
and physicians, 176–178
training for, 176–177, 181
communication channels, access to
information, 75
competency domains, in health literacy, 23
Composite Learning Index (CLI), health
literacy in Canada, 54
computer literacy, 107–108
consensus statements, for patient-centred care,
172–173
Consumer Health Information Service (CHIS), 9
continuing medical education, 99, 175
critical health literacy, 26–27
critical media health literacy (CMHL), 141
cultivation, in mass media, 128
cultural awareness, 86, 87, 89
cultural competence, 86, 87–88, 89
cultural mosaic, 91–94
cultural safety, 86, 88–89, 99
cultural sensitivity, 89
culture
    acculturation and assimilation, 84–86
    alternative medical models, 85–86
    assessment tools, 89
    definitions and concept, 81–83
    and ethnicity, 83–84, 96–98
    First Nations and Aboriginal peoples, 86,
        94–95
    and health literacy, 80–81, 94–98
    and languages, 92–93, 94–98
    multiculturalism and cultural mosaic, 79,
        82–83, 90–94

D
definition of health literacy, 2–3, 4, 13, 25
    in Canada, 28–29
    as individual issue, 22–23
    and numeracy, 24
    population perspective, 23–24
determinants of health (DOH)
    frameworks, 63–64
    and health promotion, 63
    intersectionality theory, 72–73
    literacy and health literacy, 72–75
    See also social determinants of health
        (SDOH)
development of health literacy
    in Canada, 7–10, 11–12, 28–29, 184
    information in, 21–22
    reading in, 184
    as shared responsibility, 28
digital divide, 76, 117–119

doctors. See physicians
document literacy
    and health literacy in Canada, 51–52
    IALS in Canada, 44–45
    international comparisons, 56–57
    measurement, 40
DOH. See determinants of health (DOH)
domains of health literacy, 23, 27
Downtown Eastside (Vancouver), health literacy
    interventions, 188–189
Droppin' the Flag comic book, 186–187

E
Easy Does It! training manual (CPHA), 181
education
    continuing medical education, 99, 175
    and health literacy, 44–45, 74
    health literacy interventions in, 193–194,
        195
    health professionals, 174–175
    numeracy, 50
    for provider–patient communication, 176–
        177, 181
    and science literacy, 160
Edwards, A., 157–158
eHEALS (eHealth Literacy Scale), 110, 111
ehealth and ehealth literacy
    access to computers and information, 119
    and age, 110, 119
    assessment and tools, 109–110, 111
    competencies and components, 106–109,
        119
    data use and sharing, 113–114, 116
    definition and characteristics, 105–106
    and health literacy, 108–109
    health literacy interventions, 190
    literacies needed, 119
    for older adults, 190
    and social media, 113–116
    Web 2.0 and 3.0, 115–117
    See also Internet
empowerment, 23, 63, 170
equity and equality, 11–12, 70–71, 75–76
    See also inequity and inequality
ethnicity
    in Canada, 92
    definitions and concept, 83–84
    and health literacy, 83–84, 96–98, 142–144
    and mass media, 142–144
    See also immigration and immigrants
Expert Panel on Health Literacy, 12, 13, 23,
    28–29
Eysenbach, Gunther, 104, 105